AFRICA AND GLOBAL HEALTH GOVERNANCE

T0123101

Africa and Global Health Governance

Domestic Politics and International Structures

AMY S. PATTERSON

Johns Hopkins University Press

Baltimore

Johns Hopkins University Press
2715 North Charles Street
Baltimore, Maryland 21218-4363
www.press.jhu.edu

Library of Congress Cataloging-in-Publication Data

Names: Patterson, Amy S. (Amy Stephenson), author.
Title: Africa and global health governance : domestic politics and international structures /
    Amy S. Patterson.
Description: Baltimore : Johns Hopkins University Press, 2018. | Includes bibliographical
    references and index.
Identifiers: LCCN 2017022933 | ISBN 9781421424507 (pbk. : alk. paper) | ISBN 1421424509
    (pbk. : alk. paper) | ISBN 9781421424514 (electronic) | ISBN 1421424517 (electronic)
Subjects: | MESH: Global Health | Health Policy | Health Services Administration |
    International Cooperation | Politics | Communicable Disease Control | Africa
Classification: LCC RA441 | NLM WA 530 HA1 | DDC 362.1—dc23
LC record available at https://lccn.loc.gov/2017022933

A catalog record for this book is available from the British Library.

*Special discounts are available for bulk purchases of this book. For more information, please
contact Special Sales at 410-516-6936 or specialsales@press.jhu.edu.*

Johns Hopkins University Press uses environmentally friendly book materials, including recycled
text paper that is composed of at least 30 percent post-consumer waste, whenever possible.

To Isabel, Sophia, and Neil . . .

and countless activists and health-care workers in Africa,

with love, gratitude, and hope for the future

CONTENTS

FIGURE AND TABLES

ACKNOWLEDGMENTS

What does it mean for African states to participate in the global politics of health? My experiences in Africa with people living with HIV, Ebola survivors, community health-care workers, AIDS, cancer, and tobacco-control activists, and government policymakers since the mid-2000s sometimes just did not fit with the reports, statistics, and action plans that I read from the Joint United Nations Programme on HIV/AIDS or the World Health Organization. This book investigates the relationship between what global health institutions propose, measure, promote, or assert and what African states actually do on health issues. The alignment, juxtaposition, or gap between global health governance, on the one hand, and state actions, on the other, has the potential to affect the lives of millions of Africans. Particularly, what is the role of African actors in global health diplomacy (or policy design and issue framing) and policy implementation?

I am grateful for many people who helped me in my journey to investigate this question. Jeremy Youde told me it was a good idea; Kim Dionne helped me think more deeply about AIDS institutions; Emma-Louise Anderson sharpened my thoughts on Ebola; panel members at two International Studies Association conferences sponsored by the Global Health Section forced me to think more carefully about global norms and African state structures; and Melody Crowder-Meyer explained methodological issues numerous times. Former colleagues at Calvin College supported me during the early phases of this project. My departmental colleagues at the University of the South (Sewanee) cheerfully encouraged me, while my students commiserated with me as I stayed up much too late and drank too much coffee while working on this project. Thanks also to students on the Calvin-Sewanee Ghana semester of 2017 for your encouragement and patience. Specific students served as research assistants, sorting data, transcribing interviews, and searching for documents and library resources, or as insightful questioners of my research agenda: Kiela Crabtree, Tristan Danley, Lindsey Floyd, Michelle Fraser, Madeleine Hoffman, Rachel Schuman, Harold Smith, and Brooks Young.

Funding for the fieldwork was provided by the Fulbright Commission Africa Scholars Program, a Calvin College Alumni Grant, three faculty research grants from the University of the South, and the McCrickard Faculty Development Initiative at the University of the South. Fieldwork in Liberia was facilitated by Terry Quoi, who hosted me, guided me, and arranged many interviews. His family's kindness can never be repaid. Elwood Dunn, my predecessor at Sewanee with very large shoes to fill, also was an invaluable guide and help on the Liberia research. In Ghana, individuals at the Christian Council of Ghana and the University of Ghana–Legon graciously introduced me to numerous individuals involved with health policy and mobilization. In Uganda, I am grateful to Gideon Byamugisha and the staff at Friends of Canon Gideon Foundation for their time, support, introductions, and insights. And most crucially, for being kind, generous, and inspiring friends. In Tanzania, research was facilitated by several faculty at St. John's University, Dodoma. *Asante sana* Michael Msendekwa, Andrew Ching'ole, Vice Chancellor Emmanuel Mbennah, and Alfred Sebahene. Additionally, Moritz Hunsmann helped with introductions to several health-related organizations in Tanzania, as did Njonjo Mue and Rachel Devotsu. In Zambia, faculty in the Department of Health Economics, University of Zambia, University Teaching Hospital, and Justo Mwale Theological College provided essential introductions, as did pastors with several churches, advocates with the Network of Zambian People Living with HIV/AIDS (NZP+), and staff at the Circle of Hope AIDS clinic. Observations and conversations in South Africa occurred during a 2014 workshop on churches and citizenship which was hosted at the School of Theology, University of Stellenbosch, and co-convened by Tracy Kuperus and me. The Calvin Center for Christian Scholarship financially supported this endeavor. I am grateful to external reviewers of the manuscript, who provided excellent comments, as well as Robin Coleman at Johns Hopkins University Press for his patience and insights.

I cannot express how grateful I am to the many people who discussed African state health policies, health education, community mobilization, and global health governance with me. Thank you to the scholars who took the time, the government officials who patiently explained policies, the activists who showed their passion, and, most particularly, the people who live with, are affected by, or are survivors of various diseases. Your devotion to the human right to health inspired me, and your tireless optimism about the possibilities for better health for all Africans in the future should encourage us all. Thank you for your dedication, your generosity, and your commitment to bettering the lives of millions of people.

My family deserves a prize . . . not a small prize, but a very big prize. For countless meals brought to the office, weekends as a single parent, hours spent proofreading drafts, summers conducting fieldwork, unchecked homework, missed conversations, unfolded laundry, and wretched leftovers. Thank you Isabel, Sophia, and Neil for your patience, love, hugs, intellectual curiosity, and compassion for others beyond yourselves. I love y'all.

ACRONYMS AND ABBREVIATIONS

ACT UP	AIDS Coalition to Unleash Power
AFRO	World Health Organization Regional Office for Africa
AIDS	acquired immunodeficiency syndrome
ANC	African National Congress
ART	antiretroviral treatment
ARV	antiretrovirals (medications)
BRICS	Brazil, Russia, India, China, and South Africa
CARICOM	Caribbean Community
CBO	community-based organization
CCM	country coordinating mechanism(s)
CDC	Centers for Disease Control and Prevention (USA)
CHAZ	Churches Health Association of Zambia
DFID	UK Department for International Development
ECOWAS	Economic Community of West African States
ETU	Ebola Treatment Unit
EU	European Union
EVD	Ebola Virus Disease
FBO	faith-based organization
FCTC	Framework Convention on Tobacco Control
GAC	Ghana AIDS Commission
GAVI	The Vaccine Alliance (formerly Global Alliance for Vaccines and Immunization)
GIPA	Greater Involvement of People with AIDS
GOARN	Global Outbreak Alert and Response Network
GPA	Global Programme on AIDS
HBC	home-based care
Health GAP	Health Global Access Project
HIV	human immunodeficiency virus
HPV	human papillomavirus

IDU	injecting drug user
IGO	intergovernmental organization
IHR	International Health Regulations
IMF	International Monetary Fund
IRCU	Inter-Religious Council of Uganda
LMIC	low- and middle-income countries
LURD	Liberians United for Reconciliation and Democracy
MAP	Multi-Country AIDS Program (World Bank)
MERS	Middle East Respiratory Syndrome
MODEL	Movement for Democracy in Liberia
MSF	Médecins Sans Frontières (Doctors Without Borders)
MSM	men who have sex with men
NAC	National AIDS Commission(s)
NCD(s)	noncommunicable disease(s)
NGO	nongovernmental organization
NPFL	National Patriotic Front of Liberia
NZP+	Network of Zambian People Living with HIV/AIDS
ODA	official development assistance
OECD	Organisation for Economic Co-operation and Development
OVC	orphans and vulnerable children
PEPFAR	US President's Emergency Plan for AIDS Relief
PHEIC	Public Health Emergency of International Concern
PLHIV	person or people living with HIV
PMTCT	prevention of mother-to-child transmission
PPE	personal protective equipment
SADC	Southern African Development Community
STI	sexually transmitted infection
SWAPO	South West Africa People's Organization (Namibia)
TAC	Treatment Action Campaign (South Africa)
TASO	The AIDS Support Organisation (Uganda)
TB	tuberculosis
TRIPS	Trade-Related Intellectual Property Rights
ULIMO	United Liberation Movement for Democracy in Liberia
UNAIDS	Joint United Nations Programme on HIV/AIDS
UNDP	United Nations Development Programme
UNMEER	United Nations Mission for Ebola Emergency Response

UNMIL	United Nations Mission in Liberia
WHO	World Health Organization
WTO	World Trade Organization
ZNAN	Zambia National AIDS Network

AFRICA AND GLOBAL HEALTH GOVERNANCE

chapter 1

African States and Global
Health Governance

In 2003, urged by Muslim leaders, the governors of Kano, Zamfara, and Kaduna states in Nigeria suspended an internationally sponsored polio immunization campaign, expressing fear that the vaccine contained anti-fertility agents or HIV. The action led to widespread outcry among international health experts, and the eleven-month boycott ended only after the vaccine was tested by Muslim scientists in Indonesia. The halted campaign contributed to a surge in polio cases in Nigeria by 2005, setting back progress toward the disease's eradication.[1] Yet, deeper analysis reveals reasons for the governors' actions: concern over the World Health Organization's (WHO) emphasis on polio instead of more prevalent diseases; a history of colonial health campaigns that created suspicion in local populations; the Muslim religion's focus on alms-giving that provided a way to care for people with polio; few advocacy efforts by polio survivors; and political competition between Northern Muslim officials and the Nigerian federal government led by the southern Christian president Olusegun Obasanjo (Renne 2010; Jegede 2007; *IRIN News*, April 4, 2013). The case elucidates two of this book's themes: African actors are agents in global health governance, and the complicated interplay among international, state, and societal factors contributes to this agentic behavior.

Global health policies and programs abound. The International Health Regulations (IHR) were revised in 2005 and require states and nonstate actors to report disease outbreaks that are highly contagious or that could disrupt trade and transportation (Davies, Kamradt-Scott, and Rushton 2015). The Framework Convention on Tobacco Control, the first health-related treaty, urges states-parties to regulate smoking in public, to impose taxes on tobacco products, and to limit tobacco product advertising (Youde 2012). The Joint United Nations Programme on HIV/AIDS (UNAIDS), established by the United Nations in 1996, collects HIV surveillance data from countries, provides technical support on HIV and AIDS, and coordinates

UN agency programs to address the disease. And the Pan-American Health Organization, an autonomous WHO regional office, has developed health campaigns, such as the one that led to the elimination of endemic rubella in the Americas region in 2015 (PAHO 2015). Each of these international activities requires states to design, accept, and, ultimately, implement them. This book questions why weak states, or states that lack capacity and hard power and that often receive sizeable donor resources, do or do not participate in the design and implementation of these health campaigns. In the process, it questions how global health governance is grounded in local realities.

Global health governance has been understood as the formal and informal institutions, rules, and processes by which states, intergovernmental organizations (IGOs), nongovernmental organizations (NGOs), foundations, the private sector, and other nonstate actors collectively act on health issues that cross borders (Youde 2012). Despite the focus on multiple actors, global health governance has tended to emphasize the role of donor states and IGOs and to downplay the actions of weak states (Ng and Ruger 2011; Fidler 2010). This book provides another viewpoint on global health governance: a perspective from sub-Saharan African states that are entrenched in the international system through aid, debt, migration, and representation in IGOs but are often portrayed as controlled by that very system (Whitfield 2009; Jackson 1990; Ferguson 2006).[2]

This chapter begins by providing background on Africa's health challenges. It then examines African patterns of involvement in global health governance, setting up my typology of acceptance, challenge, and ambivalence. Third, the chapter presents my hypotheses for why African states engage with global health governance in these ways. I incorporate variables from the literatures on African politics and international relations at three levels of analysis—international, state, and societal—though I recognize how these factors interact to shape outcomes. Fourth, I present a counterfactual explanation: that state reactions to global health governance depend on the nature of the disease. While I do not discount disease characteristics, this volume focuses on the politics linked to those diseases. The fifth section details my methodology for collecting data to test my hypotheses. The chapter ends with an outline of the rest of the book.

Africa: Health Problems, Health Programs

Africa has some of the most difficult and diverse health problems in the world. According to the *Global Burden of Disease Study 2015* (*Lancet* 2016), in all sub-Saharan

African countries in 2015, the leading cause of premature death was one of four communicable diseases: HIV/AIDS, malaria, lower respiratory tract infections, or diarrheal diseases. In all regions of the world except Africa, the disease burden is caused mostly by chronic diseases (or, noncommunicable diseases) and injuries, though these causes are rising in prevalence in Africa too. While sixteen sub-Saharan African countries have experienced at least a 5 percent decline in infant mortality rates since 2000, children are much more likely to die in Africa than in other regions. And while life expectancy has increased throughout the globe, this increase has occurred at a slower rate in Africa (*Lancet* 2012; Marquez 2012; WHO 2012b). One must acknowledge that there has been success in curbing premature death: since approximately the mid-2000s, deaths from HIV/AIDS have declined 37 percent in Africa, while those from malaria decreased 33 percent. These health improvements contributed to an increase in life expectancy across the continent, by as many as ten years since 2005 in South Africa, Ethiopia, Zimbabwe, and Botswana. Despite such improvements, AIDS and tuberculosis (TB) remain the leading causes of death in southern Africa. In addition, while the decline in Africa's maternal mortality rates by about one-third since 2000 should be celebrated, it is crucial to remember that most of the twenty-four countries with rates that remain stubbornly high (above 400 deaths per 100,000 births) are in Africa (*Lancet* 2016).

Africa experiences unique disease challenges: the AIDS pandemic (over two-thirds of the world's people living with HIV are located in the region); high rates of disability from neglected tropical diseases like schistosomiasis; and the highest malaria burden and TB burden of all regions (UNAIDS 2015a; *Lancet* 2016). In contrast to the conventional view that infectious diseases cause most mortality, morbidity, and disability in Africa, the continent faces both the presence of communicable diseases and a rise in noncommunicable diseases (NCDs).[3] This "double burden" has the potential to further exacerbate the continent's challenges with health care capacity (Frenk and Gomez-Dantes 2011). Commonly grouped together in one category, NCDs are chronic, long in duration, and often slow in progression. A broad collection of illnesses and health conditions, the category of NCDs includes substance abuse, accidents, road traffic injuries, mental illness, violence against women and children, dementia, seeing and hearing impairments, asthma, and epilepsy. However, 82 percent of all deaths from NCDs are caused by diabetes, cancers, cardiovascular diseases, and chronic respiratory diseases.[4] By 2030, NCDs will be the biggest cause of disability and death in Africa (Boutayeb and Boutayeb 2005); in fact, the continent's number of cancer cases is estimated to increase by

85 percent before 2020 (*Lancet* 2013). These trends are fueled by increasing prevalence of high systolic blood pressure, high body-mass index, and tobacco use, particularly among men (*Lancet* 2015, 2016).

Africa also stands out as the region with the least capacity to address these health concerns. An estimated 23,000 health-care workers from Africa migrate annually (Cooper, Kirton, List, and Bosada 2013, 6), leading to a health-care worker deficit of roughly 2.5 million doctors and nurses (Naicker, Eastwood, Plange-Rhule, and Tutt 2010). Migration results from poor pay, long hours, and inadequate working conditions as well as recruitment efforts by Western health-care providers (Hamilton and Yau 2004). Spending on health care in Africa also lags behind. In 2012, the WHO estimated that the average amount of money needed per capita to ensure basic life-saving health services was $44 per person. Fifty states in the world spent less than that amount, and the vast majority of underspenders were in Africa. For example, Eritrea spent only $12 and Burkina Faso, $21 (WHO 2012a). These facts mean that African states are not only unable to address current health challenges but also ill-prepared for the multiple NCDs they will face in the future. Dr. Masiye of the University of Zambia said, "African nations have not even begun to confront the consequences of exploding cases of mental illness, depression, pain, and the enormous burden of substance abuse that stem from those conditions" (quoted in WHO 2012b; see also WHO 2015e; *Lancet* 2011).

Because of its health challenges, Africa has been the target of many global health programs. Of the fifteen focus countries that the US President's Emergency Plan for AIDS Relief (PEPFAR) sought to address when it was first established in 2003, twelve were in Africa. By 2016, PEPFAR focused on thirty-five countries, with twenty-one of those being in Africa (PEPFAR 2015b). African states have received the highest number of grants from the Global Fund to Fight AIDS, Tuberculosis, and Malaria (the Global Fund). The region was slated to receive at least twice as much as any other global region in the 2016–2017 WHO budget. In May 2015, the WHO budget for Africa was $1.162 billion; it budgeted $186 million for Latin America and $603 million for the Eastern Mediterranean (WHO 2015h). Thousands of indigenous and international NGOs work in Africa, donating millions of dollars to health and development projects (Hilhorst 2003; Michael 2004). Given the fact that Africa has been the target of global health governance, it is crucial to examine how global programs and policies intersect with local realities.

Global Health Governance: Patterns of African Involvement

As a field of study, global health governance has suffered from "weak theorizing" and a highly normative agenda (McInnes and Lee 2012, 101). Broadly understood, global health governance involves multiple actors, disciplines, and levels, recognizes the effects of globalization on disease, acknowledges societal responses to health and health solutions, and understands the linkages between health and economics, security, and the environment (Frenk and Moon 2013). Global health governance is nonlinear, problem-based, and contested, blurring the lines of responsibility for health among many actors who compete for resources and duplicate efforts (Ng and Ruger 2011; Fidler 2010). Global health governance often emphasizes a post-Westphalian international system, or one in which state sovereignty has been undermined by globalization. Trade, transportation, and migration enable pathogens to cross national boundaries more rapidly than ever before (Kirton, Cooper, Lisk, and Besada 2014, 16). In the post-Westphalian system, nonstate actors such as NGOs or private foundations with huge budgets have the potential to undermine the sovereignty of weak states, limiting their right to noninterference in health policymaking and implementation (Zondi 2014, 57).

Global health governance scholarship has taken several paths. One trend examines linkages between security and disease (Rushton and Youde 2015). State-centric, this literature analyzes how disease undermines economic development and military preparedness, ultimately threatening state security and global stability (Price-Smith 2009). The securitization of health has tended to marginalize Africa as the place from which pathogens emerge and to discount realities of African responses to disease (Fourie 2015). Global programs on disease surveillance and control such as the IHR have the potential to overburden weak states that do not benefit from them (Rushton 2011; Calain 2007). Securitization, surveillance, and disease control reflect Western states' power and security concerns. This book does not examine health issues through a security angle, though chapter 3 does illustrate how one African state—Liberia—utilized notions of crisis, instability, and fear that are associated with this securitization in order to challenge global health governance on Ebola.

A second area in global health governance views health policymaking, organizations, and actors through a constructivist lens, or a theoretical view that moves beyond state interests as measured in material terms (e.g., economic growth, military security) to recognize the intersubjective dimension of human actions:

"Constructivism is about human consciousness and its role in international life" (Ruggie 1998, 856). Constructivism helps elucidate the cultural, social, and ethical factors that undergird the very interests that realists and neoliberals assume (Ruggie 1998; Finnemore 2003; Wendt 1999). Principled beliefs or cultural considerations can challenge states' material interests, as when African states implemented economic sanctions to punish South Africa for its apartheid policies (Klotz 1995). Constructivism does not ignore global structures; rather, it recognizes an interactive relationship between structures and actors, in which agents exhibit a capacity to independently make their own choices while being situated in larger patterns or arrangements that affect the choices and opportunities available to those actors (Wendt 1999; Stones 2005). Chapter 4, for example, shows that African states are situated in neoliberal trade structures which directly affect how they can relate to global health governance on NCDs. Increasingly, constructivism has examined how identities (of states and nonstate actors) influence power and international actions (Adler 2012). As John Ruggie (1998, 869) writes, ideas, values, and beliefs about how the world ought to be ("ideational factors") do "not function causally in the same way as brute facts or the agentive role that neo-utilitarianism attributes to interests. As a result, the efficacy of such ideational factors is easily underestimated." In chapter 3, for example, I show how Liberia's concerns over its aspirational identity as a country rebuilding from war shaped how it interacted with global health governance on Ebola.

The ideas and identities that undergird states' interests and actions must be learned and communicated. Epistemic communities, or the collection of recognized "knowledge-based experts," articulate the "cause-and-effect relationships of complex problems," help states identify their interests, and propose specific policies (Haas 1992, 2). As a distinct actor in global politics, the epistemic community holds a common set of values, shares causal understandings of phenomena, agrees on criteria by which knowledge is validated, and uses common professional practices to examine or address problems (Haas 1992; Cross 2013). As chapter 2 shows in regards to AIDS, epistemic communities, as well as activists, states, and IGOs, can frame health issues, situating them in larger discourses related to security or human rights (McInnes et al. 2012). As tools of persuasion, frames (or, as Shiffman 2009 terms them, "narratives") influence perceptions and discourses; they help target audiences understand the normative reasons why a problem should (or should not) be addressed, and they make some actions possible (or impossible). Stakeholders, advocacy groups, IGOs, and epistemic communities use frames to influence global health governance, though for frames to be effective, they must resonate with an audience and be viewed to be credible (Shiffman 2009). Yet frames are sometimes contested, as chapter 4 illustrates with regards to NCDs, and the resulting tensions can complicate policy approaches (McInnes and Lee 2012).

Frames are the foundation for global health norms, or "standard[s] of appropriate behavior for actors with a given identity" (Finnemore and Sikkink 1998, 891). Norm entrepreneurs such as activists or epistemic communities work through organizational structures to push states to accept norms, though such efforts are not always successful (Finnemore 1993; Sikkink 2011). In this process, IGOs often play a role in shaping norms, because they have their own interests, expertise, and cultures (see Kamradt-Scott 2015 on the WHO; Barnett and Finnemore 2004 and Oestreich 2007 on UN agencies). In the case of global health governance on AIDS, for example, UNAIDS helped to propagate the norm of universal access to antiretroviral treatment (ART) for people living with HIV (Kapstein and Busby 2013). In the norm lifecycle, once a critical mass of states accepts the norm it "cascades;" it then becomes institutionalized through the development of bureaucratic programs, budgets, and international law. States adopt norms because they are concerned about their legitimacy or reputations in the eyes of other states or their own populations. They wish to be part of a "club" of states that act a particular way; the adoption of some norms opens the door for particular material benefits and status (Florini 1996).

A variety of norms have emerged in global health. These include the expectation that states promote population health ("right to health" or the "right to primary health care"), the norm that people living with HIV ought to have free access to ART, and the expectation that states will report contagious disease outbreaks under the IHR (Davies, Kamradt-Scott, and Rushton 2015; Youde 2008). Norms facilitate state adherence to global health governance, but this is not always the case, as chapter 3 illustrates. In previous efforts to mobilize global action on health, "norm entrepreneurs" often prioritized human rights, using the Alma-Ata Declaration on the "right of everyone to the enjoyment of the highest attainable standard of physical and mental health" (WHO 1978). This norm was unsuccessful in the campaign to provide primary health care in the 1980s, because it competed with neoliberal discourses and because states lacked capacity to institutionalize the norm (Youde 2008). Yet in the new millennium, the right to health has facilitated action on tobacco control (Reubi 2012) and led to the scale-up in the AIDS response (Harris and Siplon 2006; Youde 2008; Kapstein and Busby 2013). But as chapters 3 and 4 illustrate, the right to health has had limited influence in global health governance on the 2014–2015 Ebola outbreak or the control of NCDs.

The literature on norms in global health governance has also tended to marginalize Africa, assuming that weak states will follow the lead of powerful states on norm acceptance and institutionalization (Finnemore and Sikkink 1998). Norm emergence is characterized as beginning in industrialized countries among social movements and epistemic communities. These movements sometimes have linkages to African partners, but these partnerships can be rooted in inequalities. In her study of global health scientific communities, Johanna Crane (2013, 94) shows how American-led scientific endeavors provided opportunities for Ugandan scholars to gain resources and connections, but ultimately led to the imposition of Western biomedicine with its "molecular gaze." Even though it incorporated African organizations such as the Treatment Action Campaign (TAC), the AIDS treatment movement of the early 2000s was dominated by advocacy groups from the West (Kapstein and Busby 2013; Smith and Siplon 2006). And while the global AIDS movement became more inclusive over time (Chan 2015), this has yet to occur with global health movements around newer health issues like NCDs.

A third trend in the literature on global health governance examines the ways that international institutions like the WHO, World Bank, International Monetary Fund (IMF), and World Trade Organization (WTO) influence health or health policies (Youde 2012; Cooper, Kirton, and Schrecker 2007). IGOs are perceived to be autonomous actors that utilize expertise, norms, and (in some cases) the backing of strong states to bolster their power and promote their own agendas (Barnett and Finnemore 2004). Yet as chapter 3 illustrates, one important global health actor—the WHO—lacks the funding, autonomy from member-states, decision-making centralization, and political savvy to bolster its influence on many health issues (Youde 2012; Kamradt-Scott 2015; Youde 2016; Gostin and Friedman 2015). Both IGO autonomy and IGO weakness have negative outcomes. For example, UN-AIDS's promotion of National AIDS Commissions throughout Africa created sites for political manipulation (Putzel 2004), while IMF-sponsored structural adjustment policies undermined Africa's health-care capacity (Gibson and Mills 1995; Pfeiffer and Chapman 2010; Benton and Dionne 2015a). Health-related IGOs can ignore cultural, logistical, and political considerations that affect program success (see, for example, Webb 2013 on malaria eradication efforts in Liberia between 1945 and 1962 and Jones 2014 on the WHO's anti-Ebola messages that blamed cultural practices). An institutional focus in global health governance has often downplayed African agency, or African actors' control over decisions made and actions taken (Bøås and Hatløy 2008, 37). Weak states do not always defer to these IGOs. For example, Tanzania and Mauritius have developed harm reduction programs to curtail illegal drug use, in direct contradiction to donor policies that stress criminalization and control (McCurdy and Maruyama 2013). Chapter 3 illustrates how Liberia challenged some assumptions that the WHO made about the Ebola outbreak.

While scholarship on global health governance elucidates security linkages, constructivist identities and norm acceptance, and international institutions, it has done little to explore how African states are agentic actors in these governance processes. To address this gap, I identify three patterns in the region's involvement with global health governance: acceptance, challenge, and ambivalence. I recognize that global health governance has two components: (1) global health diplomacy that includes framing health issues and/or designing global health policies; and (2) state implementation of such global policies. In the *acceptance* model, African states use rhetoric and actions to shape the making of global health policies; they then adopt those policies. In designing and implementing policies, they are driven by norms as well as state interests and identities. While debates around specific policies remain, there is general agreement about the need to design and implement specific health efforts around the "best practices" of global health. In *challenge*, African states attempt to reframe the narrative underlying policy design and implementation. They deny the health issue and/or its severity, or they insist on controlling the policymaking agenda. They refuse to implement policies, or they develop their own projects and programs that counter public health practices. Sometimes these challenges are explicit, while at other times, they entail obfuscation and actions around the margins (Brown and Harman 2013). *Ambivalence* is exemplified by a lack of consensus on health frames, by limited (if any) participation in debates surrounding policy design, and by states' uneven implementation of agreed-upon global health policies, institutions, and norms. Such policies receive little rhetorical or financial support. Ambivalence translates into inaction or halfhearted action, while challenge equates to words and deeds that try to change the design and/or implementation of accepted global health governance programs and norms, often by seeking to make them more palpable to African interests and identities.

Not all African states fit each pattern at a given time. Moreover, African states interact dynamically with global health governance: while acceptance can occur over time, challenge is often an initial reaction. The book examines the region at a macrolevel while also pointing to country cases that support these general patterns. In the process, it shows how the exceptions can fit within the larger explanatory framework outlined below. In all three models, African states demonstrate agency: they choose to shape, influence, speak on, accept, ignore, deny, and/or criticize global health governance policies and norms.

Why These Patterns?

Understanding why these patterns of African involvement in global health governance emerge requires assessing the political incentives that encourage or discourage such participation. These incentives exist on the international level (e.g., norm coherence and resources); they are rooted in African state structures (e.g., democratic governance and neopatrimonial patterns in decision-making); and they emerge from society (e.g., civil society mobilization). This book argues that the interplay between these three levels leads African actors to adopt particular approaches to global health governance. These approaches are issue-dependent and dynamic: states move between challenge, ambivalence, and acceptance as the political calculus changes with the emergence (or disappearance) of specific factors.

International-Level Factors

Within the international relations literature, Africa is portrayed in two opposing ways. On one hand, the conventional view sees Africa is a region of "small states," or those states perceived to have no influence in the international system.[5] Even South Africa is portrayed as lacking the economic, military, and diplomatic power of the other BRICS countries (Andreasson 2011; Dunn and Shaw 2001). Small states tend to react to initiatives from powerful states, rely on hegemons for protection and resources, and work through institutions of international cooperation to facilitate their survival (Hey 2003, 6). They can be incorporated into partnerships with stronger states, with the security and economic stability of the weak state then dependent on the international distribution of power; how willing strong states are to provide benefits to their weak partners varies based on historical ties, domestic politics, and geostrategic interests (Dunn 2009). Robert Jackson (1990) refers to African states as "quasi-states" because even though they have internationally recognized sovereignty, they lack the resources and societal legitimacy to be effective, and their dependence on donors erodes their sovereignty (Whitfield 2009; Callaghy and Ravenhill 1993; Plank 1993). On the other hand, the portrayal of African states as lacking agency is too simplistic, since African states sometimes possess sufficient agency to promote their interests and identities (Brown and Harman 2013). Global structural changes, such as the rise of regional IGOs like the African Union and the emergence of China as a major donor and trade partner to Africa, have increased African states' autonomy (Hey 2003, 1; Taylor 2008). Africa has often been a "swing region" in geopolitics (Andreasson 2011), and through political dexterity, African state leaders can align with multiple partners to protect their interests.

This book recognizes that African states are both dependent on global aid, trade, and security structures (and the powerful states that enforce these structures) and agentic in their maneuvers within those structures. (On dependent agency at the local level, see Anderson and Patterson 2017). Particular conditions increase the space in which African states can act and define global governance. First, confusion over international policies and norms allows agents to creatively reframe global health issues (Frueh 2014). The more institutionalized global health governance is, the less room that weak states will have to manipulate, challenge, or ignore that governance. Norms undergird global health governance, and if they have cascaded and become institutionalized, weaker states will find it more difficult to ignore those norms as they design or implement elements of global health governance (Sikkink 2011). Second, strong norms must also be enforced, and if norm enforcement is limited (because of a lack of funding or little interest from strong states), then weak states again have room to act autonomously (Harman 2016a). Third, since issue frames are crucial for the acceptance and institutionalization of norms, when frames compete, African states have more space in which to challenge, revamp, or ignore global health governance. And if frames around an issue undercut the very identity of African states or their aspirations, those states can seek to challenge those frames (see Ruggie 1998 on aspirational identities). Finally, when policy structures are underdeveloped or weak, African states can act. For example, when faced with donors' demands for performance-based health spending, a relatively new aid institution, some African states have theoretically accepted this component of global health governance while in fact challenging its implementation by "gaming" the system. That is, they have either set performance targets extremely high to show donors that they care about health, or they have set them especially low so that targets are easily met. In either case, the state maintains relations with donors (Barnes, Brown, and Harman 2015).

African states use two tools in these international processes: sovereignty and extraversion. In the context of foreign aid, William Brown (2013, 13) writes, "The recognition of sovereign rights of recipient states creates the basis through which the aid relationship is conducted—it defines who the actors are." Ultimately, that definition allows states to play a central role in decisions related to aid. After all, it is only the state that can sign donor agreements, allocate land for donor projects, approve the registration of international NGOs, and represent the population at international aid meetings (Englebert 2009). Sovereignty enables state officials to speak and perform, sometimes employing extraversion, or public performances in which they play to external perceptions of the continent as a weak, impoverished victim of global structures in order to gain resources (Bayart 2000; see also Ellis 2013). Nicolas van de Walle (2001) shows how in their extraversion tactics, African state elites have manipulated what William Brown (2013, 18) calls the "language of sovereignty." These states assert that international financial institutions have encroached on the state's sovereignty through their demands for neoliberal structural adjustment economic policies. International actors become convenient scapegoats to blame for a country's problems in order to win political points with constituents, a tactic that President Yoweri Museveni in Uganda has used effectively (Fisher 2013). Such extraversion claims help to rally public support or to avoid implementation of global health governance. Nonstate actors also can use extraversion: Before AIDS drugs were available in Africa, African AIDS activists gave testimonies about their difficulties living with the disease in order to get Western partners to provide them with these life-saving medications (Nguyen 2010). People living with HIV in Malawi and Zambia emphasized suffering, gender inequality, resiliency, and stigma in their performances in order to gain jobs with NGOs (Anderson and Patterson 2017.)

The literature on Africa in international relations leads to some hypotheses about global health governance. First, African states will be more likely to *accept* global health governance when the norms that undergird that governance are coherent and institutionalized. In this scenario, issue frames tend to be somewhat unified, and they do not undermine the identity of African states or populations. The result is that African states contribute to the design of policies through rhetoric and ideas that align with accepted global health norms, and they accept programs, structures, and funding mechanisms that result from those policies. Second, states are more likely to *challenge* the design and implementation of global health governance when norms have not been accepted, when there are multiple norms at play, or when norms have not become institutionalized with programs and funding. Institutions supporting those norms are politically weak and underfunded. Frames surrounding the health condition challenge the very identity of African states and populations, leading to a backlash by African states. Finally, *ambivalence* results when norms are contested or nonexistent, there are multiple and contested frames, and programs, policies, and funding are underdeveloped. In many ways, challenge and ambivalence result from the same international landscape, though in challenge, issue frames cut to the core of African state identity, generating an outward response in both global health diplomacy and policy implementation.

State-Level Factors

Given that the international and domestic realms interact to shape small state behavior (Hey 2013, 189), the international level of analysis is insufficient for explaining African engagement on global health governance. Domestic politics matter too. Here I focus on two aspects of African states: their adoption of democratic institutions and their neopatrimonial governance patterns. I chose these two variables because the literature on African politics has emphasized them as policy drivers (see Bates 1981; van de Walle 2001; Bratton and van de Walle 1997; Ake 1996; Englebert 2009), though I recognize that individual leaders can also play a role in policy adoption, as research on global AIDS policies indicates (Hey 2003; Patterson 2013; Rotberg 2012; Patterson 2006; Nattrass 2012; Lieberman 2012).[6] While leadership is mentioned in chapters 2 and 4, my analysis focuses more on the structures in which leaders operate.

Democracy surged in Africa with the end of the cold war, when many states adopted multiparty elections. While rule of law, government accountability, and citizen participation remain somewhat underdeveloped (Chabal and Daloz 1999; Bratton 2013), even in states that are only partly democratic, state officials show some concern about election outcomes and public opinion, there is some level of media freedom, and opposition parties and civil society groups seek to hold government accountable (Lindberg 2009; Cheeseman 2015). The research on the links between democracy and health is vast and somewhat inconclusive (Sen 2001; Przeworski, Alvarez, Cheibub, and Limongi 2000; Safaei 2006; Dionne 2011), but at the individual country level, democratic regimes do tend to respond to demands for social programs including health (Patterson 2006; Strand 2012). For example, Ghana, a strong democracy, established its national health insurance scheme in 2003 and continues to respond to civil society and media demands for the program's expansion and improved efficiency (*Daily Graphic*, March 30, 2017). Such government responsiveness at the country level says nothing about how democratic states engage with global health norms, institutions, or policies.

I predict that democracy will have contradictory effects on states' engagement with global health governance, and as the book's chapters indicate, this factor's explanatory power varies with the health condition. On one hand, democratic accountability and respect for rule of law, particularly in more established democracies like Botswana, Ghana, or South Africa, urge officials to participate in the design and implementation of global health governance. This outcome seems particularly likely if international norms on human rights and nondiscrimination that underlie global health governance resonate with domestic public opinion (Finnemore 2009; Fox 2014). On the other hand, short-term election concerns could lead democratic states to challenge global health governance norms and practices, particularly if health issues are highly salient to the public and global health policies contradict the perceived public interest. Democratic states remain ambivalent toward global health governance if health issues lack saliency or immediacy to those states' populations. Yet because of democracy's general weakness in many African states, its effect on state engagement in global health policy design and implementation is often limited.

The second factor that determines state actions in global health governance is neopatrimonialism, which Christopher Clapham (1985, 48) defines as "a form of organization in which relationships of a broadly patrimonial type pervade a political and administrative system which is formally constructed on rational-level lines." Neopatrimonialism interweaves notions of interdependence and community with formal state structures and bureaucratic hierarchies (Bach and Gazibo 2012), combining "features of tradition and modernity into a debilitating witch's brew" (Mkandawire 2015, 566). At its core, neopatrimonialism is rooted in reciprocal relations between, on the one hand, ruling elites, who act as patrons, and on the other hand, their clients, who reward these elites with loyalty and deference in return for benefits. Neopatrimonialism reflects several factors: (1) the "economy of affection," in which interdependence among community members in contexts of economic uncertainty creates a moral obligation to materially support one another (Hyden 1980); (2) precolonial rule in which "having people" (not land or material possessions) brought leaders legitimacy and authority (Herbst 2000; Scherz 2014); and (3) traditional authority patterns that were legitimated by charisma and cultural symbols (Schatzberg 2001). In this governance structure, "dominated [clients] understand, participate in, and even celebrate their domination" (Pitcher, Moran, and Johnston 2009, 126). Because rule occurs through informal, reciprocal relations, individual leaders (i.e., the personal ruler or big man) centralize authority, make decisions capriciously (Jackson and Rosberg 1982), and sometimes act in rapacious and gluttonous ways, literally exhibiting a "politics of the belly" (Bayart 1993). Because the lines between formal, official positions in the public realm and private interests are murky, state elites use rents from their control of state coffers and parastatals to reward supporters such as co-ethnics or to coopt opponents (van de Walle 2001; see Ekeh 1975 on the public and private realms).

Neopatrimonialism has been blamed for Africa's underperformance in socioeconomic development and democratization for numerous reasons. Some observers assert that it creates a "moral economy of corruption" which justifies the theft of state resources and makes this theft "understandable" and, at times, "acceptable" to citizens (Smith 2008; Mkandawire 2015, 571; Olivier de Sardan 1999). It discourages citizens from exhibiting exit or voice, out of a feared loss of benefits from a patron. Thráinn Eggertsson (2005, 30) portrays neopatrimonialism as static: for state elites who want to make the system more legal-rational and less personalist, "new rules clash with old" to make reform difficult. Several scholars assert that donors foster this status quo and are complicit in neopatrimonial governance when their projects and programs channel material resources and legitimacy to state elites (Uvin 1998; Clapham 1996; Barnes, Brown, and Harman 2015). Even multiparty elections have not undermined neopatrimonial practices (Kelsall 2011). Since poor countries often cannot make credible commitments to investments in public goods (Khan 2005) and since voters in poor countries act rationally to choose candidates who offer immediate, tangible benefits (Lyne 2007), candidates have an incentive to utilize short-term patronage to sway election outcomes (Chandra 2007). Political economists assert that neopatrimonialism undermines long-term investments in infrastructure, economic development, and human capital because state resources are siphoned off for short-term benefits. It creates fiscal deficits and inefficiencies that discourage capital investment; it undermines revenue collection; it fosters reactionary and disjointed policies; and it leads to a state without the capacity to promote health and development (Englebert and Dunn 2013; van de Walle 2001; Callaghy 1988; Bates 1981).

As a concept, neopatrimonialism has been criticized for being a "conceptual muddle" (de Grassi 2008); for providing a simplistic and catch-all explanation for all of Africa's problems (Therkilsden 2005; Kelsall 2011); for being reductionist (Mkandawire 2015); for downplaying African elites' ideas and actions as simply "rationalization of interests" (Mkandawire 2015, 598); for applying microlevel patterns of social behavior to macrolevel governance systems; for robbing local people of agency (Pitcher, Moran, and Johnston 2009); and for singling out Africa as a continent with clientelism, patronage, and corruption when such practices are found worldwide and are no more acceptable in Africa than any other region (Moreno 2003; Mkandawire 2015). Most crucially, though, scholars have challenged the notion that neopatrimonialism undermines economic development and growth, pointing to developmental patrimonialism in states like Botswana, Rwanda, and Ethiopia (Kelsall 2011; Matfess 2015; Mkandawire 2015; Pitcher, Moran, and Johnston 2009; Khan 2000; Levy 2010).

Despite the concept's limitations, this book takes as its starting point that neopatrimonialism is "ubiquitous throughout Africa" (Brown 2013, 9). I also recognize, though, that it is only one of several factors that drive state participation in the design and implementation of global health governance, and that states differ substantially in their level of neopatrimonialism. The relationship between neopatrimonialism and global health governance illustrates the complicated dialectic between international and domestic factors. According to the neopatrimonial model, because state elites seek rents, they look to benefit from donor health resources. These might include per diems for donor-funded workshops, health projects placed in their voting strongholds, and lucrative salaries from donor projects (Smith 2003; Giles-Vernick and Webb 2013; Vian, Miller, Themba, and Bukuluki 2012). Such resources benefit elites and/or the clients in their patronage networks. One might speculate that such material benefits would lead elites to accept global health governance, since its programs and projects would enable these elites to gain needed resources for their networks. In each of the case studies below, though, neopatrimonial states react differently to global health governance. These actions vary in three ways.

First, the neopatrimonial logic rests on the idea that state elites seek global resources which can be used for rents. But what if these resources are limited or nonexistent, thereby creating no incentive for state action? As chapter 4 illustrates, multilateral and bilateral donors have committed few resources to combatting various NCDs globally. For states with an interest in rent generation, there is little to be gained from accepting global health governance on NCDs. As that chapter illustrates, this pattern of ambivalence is evident for some states, though others have adopted some policies on NCDs for reasons not linked to neopatrimonial interests. Because resources might be forthcoming if donors' priorities change, many states hedge their bets, sometimes adopting minimal actions or only half-heartedly implementing the policies they have adopted. They exhibit a long time horizon in their ambivalence.

In the second pattern, a state's neopatrimonial search for rents urges it to challenge global health governance in order to gain resources. The impetus to do so is particularly acute in states with high levels of corruption and decentralized patronage networks, where access to resources is a highly competitive free-for-all that is controlled by state or societal gatekeepers (Beresford 2015; Utas 2008; Reno 2000).

The decentralized, winner-take-all nature of such networks drives actors to embrace a short time horizon that undermines long-term investments, inclusive decision-making, and the curtailment of corruption (Kelsall 2011). Perceiving they have nothing to lose, these neopatrimonial states challenge global health governance norms, structures, and programs. Chapter 2 illustrates this pattern using the cases of South Africa and The Gambia, who challenged biomedical approaches to AIDS, while chapter 3 shows how competition between neopatrimonial networks in Liberia shaped that country's reactions to Ebola governance.

In the third model, neopatrimonialism and global health governance are dialectically linked. While the neopatrimonial objective of resource acquisition urges the state to accept global health governance in the first place, the very programs, policies, and resources of global health governance then push the state to continue that acceptance. This occurs when global health governance institutions are coherent, rooted in accepted norms, and well-financed. They then feed the state's long-term development goals and urge the construction of centralized state institutions to manage health policies. The resulting state structures have the ability to create, gather, and distribute rents; they also are rooted in a long time horizon, which urges leaders to curb corruption excesses, to build long-term investments, and to foster positive development outcomes. These institutions are relatively inclusive, which allows rents to be "shared around sufficiently so that no important groups feel completely excluded" (Kelsall 2011, 82). Ultimately, these structures generate control over rents for the state, create buy-in for global health governance, and increase state legitimacy. Chapter 2 illustrates this pattern in the context of AIDS.

To summarize, I predict that democracy will have various effects on state engagement with the design and implementation of global health governance. Democratic states will accept global health governance that aligns with their own democratic values, though short-term election pressures may cause these states to challenge global health policies. Ambivalence results in democracies when civil society mobilization is limited (see below). Neopatrimonialism's influence on state engagement with global health governance will be context-specific, based on the availability of resources that undergird global health policies and the level of centralization of state structures to distribute those resources.

Societal-Level Factors

While democracy and neopatrimonialism can affect how African states interact with global health governance, bottom-up pressures from civil society matter too.

Civil society is the collection of groups which are formed around a common interest and which lie between the family and state. With ideological attributes that link the concept to neoliberalism and sustainable development (Chabal and Daloz 1999, 22; Scherz 2014; Ferguson 2009), civil society has tended to be viewed by donors (including international health officials) as an organized force that counterbalances the state, demands good governance, provides social services, and teaches participation (Cheeseman 2015; Putnam 1994; Rothchild and Chazan 1988). While some African civil society groups play these roles, others are under-resourced, internally divided, lacking in transparency and accountability, hierarchical, and discriminatory (Michael 2004; Gyimah-Boadi 2004; Chabal and Daloz 1999). Civil society is often more fluid than organized. In the African context, participation in groups outside of religious organizations is low (Afrobarometer 2012), and ethnic, traditional, and religious groups sometimes demand state policies and resources that benefit solely their own constituencies (Chabal and Daloz 1999; Migdal 1988). As this chapter's opening vignette illustrates, civil society actors like the Muslim leaders in northern Nigeria have the potential to influence policy, if they tap into social attitudes such as distrust of the state and suspicion of biomedicine, and if they command their followers' loyalty.

Victor Azarya (1988) describes two models for state-civil society interactions in Africa: incorporation and disengagement. In the former, civil society actors are often coopted into state institutions using the aforementioned patronage resources or rent-managing institutions. Dependent on state resources to pay for programs, to bolster their legitimacy, to obtain legal recognition, and, ultimately, to ensure their survival, these organizations cannot effectively challenge the state (Englebert 2009). In this model, local people become "quiescent and complicit in their own exploitation" (Mkandawire 2015, 571), though Nic Cheeseman (2015, 69) points out that "few governments [are] powerful enough to wholly subordinate." In Azarya's disengagement model, civil society avoids the state: villagers conveniently "forget" to pay their taxes, and they grow food crops instead of cash crops that generate foreign exchange (Bunker 1987); urban populations engage in the informal (and untaxed) economy; women develop intricate global trade networks on the margins of the law (MacGaffey and Bazenguissa-Ganga 2000); and African religious leaders and believers turn to spiritual power for assistance in the material world (Ellis and ter Haar 1998). The incorporation and disengagement models, however, ignore a middle position of state–civil society interactions: civil society opposition to the state. At crucial moments, such as the democratic transitions of the early 1990s, society has engaged in protest. Such activities are the work of both

organized groups—labor unions, student groups, human rights organizations—
and relatively unorganized, disenfranchised urban youth who deeply distrust the
state and its institutions. Through their sheer numbers in cities even the marginalized have at times influenced politics (Branch and Mampilly 2015; Bratton and van
de Walle 1997).

I assert that what Donald Rothchild and Naomi Chazan (1988) term the "precarious balance" between the African state and civil society shapes Africa's engagement with global health governance. State incorporation of civil society facilitates
the pattern of acceptance, because it enables the state and civil society to act in a
unified manner within the context of global health policy design and implementation. Yet for states to "get to acceptance," it is often necessary for civil society to oppose the state, sometimes empowered by transnational advocacy networks (Keck
and Sikkink 1998). State ambivalence toward global health governance results
from civil society disengagement from the state; this disengagement is not always
by choice but rather results from limited resources, weak leadership, or lack of coordination. Disengagement means the state feels little pressure to act. Challenge in
global health governance reflects an oppositional civil society, one that mobilizes
in public and private ways against state authority. In order to preserve its legitimacy and maintain its control over civil society, the state opposes global health
governance norms and institutions, particularly if these appear to undermine the
core identities that civil society organizations support. Chapters 2 and 3 illustrate
how these patterns of state–civil society interactions have led states to challenge
the rhetoric, policies, institutions, and policies of global health governance in both
the design and implementation phases.

To summarize my predictions about African state participation in global health
governance: First, *acceptance* results when international norms are coherent and
institutionalized in programs and resources. Issue frames do not undermine state
identities. African elites participate in policy design, voicing their opinions and
shaping norms and narratives in global health diplomacy. These elites recognize
the potential material and legitimacy benefits of acceptance and, using a long time
horizon, develop inclusive institutions that centralize management of the rents
that emerge from a well-entrenched system of global health governance. For democratic states, acceptance is partly a reaction to civil society mobilization or global
norms, and acceptance helps to increase state legitimacy. As global health governance becomes accepted, civil society groups become incorporated into state institutions that manage that governance. The very implementation of global health
governance policies and programs then generates new or different neopatrimonial

benefits for the state. Over time, civil society plays not a challenging role but a legitimating one as it urges states to continue to accept global health governance systems.

Challenge results when global norms and programs surrounding health are underdeveloped or contradictory. Through global health diplomacy and policy implementation, state elites contest, underenforce, or ignore norms. Perceiving that the frames around health issues undermine the aspirational identities of African actors, elites engage in backlash. In search of resources for short-term gain, neopatrimonial states, particularly those with high levels of corruption and exclusive, winner-take-all networks, engage in challenge. For democratic or partially democratic states, immediate election concerns urge state leaders to challenge global health governance. Civil society opposition, perhaps rooted in a history of distrustful relationships with the state, also leads state elites to challenge global health governance. This pattern is more likely if civil society is led by groups with their own power base, such as ethnic, religious, and traditional associations that rely on moral, spiritual, and symbolic power.

Ambivalence reflects limited political incentives, though it also shows how states hedge their bets about future global health actions. States reflect ambivalence when global health structures and policies are in flux, often vaguely articulated, unfunded, or lacking institutional homes. Norms are contested or nonexistent, and frames around the health issue are numerous. Because international resources are few, state elites are relatively unconcerned about developing rent management institutions that reflect a long time horizon, centralize decision-making, and include major stakeholders. Most leaders do not oppose global health policies and programs, but they also are not motivated to be proactive. This ambivalence is evident in weak participation in global health diplomacy and norm articulation. Ambivalence reflects weak civil society mobilization, or organizations that are disengaged from the state because of their own divisions or lack of resources. Ultimately, state commitment to global health governance is not embedded in larger political strategies for state elites; that is, engagement with global health policies does not bring leaders political legitimacy, resources, or positive relations with important civil society actors.

An Incomplete Explanation: Disease Characteristics

This volume focuses on political factors such as framing, norm acceptance, international health institutions, state characteristics, and the state–civil society dialectic that determine if African states accept, challenge, or show ambivalence toward the design and implementation of global health governance. I do not discount that the very nature of a health issue—its severity, tractability, and the people it affects—could provide a partial explanation for state actions (Shiffman and Smith 2007; McInnes and Lee 2012; Shiffman 2010; Tomlinson and Lund 2012; Shiffman et al. 2016; on qualities of non-health issues, see Keck and Sikkink 1998). First, disease severity does matter, as the magnitude of the AIDS crisis illustrates. By the new millennium, some African states faced high HIV rates and a growing number of deaths from the epidemic. One interviewee said about Zambia, a country with a 12 percent HIV prevalence: "The government just had to do something. There was such a high level of mortality, funerals all of time. At that church across the street, [there were] funerals every day. And then two or three people in a hospital bed" (interview, multilateral donor official, Lusaka, February 23, 2011; UNAIDS 2015a). As chapter 2 illustrates, the increased number of deaths led African states to collectively address the issue in 2001. Yet severity alone does not explain this action, since some states with very high HIV rates have not necessarily adopted more global AIDS structures than states with low HIV rates. More broadly, if disease severity is a crucial driver of action, why have African states not done more to address some NCDs such as heart disease and cancers, which kill millions of Africans and cause high rates of morbidity?

Disease severity only partly determines policy outcomes because of limited information about the incidence, morbidity, and mortality rates of many health conditions in Africa. Health-related data remains woefully inadequate. Data collection challenges range from stigma surrounding diseases to poor access to health-care institutions, where disease statistics might be recorded (*Lancet* 2016). Global and state actions on AIDS were facilitated by data about HIV prevalence and AIDS deaths, statistics collected through years of UNAIDS's surveillance programs (UNAIDS 2015a). Advocates working on NCDs point out that the severity of cancer, diabetes, mental illness, and hypertension in Africa is unknown, as many cases go undiagnosed and unreported (*Devex News*, June 3, 2016; interview, advocate on NCDs, Lusaka, June 12, 2014). In the case of neglected tropical diseases such as schistosomiasis or hookworm, many people never seek treatment, and thus prevalence rates are merely estimates (Hotez, Asojo, and Adesina 2012). Even the process of defining some conditions as a disease can undermine data collection, as has been the case with some mental illnesses (Tomlinson and Lund 2012; Bird et al. 2011).

A second incomplete explanation for state engagement in global health governance is tractability, or the presence of solutions for a particular health issue. If solutions do not require policymakers to address economic, political, or social structures, the issue is more tractable and has the potential to receive attention (Shiffman et al. 2016; Stone 1989). The availability of technically focused solutions like immunization campaigns to reduce child mortality rates or the distribution of insecticide-treated bed nets to prevent malaria makes it easier for states to accept global health governance on those issues. In contrast, the perception that surgery is costly has led to the underprovision of basic surgical procedures to alleviate broken bones, obstructed labor, or appendicitis for millions of people in the Global South. Without tractability, global surgery has not gotten political attention (Shawar, Shiffman, and Spiegel 2015). The perception that easy-to-implement and acceptable solutions exist often matters more than the actual presence of such solutions, since addressing almost all health conditions requires a mix of biomedical and social approaches. For example, bed net distribution does not ensure that people will use those nets (Shah 2010); provision of free ART does not address the cultural, social, or economic reasons that some people do not adhere to the treatment regimen (van Dijk, Dilger, Burchardt, and Rasing 2014; Smith 2014; Burgess and Campbell 2014; Patterson 2015); and the rise of the antivaccine movement in the West indicates that even well-established solutions can be questioned (Kirkland 2012; Kata 2012). While tractability matters, it does not explain why African actors challenge or remain ambivalent toward relatively tractable solutions to health issues, such as immunizations, anti-smoking campaigns, and condom distribution for HIV prevention.

A third insufficient explanation for African state reactions to global health governance is that the state acts because of the people a disease affects. Identifiable groups, groups that inspire sympathy because they are perceived to be "innocent" or "deserving," or those who can mobilize for their own cause have been more likely to generate policy responses (Shiffman et al. 2016; Schneider and Ingram 1993). For example, donors' attention to AIDS in Africa after 2000 partly reflects the fact that women were the majority of people living with HIV and were viewed to be higher up in the "hierarchy of deservedness." In contrast, the fact that AIDS first affected gay men contributed to a slow government AIDS response in the United States in the early 1980s (Siplon 2002, 2013). Yet the limited attention to maternal mortality until the mid-2000s or to breast and cervical cancers until the present shows that women (and their health issues) are not always perceived to be deserving (Shiffman and Smith 2007; Confortini and Krong 2015; Livingston 2012). While I do not discount that disease characteristics—severity, tractability, and population affected—matter in global health governance, disease qualities are not a sufficient explanation for African state acceptance, challenge, or ambivalence to global health governance. Partly this is because IGOs, epistemic communities, advocates, and state officials themselves shape how these qualities are viewed. In addition, these disease attributes affect policy views and actions of all global health actors, not just African states; thus they cannot explain unique African state actions (McInnes et al. 2012; Shiffman et al. 2016; on activists and framing NCDs, see Geneau et al. 2010).

Methodology

To analyze these patterns, I use three health conditions: the AIDS pandemic; the 2014–2015 Ebola outbreak in West Africa; and the increasing prevalence of NCDs. The goal is not to focus on the global health campaigns linked to these diseases but rather to use the health issues as a way to explore how weak states engage in global health governance. I recognize the danger of a disease focus, as it places health conditions in "silos" without acknowledging the linkages between them. Yet, because global health governance has tended to focus on vertical programs (see Benton 2015), my approach emulates empirical reality. In order to minimize the number of variables that shape African state reactions, I have chosen issues that are similar in terms of the attention they have received from global health institutions (although attention has not always translated into programs and resources), their unprecedented mortality and morbidity rates, and the ways that society has reacted to them. The choice of these health conditions also enables me to compare African state reactions to global health governance over a long period (with AIDS), during a crisis (with Ebola), and for an emerging health issue (NCDs). I do, however, acknowledge that these health conditions differ: AIDS and Ebola are caused by viruses; Ebola rapidly causes morbidity and, in approximately 40 percent of cases, mortality (CDC 2016), whereas most NCDs are chronic and slow in progression.

There is more overlap between these health conditions than conventional wisdom suggests. Access to ART has made AIDS a chronic condition, with some Africans who live with HIV actually dying of some NCDs like cancer and diabetes (Mendenhall and Norris 2015; Livingston 2012). Ebola was a crisis, but AIDS also was portrayed as a crisis and an "emergency" (Patterson 2006). An estimated 15 to 20 percent of cancers—one category of NCDs—are caused by viruses, including some liver cancers, cervical cancer, and some forms of leukemia (Liao 2006). In terms of attention, AIDS is unprecedented in the amount of media coverage and donor money it has attracted (Kenworthy and Parker 2014). The Ebola outbreak led to panic in the West, widespread media attention, and new reform proposals for emergency responses at the 2015 World Health Assembly (Specter 2015; *Guardian*, May 18, 2015). And the UN General Assembly held High-Level Meetings to discuss both AIDS and NCDs.

All of these health conditions are associated with high morbidity and mortality rates. In 2014, there were 36.9 million people living with HIV, with over 70 percent of those individuals living in Africa. In the same year, 1.4 million new HIV infections occurred in the region, and an estimated 800,000 Africans died from AIDS-related complications (UNAIDS 2015a). According to the US Centers for Disease Control and Prevention (2016), as of April 2016, the world's largest Ebola outbreak had led to 11,310 deaths and 28,616 probable, suspected, and confirmed cases in the affected states of Liberia, Guinea, and Sierra Leone.[7] And NCDs kill over 36 million people annually, with most of these deaths occurring in low- and middle-income countries (Manyema 2013). Societies have reacted in similar ways to NCDs, Ebola, and AIDS, exhibiting a mixture of stigma, fear, ignorance, and compassion. The high-level attention and magnitude of AIDS, NCDs, and Ebola, as well as shared societal reactions to these health challenges, makes them ideal issues in which to observe how African states engage with global health governance. But it is important to recognize that even though I have chosen specific diseases (or in the case of NCDs, a collection of diseases) in order to exemplify these patterns, in reality, no single health condition fits completely into one response category.

My investigation uses both qualitative and quantitative data to discern patterns in African state interactions with global health governance. In addition to consulting the secondary literature in political science, anthropology, public health, and sociology on various NCDs, Ebola, and AIDS, I conducted key informant interviews with almost two hundred donor and African state officials, local and international NGO representatives, African and global health activists, and local people living with (or surviving from) one of the three health conditions. Interviews were conducted during research trips of three weeks to six months in duration, which occurred between 2005 and 2017. This long time frame enables me to see changes in Africa's involvement in global health governance, particularly on the AIDS issue. This includes fieldwork in Ghana (forty interviews), Uganda (twelve interviews), Tanzania (eleven interviews), Liberia (twenty-five interviews), Zambia (sixty-two interviews), and the United States (fifty interviews). While I sought to include multiple health topics in the discussions, Zambian interviews focused on AIDS and the NCDs of diabetes and cancer, as well as tobacco control; Ghanaian interviews on AIDS, tobacco control, mental illness, and NCDs (as a collective unit); Tanzanian and Ugandan interviews on cancer, tobacco control, and NCDs (as a collective unit); and Liberian interviews on Ebola.[8] In the United States, I spoke with global health activists, UN officials, US government officials, African government representatives, and international NGO workers on all of these health conditions. Interviewees were identified through the organizations that they represent, media stories, online organizational reports, recommendations from health experts, and snowball sampling. Themes of interviews included government policies on AIDS, NCDs, and/or Ebola; challenges and effectiveness of African civil society groups in health advocacy; relations between African actors and international health institutions and global health activists; changes over time in program priorities on AIDS and NCDs; challenges in African responses to health issues; and societal and state perceptions of health issues. Interviews utilized open-ended questions. In order to encourage honest responses, interviewees were assured of their anonymity in all written documents. Interviews were either audiotaped (if permission was granted) or summarized in notes. Interviews were transcribed, read for accuracy, and sorted using NVivo to discern particular themes, such as health and security norms, global cooperation, and resources.

In 2011, I conducted fifty-seven focus group discussions with support groups for people living with HIV as well as groups of caregivers who help both people living with HIV and also AIDS orphans in the poor neighborhoods of Lusaka, Mumbwa, Kabwe, Livingstone, Ndola, and Kitwe in Zambia. These groups had been established by AIDS clinics, churches, or communities between 2001 and 2011. I was introduced to groups through informants at various churches and from the Network of Zambian People Living with HIV/AIDS (NZP+), who then accompanied me for discussions. Focused discussions examined these groups' interactions with donors and state officials, their health and development projects, the challenges they faced, and their group achievements. Interviews also investigated the role of stigma and religion in the AIDS response. Findings from these discussions undergird the examination of civil society mobilization on AIDS (see also Patterson 2015, 2016; Anderson and Patterson 2017). In addition, lengthy periods of fieldwork in Ghana (four months in 2008 and six months in 2017) and Zambia (six months in 2011), as well as two research trips to Tanzania and three to Uganda, facilitated my observations of African community health mobilization efforts. These observations varied from watching meetings of support groups for people living with HIV in Zambia, to listening to Ghanaian pastors share health messages during worship services, to documenting conversations about tobacco use among Tanzanian and Ghanaian university students and professors. These observations undergird many of my conclusions regarding civil society mobilization. The research protocols for my fieldwork were approved by the Institutional Review Boards at the University of the South, Tennessee (my current institution), and Calvin College, Michigan (my former institution).

To ascertain state interest in particular health topics, I conducted content analysis of African leaders' statements on health issues in the media and international forums such as the UN Special Session on HIV/AIDS in 2001 and the UN High-Level Meeting of the General Assembly on the Prevention and Control of Non-Communicable Diseases held in 2011. Chapters 2 and 4 use this material; for both, I searched these leaders' speeches for particular themes around which the health issue (AIDS or NCDs) had been framed such as human rights. I used NVivo to categorize and sort speeches. In the case of Ebola, I also examined thirty newspaper articles from Namibia on that state's reaction to the outbreak, and I read news articles from Liberian newspapers online, particularly the *Observer* and *FrontPageAfrica*. In addition, my research assistant and I classified over 180 news articles on Ebola published in the *New York Times*, the *Washington Post*, and the *Guardian* between January 1, 2014, and August 31, 2014, to discern major themes in coverage before and during the early days of global attention to the outbreak.

In terms of quantitative data, I constructed databases using WHO and UNAIDS reports on health indicators and African states' acceptance of global health policies related to AIDS and NCDs, as chapters 2 and 4 illustrate. I compiled data from the World Bank's socioeconomic development indicators and state capacity measures in order to discern the relationship between these factors and state design and implementation of global health governance (World Bank 2014c, 2015d). Data from Polity IV were used to classify countries by regime type to discern how democracy relates to states' participation in global health governance (Marshall and Cole 2014, 20–21). The use of various data sets to explore how African states act on global health governance is detailed in each of the chapters.

This multi-method examination enables me to develop a better understanding of how international factors such as donor health programs interact with domestic political considerations and local mobilization to shape Africa's involvement in global health governance. Such investigations elucidate general patterns that can inform global health policymaking and implementation. Yet because context matters for the dynamic interplay among these drivers of participation in global health governance, I utilize case studies to illustrate patterns (see Brett 2006, 4 on contextual factors and African development). Chapter 3, for example, uses a case study of Liberia's response to the 2014–2015 Ebola outbreak, in order to trace causal mechanisms that drove state actions. The methodology of process tracing enables a "within-a-case" examination that uses thick descriptions and sequential analysis of variables to elucidate causal relationships (Collier 2011). Chapter 4 explores the case studies of South Africa, Ghana, Zambia, and Eritrea to highlight the causal variables that affect state ambivalence toward global health governance. Though similar in their engagement with global health governance on NCDs, the cases differ in regime type, government effectiveness (as a measure of neopatrimonialism), income level, and severity of disease burden for NCDs. The cases elucidate the context-specific factors that shape action; their broader themes are echoed in an aggregate analysis of states that have adopted WHO-endorsed policies on NCDs.

Plan of the Book

In chapter 2, I analyze Africa's move from challenge to acceptance of global health governance on AIDS. These patterns are evident in both the design and implementation of global AIDS governance. The chapter concentrates on the pattern of acceptance, which became the predominant pattern after the early 2000s, though it does analyze two exceptions to this rule with the cases of South Africa under former president Thabo Mbeki and The Gambia under former president Yahya Jammeh. In spite of the two exceptions and even though debates remain on some specific AIDS policies, such as HIV prevention, norms about the need to address AIDS and to provide universal access to ART have cascaded and been institutionalized. Most African states have provided free access to AIDS drugs and eliminated health-system user fees in order to institutionalize this norm (Youde 2008). Acceptance was possible because international norms and structures on AIDS have been coherent and institutionalized; in policy design and issue framing, African states helped to shape and articulate these norms (Kapstein and Busby 2013). In the implementation phase, African states established institutions like national AIDS commissions and country coordinating mechanisms, structures that helped to centralize a long time horizon on rent dispersal for AIDS responses and create state and civil society acceptance for AIDS policies. While during the early period of challenge of global health governance civil society was disengaged from the AIDS issue, it then began to oppose the state in the late 1990s and early 2000s, pushing many states to act. Civil society became incorporated into AIDS institutions, giving the state a reason to continue AIDS governance (Patterson 2006; Mbali 2013). African states have benefited from resources and the increased domestic legitimacy they have gained through AIDS actions (Fox 2014). As such, global health governance on AIDS has been a driver of new types of neopatrimonial governance patterns.

Chapter 3 examines the Ebola outbreak in West Africa as an example of challenge. As the first large-scale epidemic of an extremely deadly contagious disease to emerge from Africa since the revisions of the IHR in 2005, Ebola highlights how African states reacted to global health policies on disease surveillance and control. Challenge was evident at two levels. First, over half of African states established travel restrictions despite the WHO and UN Security Council statements against such actions. Second, affected states acted in challenging ways: Guinea and Liberia downplayed the epidemic in early 2014, for example. In the policy design process, Liberian officials confronted and utilized global health framing to their advantage. These challenges occurred because of weak, underfunded international health institutions that could not (or would not) enforce the norm of IHR adherence (see Davies, Kamradt-Scott, and Rushton 2015; Kamradt-Scott 2016). Global action was not rooted in clear norms, such as health as a human right. The disease was framed in light of neglect and crisis, both of which emphasized Ebola's emergence from "backward" Africa. This frame challenged the aspirational identity of the affected states, all three of which sought to remake themselves after protracted conflicts and refugee crises (Wilkinson and Leach 2014).

At the state level, for nonaffected states that implemented travel restrictions, location mattered: many of those close to affected states put into place some limitations. Yet many states with upcoming elections, regardless of proximity to an affected state, also challenged global health governance, as did states with a heavy reliance on tourism for resources. In the process, these states sought to distance themselves from the framing of Africa as a site of deadly outbreaks. In the specific case of Liberia (the focus of chapter 3), the crisis nature of the issue meant that state leaders did not develop a long time horizon; instead, the state sought to control decision-making and use global health frames of crisis and neglect to gain resources. The country's decentralized system of rent dispersal and rule through networks benefited from short-term funding and attention to Ebola, but global health governance patterns did not deepen institutions and programs that might generate long-term political legitimacy around health. Civil society also led the state to challenge global heath governance, as it mobilized along traditional and religious lines and its actions were rooted in distrust of state institutions (Specter 2015; WHO 2015d, 2015f). In the process, it pushed state elites to react, particularly to policies in global health governance that discounted culture and tradition.

In chapter 4, I investigate actions on NCDs (as a collection of health conditions) to exemplify the ambivalence pattern. With a few exceptions (particularly, South Africa), African states have been notably absent in global health governance related to the prevention and treatment of NCDs. When African actors speak about these health conditions and their impact on African development, such statements rarely move beyond generalities. In terms of policy implementation, the majority of African states have adopted few WHO-suggested policies on tobacco control, alcohol use, or the promotion of healthy lifestyles, programs which are intended to decrease the risk of the most prevalent NCDs—cardiovascular diseases, cancers, diabetes, and chronic respiratory diseases. Additionally, many African states have yet to develop multisectoral plans to combat any NCDs, despite encouragement from the WHO. Yet African states do not publicly refuse to act on NCDs; they do not speak against programs or policies. Rather, they engage in foot dragging, adopting some policies but not all. The chapter argues that ambivalence reflects the nascent aspect of this health issue: the international community itself has been slow to act on NCDs, with institutional development and funding being largely absent. With few resources and low political saliency for the issue, state elites have little incentive to establish global health governance policies or institutions. For neopatrimonial leaders who wish to reward particular groups, identifying such populations is difficult since NCDs are a variety of diseases, they affect disparate groups in society, and their chronic nature and slow progression from diagnosis to death make it difficult to keep the public and politicians interested. There is also limited short-term payoff for acting for democratic regimes, because the health benefits from policies enacted today accrue many years later. Civil society mobilization on NCDs has been weak, exhibiting a certain level of disengagement beyond caregiving for people with these health conditions.

The case studies illustrate a level of dynamism between these patterns as political conditions change. This mutability is most evident with state responses to AIDS governance: most African states initially challenged global AIDS policies through denial. But as international, state, and societal factors changed (e.g., international structures emerged and community AIDS mobilization occurred), states (including South Africa after Mbeki's presidency) accepted global AIDS governance. In the case of Ebola, I illustrate how challenge, as a short-term reaction, has little long-term effect on global health governance, particularly if challenge occurs in the context of a crisis which ultimately fades. In the case of NCDs, the issue is "too new" to observe this dynamism in state actions. Yet I argue that part of the reason African states are ambivalent on the global health governance of

NCDs is because the future may bring new opportunities, resources, and saliency to the issue. Indeed, some states that have done more to address NCDs, such as South Africa and Ghana, seem to recognize this fact.

After summarizing the book's findings, the conclusion draws out lessons for African agency in global health governance. First, I argue that African agency itself shapes global health governance because governance processes are dialectical and dynamic. African states' expertise on particular issues gives them voice, enabling them to not be silent bystanders but movers and shakers in global health politics. Second, I question if African agency might help global health governance focus less on vertical (or disease-specific) programs and more on strengthening health systems. I conclude by arguing that African state actions in global health governance—the patterns of challenge, acceptance, and ambivalence this work details—have implications for the health of millions of Africans.

[chapter 2]

When All Factors Align
Acceptance of Global AIDS Governance

When I came [to this clinic] I was very sick, but I got medicine. Today I am not 100 percent, but I am doing okay. I am doing my work. You know, before [the government ART program] there was this medicine, but no one had money for it. Now they are giving it for free. It has saved many lives. It has saved my life. I am grateful. Thank you.
(Interview, person living with HIV, Lusaka, March 2, 2011)

I was in Copperbelt and my husband died with AIDS. . . . So I was thinking I would be the next victim. I moved here [Lusaka] and found help at the clinic and in this support group.
(Focus group discussion, group of people living with HIV, Lusaka, March 23, 2011)

When I tested HIV positive, the first thing I thought was suicide. I was put on medication, but I am married. I thought that if my husband finds out that I am HIV positive, there will be no more marriage. So I decided to take the medicine and hide it somewhere. So I would be sleeping with my husband, while the medicine was somewhere else. But then a counselor helped me to break the news to my husband. We are still together. I have been on medication for six years and my husband is still HIV negative. I thank God every day.
(Interview, person living with HIV, Chawama, March 23, 2011)

We people living with HIV educate the community about AIDS. We tell them how we were back then—sick, no one cared for us, left to die. . . . And some don't even believe our story. They say, "Wow. You are joking," when we tell them we are on AIDS drugs.
(Focus group discussion, group of people living with HIV, Lusaka, May 10, 2011)

Most of us were bedridden. Now we are strong. We have hope. We are here to stay. Yes, we are here to stay.
(Focus group discussion, group of people living with HIV, Lusaka, May 5, 2011)

These statements come from focus group discussions and interviews with Zambian people living with HIV in 2011, six years after the Zambian government (with funding from international donors) committed to free ART and a ramped-up AIDS response. The respondents' comments illustrate the profound losses—death

31

of a spouse, communal ostracism, diminished health, psychological depression—
and the huge triumphs—physical survival, intact marriages, ascendance to community leadership, return to work, renewed hope—that have accompanied the
pandemic. As Lawrence Gostin (2016) writes, "There is no story in global health as
transformative, awe-inspiring, and yet as tragic as the AIDS pandemic." Indeed,
the magnitude of the pandemic is great: In 2015, UNAIDS reported that there were
36.9 million people living with HIV, with over 70 percent of those individuals (and
88 percent of all children living with HIV) located in sub-Saharan Africa. In the
same year, 1.4 million new HIV infections occurred in the region, and an estimated 800,000 Africans died from AIDS-related complications (AMFAR 2015;
UNAIDS 2015a). The region's average HIV rate (or the percentage of people fifteen
to forty-nine years old who are estimated to be living with HIV) is 4.6 percent,
though it varies from a high of 27 percent in Swaziland to less than 1 percent in
Mali, Niger, Burkina Faso, Cape Verde, Eritrea, Madagascar, Senegal, and São Tomé
and Príncipe (UNAIDS 2014b).

No health issue has received as much attention from donors, states, and civil
society activists as AIDS has (Morfit 2011; Dionne 2012; Watkins and Swidler
2012). In one sense, this attention is somewhat surprising, given the complexity of
responding to the disease. There are significant obstacles to the design and implementation of global AIDS governance: the virus's transmission through sexual
behavior, intravenous drug use, and pregnancy; the disease's long asymptomatic
period; the lack of an AIDS cure or vaccine; the disease's intersection with religious beliefs and patriarchy; the social stigma surrounding AIDS; and the fact that
the first AIDS cases emerged among marginalized populations of men who have
sex with men, sex workers, and people who inject drugs (Hunter 2003; Guest 2001;
Patterson 2006; Anderson 2015; Van Dijk, Dilger, Burchardt, and Rasing 2014;
Chazan 2015; Green and Ruark 2011; Trinitapoli and Weineb 2012; Kalipeni,
Craddock, Oppong, and Gyosh 2004). On the other hand, the magnitude of the
pandemic, the political activism that has accompanied it, and scientific advance-
ments help explain this global commitment (Epstein 2007; Smith and Whiteside
2010; Smith and Siplon 2006; Chan 2015). From the emergence of the region's first
cases in the mid-1980s, African state approaches to global health governance on
AIDS have changed from challenge through the 1990s to overall acceptance in the
new millennium, though South Africa and The Gambia presented significant challenges throughout the 2000s (Patterson 2006; Harman 2009; Cassidy and Leach
2009; Nattrass 2012). This transformation has been possible because of the align-

ment of factors at the international, state, and societal levels. The evolution of strong, well-funded global institutions undergirded by accepted norms and issue frames that reinforce African states' aspirations coincides with African states' development of centralized, neopatrimonial AIDS institutions, incorporation of civil society organizations, and African democracies' willingness to accept many norms underlying the AIDS response. These factors led African states to accept global AIDS governance, through participation in both the policy design and implementation phases.

The chapter examines this transformation in state approaches, and as such, it is divided into two parts—one on challenge and one on acceptance. To be clear, acceptance of global health governance on AIDS does not mean that African states as sovereign entities with unique histories and cultures do not present some challenges on select issues. Acceptance also does not necessarily translate into individual-level behaviors that decrease infections, overcome stigma, or ensure adherence to AIDS treatment plans. Yet in comparison to Ebola (chapter 3) and NCDs (chapter 4), African states have accepted much of global health governance on AIDS: They have articulated norms and policy ideas in global health diplomacy, and they have implemented structures, policies, and programs suggested by global AIDS experts.

In this chapter, I first examine the initial challenges that African states presented to global health governance on AIDS during the 1980s and 1990s, and I explain the reasons for those challenges. I then detail the institutions and funding mechanisms of global health governance on AIDS in the new millennium as well as their roots in accepted global norms. The third section provides evidence that African states have accepted these institutions and norms, though it also illustrates that acceptance is not absolute. I illustrate acceptance in two ways—in the narratives and policy ideas espoused by African leaders in global health diplomacy and in the implementation of AIDS structures, policies, and programs. The fourth section examines the exceptional cases of South Africa and The Gambia. The fifth section analyzes how state-level characteristics and civil society incorporation, as well as international coherence in the AIDS response, drove state acceptance of AIDS governance. It uses these three levels of analysis to explain the challenging actions of South Africa and The Gambia too. The conclusion highlights the potential dangers of acceptance, which, while giving states a stake in global health governance, can become so entrenched that the state cannot incorporate marginalized groups.

African Challenges to Global Health Governance on AIDS: The 1980s and 1990s

The first cases of AIDS emerged in the United States in 1981 among homosexual men, though by the mid-1980s cases were reported worldwide. Between 1981 and 1987, international action on AIDS was slow to develop. The first international AIDS conference among scientists and health officials occurred in 1985, and most activism, led primarily by gay communities, focused on domestic policies in post-industrialized countries (Siplon 2002; Gould 2009). In 1987, the WHO established the Global Programme on AIDS (GPA) to develop biomedical standards for diagnosing cases, to conduct surveillance, and to mobilize societies for AIDS prevention programs. Directed by Jonathan Mann, the program worked directly with governments and grew in staff and funding between 1987 and 1990, with over two hundred experts and a $90 million budget by 1989 (*Washington Post*, December 26, 2000). But by the early 1990s, the United States (the program's biggest contributor) lost interest due to declining fear that AIDS would become a heterosexual epidemic, the rise of health NGOs in the United States that started to work on the issue, and infighting within the WHO over the program's budget and priorities (Patterson and Cieminis 2005, 172; Will 1991; Gordenker, Coate, Jönsson, and Söderholm 1995; Behrman 2004, 51–56).

The early global health governance on AIDS also suffered from competing issue frames. Most scientists and health experts emphasized a biomedical frame, which led to technical solutions like data collection and surveillance. In contrast, Mann and AIDS activists stressed a human rights frame. They asserted that violations of socioeconomic and political rights make individuals more vulnerable to HIV infection and that AIDS, because of its lethality and stigma, undermines the basic right to dignity, safety, life, health, work, family, and education for people living with HIV. In addition, the people most vulnerable to HIV infection are poor and disenfranchised, making their health situation the outcome of the political, economic, and social structures that marginalize them (Mann 1999; Davies 2010, 73). Incorporating human rights into AIDS work required recognition of the right to health information, gender equality, nondiscrimination, and medical care (Davies 2010, 73). This human rights frame demanded social mobilization and state commitment; essentially, AIDS needed to become politicized (Patterson 2007).

By the mid-1990s, GPA was essentially defunct; only four staff members at the WHO worked on AIDS. And though the United States had some HIV prevention and surveillance programs in a few African countries, in the first post–cold war decade, other development priorities such as democracy promotion and economic development dominated. In what Greg Behrman (2004) describes as a period of "quiescence," the United States dramatically cut foreign aid programs and US Department of State positions in Africa, and it refused to intervene to prevent mass atrocities in the Liberian civil war or the Rwandan genocide (van de Walle 2010). Every year during the 1990s the United States spent over $10 billion on the domestic AIDS response but only $100 million on the global pandemic (Behrman 2004, 78).

This retreat from AIDS was set within a broader frame that portrayed Africa in a hopeless light and that justified the continent's neglect. A popular read with US policymakers, Robert Kaplan's 1994 article "The Coming Anarchy" emphasized war, ethnic conflict, disease, corruption, and suffering in Africa. Stories about child soldiers amputating the arms off villagers in Sierra Leone or raping young girls in Liberia, all while high on drugs, contributed to this imagery (*NBC News*, August 4, 2003; *New York Times*, February 14, 1999; *Reuters*, June 2, 2007; on child soldiers in Africa, see Honwana 2005). The Rwandan genocide, with the brutal murders of over 800,000 people, added to the view of Africa as chaotic and violent (Mamdani 2001; Des Forges 1999). In this context, AIDS was just one more horrific problem. This framing also blamed Africans' cultural practices like polygyny and alleged sexual promiscuity for the disease's massive spread (Caldwell, Caldwell, and Quiggin 1989; UNFPA 1999).[1]

During this period, African states were not merely ambivalent about AIDS governance; some presented outright challenges to global AIDS efforts.[2] In the early stage of global AIDS diplomacy, some African states refused to acknowledge the disease, all but hampering policy design. Goran Hyden and Kim Lanegran (1993, 51) write: "Governments do not put it very high on their policy agenda; if anything, they try to hide the issue from public attention." In 1985, then Kenyan president Daniel arap Moi said that the foreign press was conducting a hate campaign against his country when it reported that there were twenty AIDS cases in Kenya (Fortin 1987). Officials in apartheid South Africa said that most cases of AIDS were among people from "countries to the north" or gay men, denying the real magnitude of the epidemic and curtailing action to address it (Furlong and Ball 2005, 130). These attitudes, as well as limited scientific engagement with AIDS in Africa, meant that Western scientists dominated international AIDS conferences, where they pushed a biomedical agenda to develop HIV tests and therapeutics (Crane 2013). Similarly, when AIDS activists pushed to establish the Greater Involvement of People with

AIDS (GIPA) Initiative in 1983, the vast majority of these activists were from Western AIDS organizations like the AIDS Coalition to Unleash Power (ACT UP) (Gordenker, Coate, Jönsson, and Söderholm 1995). (See below on GIPA.)

In AIDS policy implementation, some ministries of health worked with GPA to put data collection and blood supply safety programs in place, but these activities required African states to devote few if any political or financial resources to AIDS (Will 1991). For example, the Zambian government quickly mobilized funds to address the country's 1992 drought but did not do the same for AIDS, even though the disease was eroding local capacity to survive the agricultural crisis (G. Scott 2000; de Waal and Whiteside 2003). There were no national AIDS councils to oversee government policies and few forums in which leaders spoke to educate the public on the issue.

African states' challenge occurred for several reasons. At the international level, funding was inadequate, the WHO was divided about AIDS policies, GPA was a weak institution, human rights and biomedical frames competed, and the United States backed away from its AIDS commitment. No norm coherence emerged to push institutional development, partly because what Charles Epp (1998) terms the "human rights revolution," or the rise of human rights advocacy and human rights law, was just becoming institutionalized (see also Sikkink 2011). And when AIDS became symbolic of all of Africa's problems, African state identity was challenged. Instead of emphasizing the AIDS pandemic, or "just another African disaster" (Behrman 2004, 67), African state leaders preferred to herald their efforts to promote democracy, human rights, and neoliberal economic development, and their identity as a continent experiencing a renaissance (on the African Renaissance, see Ajulu 2001).

At the state level, the transitions that led to multiparty elections in the early 1990s in most states had the potential to make new democracies more accountable on AIDS policies (Cheeseman 2015). While not all of these elections were competitive or led to alternation of power, in states where there was more competition, newly elected regimes faced a host of popular demands, and, because of the high stigma against AIDS, state officials felt little pressure to act on AIDS (Justesen 2015; Dionne 2011; Patterson 2006). Democracy seemed to matter little for state action on AIDS, since both democratic and nondemocratic states challenged global health governance with their silence and inaction. Neopatrimonial objectives could have urged some action in global AIDS governance, but the lack of long-term global commitment to AIDS resources led to the underdevelopment of AIDS institutions. GPA also urged states to develop short time horizons of six to twelve months for achieving results, leading to a frantic pace in establishing surveillance and control programs (Berhman 2004, 49). These were often situated in ministries of health, which in most African countries tend to be under-resourced and politically marginalized (interview, multilateral donor official, Accra, October 8, 2008). One respondent said: "Health ministers, they are at the end of the line in the cabinets. Down there with environment. The last positions to be filled and with little political clout" (interview, multilateral donor official, New York, October 1, 2015). Decision-making focused on technical debates and rarely included civil society representatives; neopatrimonial states and their networks benefited little.

Even if state institutions had tried to include civil society, community mobilization on AIDS was limited. Jennifer Chan (2015) describes the period of the 1980s and 1990s as one during which most Western AIDS advocacy groups and professional health-related organizations emerged. In Africa, a few organizations such as The AIDS Support Organisation (TASO) in Uganda were established at this time, but they focused on care for people infected with or affected by HIV, not advocacy (Patterson 2006, 31). (Later, TASO would effectively engage in advocacy too.) In Zambia, the Catholic Church developed home-based care programs to assist the dying in 1991 (Patterson 2011, 54; see also Iliffe 2006), but the Network of Zambian People Living with HIV/AIDS (NZP+), an advocacy organization, did not form until 1996. And Africa's most well-known AIDS activist organization—the Treatment Action Campaign (TAC) in South Africa—did not form until 1998 (Patterson 2006, 97). Some international NGOs supported community-based AIDS care, but many had yet to turn their attention to the pandemic (interview, international NGO official, Washington, DC, March 18, 2005). Stigma dissuaded mobilization because it made suffering from AIDS a private problem rather than a public issue. One Ghanaian respondent explained, "PLHIV [people living with HIV] were not dying because of AIDS but because of the stigma. The loneliness and isolation were killing them" (interview, AIDS NGO official, Accra, October 22, 2008). The deaths of group members and leaders made it problematic for AIDS advocacy organizations to build capacity, forge institutional memory, and sometimes, continue their activities (Whiteside, Mattes, Willan, and Manning 2002). These nascent groups also lacked global allies: it was only in the late 1990s that AIDS advocates in the West developed a transnational agenda (Behrman 2004; Smith and Siplon 2006). Civil society's disengagement permitted the state to challenge global health governance on AIDS, particularly because that governance itself was weak. The next two sections show how this dynamic changed.

Deepening Global Health Governance on AIDS

According to Jeremy Shiffman and Stephanie Smith (2007), a health issue has become a global priority when leaders speak on it publicly and privately, policies and programs address the problem, and resources are provided that are commensurate with the need that the issue poses. By those three indicators, AIDS became a global health priority in the early 2000s. This section illustrates the development of norms that undergird this commitment and the establishment of global, national, and subnational institutions, including UNAIDS, national AIDS commissions (NAC), and country coordinating mechanisms (CCM). Finally, I indicate that the international community has generated large amounts of funding for AIDS. The outcome has been what Susan Watkins and Anne Swidler (2012) term the "AIDS enterprise," or a hierarchy of donor agencies, governments, and NGOs that are interconnected and well funded, all with the long-term interest of continuing the AIDS response.

Noncompeting Frames and Cascading Global Norms

Global interest in AIDS re-emerged in 1996 with the formation of UNAIDS, an agency that sought to coordinate other UN agencies' responses to AIDS, to build political commitment to the disease, to provide states with surveillance data, and to develop best practices in the AIDS response. In 2000, the United States led a special session of the UN Security Council that discussed AIDS, generating attention to the disease (McInnes and Rushton 2010; Elbe 2006), and in 2001, the UN General Assembly held a special session on AIDS. Attended by most heads of state, the 2001 Special Session on HIV/AIDS generated significant media attention and activism from human rights and women's rights advocates, AIDS activists, and health and development NGOs. It resulted in the *Declaration of Commitment on HIV/AIDS,* a document which guided the establishment of AIDS institutions and funding mechanisms (UN 2001; Patterson and Cieminis 2005).

To build support for AIDS efforts, bilateral and multilateral donors framed the disease as "an unprecedented emergency with global consequences" (Watkins and Swidler 2012, 198). AIDS was securitized, being portrayed as a threat to African economies and militaries and, ultimately, as a contributing factor to economic stagnation, internal turmoil, and failed states (Price-Smith 2009; International Crisis Group 2001). These arguments took on greater sway in a post–9/11 world, especially since Osama bin Laden planned his attacks from hideouts in the "failed states" of Sudan and Afghanistan. Though securitization was most ardently supported by the United States (McInnes and Rushton 2010), UNAIDS officials also framed AIDS as an "exceptional" health problem because HIV prevalence seemed to have "no plateau in sight." The great "severity and longevity of its impact" and the "special challenges [that] it poses to effective public action" demanded immediate and unprecedented attention (former UNAIDS director Peter Piot quoted in Benton 2015, x).

In addition to the security frame, AIDS advocates articulated a human rights frame more strongly than they had in the past (see Farmer 2005; Davies 2010, 66; Gruskin 2005). While at times the security and human rights frames collided (particularly because the security frame had the potential to stigmatize people living with HIV), the use of multiple frames for AIDS helped to bolster support from different policymaking realms (McInnes et al. 2012; McInnes and Rushton 2010). This situation was unlike in the early 1990s when competing frames undermined programs. Activists with ACT UP, the Global AIDS Alliance, Health Global Access Project (Health GAP), Human Rights Watch, and Médecins Sans Frontières (MSF) joined together with women's groups and some faith-based organizations (FBOs) to assert that the right to health that is codified in such documents as the Universal Declaration of Human Rights, the Alma-Ata Declaration, the Convention on the Rights of the Child, the International Covenant on Economic, Social, and Cultural Rights, the Convention on the Elimination of All Forms of Discrimination against Women, and the Millennium Development Goals necessitated well-funded, institutionalized AIDS programs. While health as a human right remains highly contested, particularly in terms of the state's legal obligation to promote and protect this right (Davies 2010, 68; Mold and Reubi 2013), the rights discourse did pressure states to act on AIDS in the face of normative discourses and moral messages (see Johnson 2006; Friedman and Mottiar 2004; Youde 2008; Kapstein and Busby 2013). Below I will focus on three issues related to human rights norms: inclusive decision-making, nondiscrimination of marginalized populations, and access to HIV treatment.

First, the norm of inclusive decision-making undergirds many global AIDS initiatives, because inclusion is believed to be essential for the achievement of the right to health. Inclusive decision-making brings together representatives from donor agencies, governments, civil society, and affected communities. With the aforementioned GIPA Initiative of 1983, activists demanded a move from tokenism to full incorporation of people living with HIV into decision-making on AIDS policies and resources (Smith and Siplon 2006; Mbali 2013; Chan 2015; Patterson 2006). GIPA resulted in funders demanding that decision-making institutions have representation of people living with HIV and civil society organizations, a policy I analyze below.

Second, the norm of nondiscrimination underlies much of human rights law; all individuals by virtue of being human should have equal access to health-care services regardless of personal characteristics like economic status, race, gender, or nationality. Health issues that affect only some populations—such as racial or sexual minorities—cannot be ignored if health is a human right for all. Non-discrimination is particularly important for the AIDS response because some key populations affected by AIDS have been highly marginalized in society, including men who have sex with men, sex workers, and people who inject drugs (Csete 2007).[3] Some key populations also engage in behavior that is criminalized (such as drug use or sex work), making it difficult to protect their human right to health. Tensions between providing health services to people engaged in illegal activities, on the one hand, and the norm of nondiscrimination, on the other, complicate the institutionalization of nondiscrimination (Mold and Reubi 2013, 5)

Third, activists argued that health as a human right necessitated universal access to ART (Youde 2008). In the early 2000s, activists emphasized that pharmaceutical companies used patents protected under World Trade Organization (WTO) agreements in order to set high prices for antiretrovirals (ARVs), effectively denying access to affordable, life-saving drugs for millions of Africans. The norm of universal access to ART became acceptable because activists emphasized women and children ("innocents") and because this norm challenged unjust structures (Kapstein and Busby 2013; see also Keck and Sikkink 1998). The norm of universal access to ART appeared to have cascaded when UN member states signed the 2001 Declaration of Commitment on HIV/AIDS with its call for ARV access and when world leaders such as former US president George W. Bush promoted access to HIV treatment (Youde 2008; Bush 2003). Unity within global health epistemic communities also played a role: increasingly, scientific studies showed that access to ART encouraged people to get tested for HIV, and testing was essential for preventing new HIV infections (Patterson and Cieminis 2005). A major pilot project by MSF in Khayelitsha, a poor urban community in South Africa, illustrated that Africans would adhere to the treatment and that logistical challenges surrounding drug distribution could be overcome (Coetzee et al. 2004). In 2011, a major study showed that ART suppresses viral load, making the transmission of the virus 96 percent less likely for people taking ART than for those not taking the medications (Cohen et al. 2011). Among Africans on ART, 76 percent had achieved this "viral suppression" by 2013 (UNAIDS 2014d). The norm of ART access became institutionalized through funding mechanisms (see below) and the WHO's 3 by 5 Initiative that aimed to place three million people living with HIV who needed ART on medication by 2005. There were positive results: In 2002, only one million people living with HIV globally (and only 300,000 in low- and middle-income countries) had ART access (UNAIDS 2013; UNAIDS 2015a; WHO, UNICEF, and UNAIDS 2013). By 2014 the number was 14.9 million globally. While in 2016 this number remained less than half of the approximately 36 million people living with HIV in the world, it was a significant increase since the early 2000s (UNAIDS 2015a).

Building Institutions, Funding the Response

Because AIDS was framed as an exceptional disease in terms of its security and human rights implications, it required its own institutions and funding sources, an approach that led to vertical, or disease-specific, programs that often addressed AIDS in isolation from larger health issues (Benton 2015). Institutions at the international and state levels oversaw these programs, and their establishment was intended to indicate states' political commitment to the AIDS response. In addition to UNAIDS (see above), the World Bank set up the Multi-Country AIDS Program (MAP) in 1999 with the goal of providing states with funds and technical advice on the establishment of the NAC (World Bank 2000). Each state's NAC, with a membership that included people living with HIV and civil society representatives, established a long-term AIDS strategy that incorporated multiple sectors and societal groups. These ranged from agricultural production and food security for rural people living with HIV to HIV prevention among military recruits. Using this "multisectoral approach," the NAC dispersed funding to district AIDS committees and civil society groups that then mobilized society for HIV prevention, care, and support (World Bank 2000, 2–3). NAC monitored results in order to document successful programs and to reform (or eliminate) unsuccessful ones. As one NAC member said, "They [World Bank, UNAIDS] want easy access to reporting, because they want data to flash around because donor governments want to show results to those who allocate money" (interview, GAC official, Accra, October 10, 2008).[4] To demonstrate that political leaders supported these efforts, most states situated the NAC in the president's office (Harman 2009), and high-level government or civil society leaders chaired these efforts. For example, Senegal's prime minister led the country's first commission, and a prominent Pentecostal pastor chaired Zambia's (Putzel 2004; Patterson 2011). As indicated below, these institutional arrangements increased national-level buy in, though the World Bank's adoption of this "cookie cutter" approach has been criticized for ignoring local realities (Putzel 2004; Harman 2009).

The other national-level institution that emerged in the mid-2000s was the CCM, a committee required for any country that applied for grants from the Global Fund (see below). Composed of representatives from civil society, the national government, donors, groups of people living with HIV, and the private sector, the CCM writes grant proposals to the Global Fund and then administers funding that the country receives (Patterson 2006). The Global Fund recommends that 40 percent of CCM members be from civil society, and it requires that populations affected by malaria, AIDS, and/or TB be represented. The Global Fund structures seek to "operationalize human rights principles that include non-discrimination, general equality and participation of key affected populations" (Global Fund 2013). In reality, the inclusiveness and transparency of the CCM have varied widely, as has their autonomy. In Tanzania and Uganda, the CCM was situated within the NAC (Harman 2009), increasing the NAC's control over resources while also leading to increased coordination challenges.

In addition to new institutions, new funding mechanisms characterized global health governance on AIDS. The Global Fund was established in 2002. It raises and invests roughly $4 billion each year in grants to low- and middle-income countries. As of 2015, it had dispersed over $27 billion, with its monies being used to purchase ARVs, TB medications, insecticide treated bed nets to prevent malaria, and health-education programs (Global Fund 2016a). A second was the US President's Emergency Plan for AIDS Relief (PEPFAR), which, as of 2016, had given away $57 billion since its inception in 2003 (PEPFAR 2016). While it initially worked in only fifteen countries (twelve of which were in sub-Saharan Africa), the program has expanded to thirty-five countries and geographic regions, with twenty-one being in Africa (PEPFAR 2015a). In 2015, the United States contributed two-thirds of donor government funding for AIDS. The United Kingdom was the second-largest donor (13.0 percent), then France (3.5 percent), Germany (2.7 percent), and the Netherlands (2.3 percent) (Kaiser Family Foundation and UNAIDS 2016). Both the Global Fund and PEPFAR have given substantial funding to African states (as indicated below), but they differ in their management. PEPFAR provides grants to subrecipients, the vast majority of whom are US-based NGOs and FBOs (e.g., Catholic Relief Services, Family Health International), US government agencies (e.g., US-AID), and US universities (e.g., Baylor University Medical School). These entities then provide subgrants to local partners, such as indigenous NGOs and FBOs. For example, in fiscal year 2015 Botswana received $38.9 million, though all but $1.65 million went to US NGOs, universities, and government agencies (PEPFAR 2015a). In contrast, most principal recipients of Global Fund money are African state ministries and civil society organizations.

The global health governance of AIDS has received an unprecedented amount of funding (see Smith and Whiteside 2010; Nguyen 2010, 13; Dionne, Gerland, and Watkins 2013), a pattern that has had unclear effects on other health programs such as health system strengthening, infectious disease control, and reproductive health (Shiffman, Berlan, and Hafner 2009). Though in 2016 AIDS experts asserted that funding for the pandemic remains insufficient (UNAIDS 2016), money for the response increased from $200 million in 1996 to roughly $8.6 billion in 2014. The biggest increase occurred between 2001, when $1.2 billion was spent, and 2008, when $7.8 billion was spent. With the global financial crisis of 2008, funding stagnated in 2009 and then decreased to below-2008 levels until 2013. In 2013, funding increased to $8.5 billion, but in 2014 it was only marginally higher ($8.6 billion). In that same year, money from nine of fourteen donor governments declined, while donations from the United States and Germany remained flat (Kaiser Family Foundation 2015b). In 2015, global monies dipped to $7.5 billion, the first time in five years that funding levels decreased (Kaiser Family Foundation and UNAIDS 2016). Despite this decline, AIDS continues to dominate global health funding. For example, roughly 57 percent of the US global health budget in 2016 was allocated to HIV (and 71 percent if US donations to the Global Fund are included) (Wexler and Valentine 2015).

In summary, the new millennium has witnessed the development of well-defined institutions like UNAIDS, World Bank MAP, the Global Fund, and PEPFAR to coordinate an AIDS response and to provide funding and technical support to countries that need assistance. These outcomes have been possible because the issue was framed as a security threat and a human rights issue, a strategy that drew in two different constituencies and made it easier for states that had low interest in the disease to develop (or redevelop) that interest. Global health governance on AIDS became increasingly embedded in a growing norm that health care access is a human right, a norm that emphasizes inclusion of civil society and people living with HIV in decision-making, nondiscrimination in services, and universal ART access.

African Acceptance of Global AIDS Governance

In the new millennium, most African states accepted global health governance on AIDS, though as Ashley Fox (2014) indicates, some states such as South Africa under President Thabo Mbeki (1999–2008) and The Gambia were policy laggards. (See below on these two cases.) Here I detail this general acceptance in four areas: (1) participation in policy design through shaping the AIDS narrative and policy options; (2) support for and formation of national AIDS institutions; (3) policies and structures to implement norms of inclusive decision-making, nondiscrimination, and access to ART; and (4) state spending on AIDS.

This section relies on three data sources: interviews with participants in AIDS efforts; African state leaders' public statements at the 2001 UN Special Session on HIV/AIDS; and the 2012 and 2014 National Commitments and Policies Instrument for forty-one African countries (UNAIDS 2012a, 2014a). A questionnaire administered by UNAIDS and completed by state, donor, and NGO officials in a specific country, the Instrument includes yes/no questions about political commitment; civil society involvement in policymaking; and the efficacy of programs for treatment, HIV prevention, and care of orphans and vulnerable children (OVC). UNAIDS validates responses for internal consistency and completeness, correcting for illogical and missing data in order to minimize the problems of self-reported data. While there could be the inclination for African respondents to overstate HIV problems in order to gain resources, this action is less likely because UNAIDS itself is not a funding agency. Additionally, because government and civil society representatives independently answered the questionnaire, it is less likely that civil society groups will be pressured by state officials to respond in a particular way.

Designing Policy Options: A Role in Global Health Diplomacy

African states' participation in the global health diplomacy on AIDS can be interpreted in two ways. In the first, African states lack agency; they followed the initiative of UNAIDS, whose officials galvanized political support in the years before the 2001 UN Special Session on HIV/AIDS (phone interview, multilateral donor, October 15, 2002; Patterson and Cieminis 2005). In 1998, UNAIDS worked with African state leaders and the World Bank to establish the International Partnership against AIDS in Africa, a program that developed objectives for combating the disease and eventually led to the 2001 African Summit on HIV/AIDS, Tuberculosis and Other Related Infectious Diseases in Abuja, Nigeria.

In the second perspective, while still dependent on UNAIDS public leadership, African states exhibited agency in this diplomatic process. In the Abuja Declaration, leaders used strong language, asserting that AIDS was "a state of emergency" and pledging to "take personal responsibility and provide leadership." They promised to "place the fight against HIV/AIDS at the forefront," to end the stigma against people living with HIV, and to involve them in policymaking. As evidence of their commitment, they pledged to devote 15 percent of their national budgets to improving health care (OAU 2001; *Africa Recovery*, June 2001). This promise was rooted in the recognition that donors demanded an African commitment to health before they would support the establishment of the Global Fund (phone interview, multilateral donor official, October 15, 2002; see also Patterson and Cieminis 2005). The pledge had an impact: one donor official said, "After years of denial, it appeared that African officials were finally willing to take a leadership role on AIDS" (phone interview, bilateral donor, October 21, 2002). The pledge helped to pressure donors to commit greater resources to AIDS.

African states also shaped the narrative surrounding the disease at the 2001 UN Special Session on HIV/AIDS. While UNAIDS officials negotiated behind the scenes (e-mail conversation, UN representative from EU state, October 1, 2002), African leaders' public pronouncements helped to move the agenda forward and gain Western media attention (on media coverage of AIDS after 2000, see UNAIDS 2004; Moeller 2000). Many African heads of state attended the meeting, and several emphasized the magnitude of the epidemic. The King of Swaziland began: "Today we speak not of the hopes for the future generations, but in terms of their very survival." His dire prediction was echoed by leaders from Ethiopia ("The impact of the disease on the economic and social sector is severe"), Ghana ("Our social security and economic development are being undermined"), and Mozambique ("Every day the infection and death toll grow"). Other leaders echoed underlying norms of AIDS governance: The Nigerian president asserted the human right to ART access, the Rwandan president pointed to the vulnerability of women and children to HIV infection, and the Ugandan president praised the involvement of people living with HIV in his country's AIDS response (presidential speeches are available at UNGA 2001). These acts of extraversion heightened attention to the need for global AIDS governance.

In addition, the policies of Botswana and Uganda influenced global AIDS governance. In 2000, the Botswana government formed a public-private partnership with Merck Pharmaceuticals and the Gates Foundation in order to distribute free ART. The Gates Foundation provided $50 million over five years to the project, the Merck Foundation gave $50 million, and the Merck company donated the ARVs of Stocrin and Crixivan. The government pledged to purchase other AIDS medications that were not donated (Austin, Barrett, and Weber 2001). The partnership was a key step in reaching the government's goal of providing universal ART.

The program demonstrated Botswana's agency in several ways. First, during initial negotiations, the country demanded that the partners commit to develop the country's health-care capacity. Second, the government—not donors—made the ultimate decision to establish a universal ART access program in 2001 (Ramiah and Reich 2005). Third, when uptake on ART was slow to occur because the AIDS stigma discouraged people from testing for HIV, the government announced that all clients at public health-care centers would receive an HIV test unless they specifically opted out. The routine testing policy led to earlier identification of people living with HIV and increased survival rates. As the first African country to introduce this testing model, Botswana had to innovatively develop its own guidelines and protocols (Steen et al. 2007). Through the public-private partnership and the routine testing policy, Botswana played a leadership role in AIDS policymaking. Its actions provided a treatment model to low- and middle-income countries.

Uganda also influenced global AIDS governance, because it was the first African country to experience a decline in HIV prevalence. From 1990 to 2001 its HIV rate dropped from 15 percent to 5 percent (Murphy, Greene, Mihailovic, and Olupot-Olupot 2006). Debates about the reasons for this decline are heated. These reasons include proactive political leadership, the mobilization and empowerment of women, the implementation of village projects that punished young people for premarital sexual activities, country-wide programs to fight stigma, widespread condom distribution, delay in young people's first sexual experience, what President Yoweri Museveni termed "zero grazing" (or sexual fidelity), and death (Murphy, Greene, Mihailovic, and Olupot-Olupot 2006; Parkhurst 2012; Epstein 2007; Wawer et al. 2005). These debates created room for Ugandan officials to shape AIDS policies. They have insisted that the country's success revolves around its ABC Policy— abstinence, being faithful, and consistent and correct use of condoms (Okware et al. 2005; Sinding 2005; Wakabi 2006), even though this policy was not mentioned in Uganda until 2003 (Parkhurst 2011; Slutkin et al. 2006). By stressing ABC, the Ugandan government gained favor with the Bush administration and the Republican Congress that established PEPFAR in 2003. The Ugandan government also could tap into funding from evangelical Christian FBOs. The ABC policy shaped PEPFAR's design, which required that one-third of funding for HIV prevention programs be used to teach abstinence and fidelity messages (Patterson 2006; Green and Ruark 2011). PEPFAR supporters asserted that ABC was an "African solution" to the AIDS problem, while critics said it lacked a comprehensive approach and it made inaccurate assumptions about women's power to insist on abstinence or fidelity (Murphy, Greene, Mihailovic, and Olupot-Olupot 2006; Epstein 2007;

Parkhurst 2012). Regardless of its impact on HIV transmission, Uganda's ABC policy influenced the United States' HIV prevention efforts in Africa, and it illustrated African agency in global health governance.

Acceptance through Implementation: Demonstrating Political Commitment and Forming Institutions

In addition to shaping the debate on AIDS and influencing some prevention and treatment policies, African states also showed acceptance through political commitment to AIDS and the establishment of AIDS institutions. States have accepted these institutions regardless of their HIV rates, indicating that disease severity had little effect on AIDS policy decisions. Building political commitment has been one of UNAIDS's primary objectives, but the notion of political commitment has conflated political leadership with particular institutional arrangements (Putzel 2004, 1133). To address this problem, UNAIDS asks questions in the Instrument on both individual leaders' actions and state institutions. In terms of leaders' actions, all countries that completed the National Commitments and Policies Instrument said that high-level national officials have spoken "publicly and favorably" on AIDS in "major domestic forums at least twice a year" (UNAIDS 2014a). AIDS activists and experts have stressed the value of public discourse on the disease, with many interviewees commenting, "We need leaders to speak out"; "When leaders talk it decreases the AIDS stigma"; or in some cases, complaining, "No one at a high level has been open about their AIDS experiences" (interviews, AIDS NGO officials, Lusaka and Accra, August 17, 2007, August 20, 2007, and September 24, 2008). And because the discourse of nonstate officials is also important—"If the community leaders don't talk about it then you don't know yourself if it is okay to disclose your [HIV] status. You don't know if you will be accepted" (interview, leader of group of people living with HIV, Lusaka, August 14, 2007)—UNAIDS asks about the speech acts of leaders at the subnational level. Again, 100 percent of states reported that local leaders had spoken "positively and favorably" on AIDS. This public discourse contrasts with the silence among most African state and civil society leaders during the 1980s and 1990s.

African states also have illustrated institutional commitment, with 100 percent establishing a NAC and 100 percent designing a multisectoral AIDS strategy. They use donor-derived language to frame the NAC's work, emphasizing the involvement of civil society and the commitment to monitor results. One official with the Ghana AIDS Commission (GAC) explained:

GAC is . . . a supra-ministerial body that is under the president's direction. We coordinate the response to AIDS across the ministries. We form policy and deal with all of the policy issues that arise around AIDS. We mobilize resources, so this means dispersing funds to civil society groups and to other implementing agencies. And we monitor and evaluate how the programs are helping us meet our goals with the national response. We make sure we are implementing relevant programs that work within the national policy. (Interview, GAC official, Accra, October 10, 2008)

While this description highlights how the national commissions are theoretically supposed to work, the reality was often more complicated. The establishment of the NAC could sideline state agencies and NGOs that had already been working effectively on AIDS, something that occurred in Senegal and Uganda. The resulting resentment and interagency competition complicated consensus building, particularly when governments took resources from other ministries to set up the NAC (Putzel 2004). There also were questions about the NAC's power because of its lack of institutional rootedness and its financial dependence on the World Bank MAP. One Zambian respondent showed this confusion about the NAC's role:

Structurally, where does NAC really belong? How does it engage the line ministries like Ministry of Health? The structure is that NAC isn't within the Office of Vice President or President, and then it cannot be the one to hold the other line ministries accountable. So there is constant jostling within institutions. Should [NAC] be a command and control center or an information hub? (Interview, NAC official, Lusaka, August 15, 2007)

The quote shows the ambiguous position of Zambia's NAC. Because it was a presidential creation, it had no enforcement power for its policies. One outcome was that even though Zambia's NAC pushed the national parliament to pass policies related to housing and nondiscrimination for people living with HIV, it had no way to implement those laws (interview, AIDS NGO official, Lusaka, August 14, 2007).

Additionally, even though donors had pushed the establishment of NAC, they continued to work through multiple actors, spreading funds widely. These national institutions were expected to achieve much, but many of their members did not think they were given sufficient resources to do so. One GAC official explained:

Only 30 percent of the [GAC] money is from donors. Donors give most of their money to civil society directly. But, we as GAC are responsible for AIDS programs and policies. They say they want to support GAC but when we don't reach our goals, they blame us. But they haven't made it possible for us to reach our goals because they haven't given us the resources and they have given them to civil society groups instead. (Interview, GAC official, Accra, October 10, 2008)

The respondent shows that donors have a somewhat ambiguous relationship with NAC. More broadly, the respondent illustrates the complex web of actors involved in global health governance of AIDS and how that complexity can generate tension between the state (which ultimately is responsible for results on AIDS) and civil society groups (which get donor funds).

Some of the challenges that NAC face are reflected in answers to the National Commitments and Policies Instrument (UNAIDS 2014a), which asked respondents to rank political commitment in their country on a scale of 0 to 10, with 0 being low and 10 being high. The average for the thirty-nine states that answered this question was 7.3, with one state (Côte d'Ivoire) giving itself a 10 and six states (Democratic Republic of Congo, Djibouti, São Tomé and Príncipe, Seychelles, Somalia, and Togo) rating themselves with a 5. (No state rated itself below 5.) Here is a case where disease magnitude affects commitment for some states, though not all. On one hand, all states with an HIV prevalence of greater than 10 percent gave themselves a score of at least 8.[5] In contrast, many countries that gave themselves the lower grades have HIV rates of 1 percent or less. On the other hand, these very low HIV prevalence countries tended to rate themselves higher than states with HIV rates between 1 and 10 percent; only one-third of states in the 1–10 percent group had political commitment scores of at least an 8, compared to two-thirds of the states in the very low HIV prevalence category. States such as Kenya, Tanzania, Nigeria, and Ethiopia in the 1–10 percent group have millions of people living with HIV, so if epidemic magnitude were the sole driver of acceptance of global AIDS governance, one might expect greater scores within this group. Instead, it appears that other factors matter: AIDS must compete with other health conditions for the interest of state officials and the population. The "passing grade" of 7.3 also indicates that the term "political commitment" has been interpreted to mean technical competence or, as illustrated above, leaders' speech acts, not institutional structures or policies (Putzel 2004, 1133; see Bor 2007 on leadership).

Implementing the Norms of Inclusion, Nondiscrimination, and Treatment Access

I now investigate if African states have accepted the norms undergirding global health governance of AIDS, particularly the norms of inclusive decision-making, nondiscrimination of key populations, and treatment access. In terms of inclusion,

I looked at participation of civil society and people living with HIV in NAC, since UNAIDS, donors, and activists have emphasized that affected populations should be involved in decision-making and resource allocation. Of the countries that completed the National Commitments and Policies Instrument in 2012 or 2014 (UNAIDS 2012a, 2014a), 93 percent include civil society representatives on the NAC, while 95 percent include people living with HIV. Nominating civil society representatives to NAC is a relatively easy way to show commitment to human rights, though, as indicated below, "having a seat at the table" says nothing about the quality of that representation. In the Instrument, countries were asked to evaluate the quality of civil society's involvement using a scale of 0 to 5, with 5 signifying high levels of involvement. The resulting average for the forty-one reporting countries was 3.36. Ghana and Mali reported a 5, while São Tomé and Príncipe and Swaziland reported a 2. I return to the issue of civil society inclusion and the quality of representation below.

Second, I examined policies or structures to address discrimination, particularly responses to the Instrument question: "Is there a mechanism to record, document and address cases of discrimination experienced by people living with HIV, most-at-risk populations and/or other vulnerable subpopulations?" (UNAIDS 2014a) While all countries said they include human rights protection in their national strategies, only 61 percent said they had specific mechanisms for reporting and addressing human rights violations that are linked to AIDS. As another point of data, country representatives were asked: "Overall, on a scale of 0 to 10 (where 0 is 'Very Poor' and 10 is 'Excellent'), how would you rate the policies, laws and regulations in place to promote and protect human rights in relation to HIV in 2013?" (UNAIDS 2014a) The average for thirty-eight reporting states was 5.3, two points lower than the average for the above-mentioned "political commitment" question. These two measures indicate that, while the global norm of human rights promotion in the HIV response exists, its acceptance remains somewhat aspirational.

As another way to examine nondiscrimination, I looked at policies for HIV prevention, care, support, and treatment for the key populations of men who have sex with men and people who inject drugs, groups that UNAIDS has increasingly tried to incorporate into the AIDS response (McKay 2016). Seventy-six percent of reporting states said they had programs for men who have sex with men in their strategies, while only 46 percent said they have such policies for people who inject drugs. Men who have sex with men have become more incorporated into African HIV policies, partly because of global advocacy efforts and partly because they have been less difficult to reach than people who inject drugs (though people who inject drugs and men who have sex with men could be the same individuals). But just because there are policies for men who have sex with men does not mean these policies are adequately implemented. A lack of data on the sexual behavior of men who have sex with men and political opposition lead to underimplementation (McCay 2016). For example, one Ghanaian official argued against donors' focus on key populations in that country's AIDS response:

> Donors have started giving to groups working with at-risk populations: MSM [men who have sex with men], IDUs [injecting drug users], and prisoners. But, it is really difficult to affect major change in these groups. It is not that I object to funding some programs for these groups. We need prevention there. But, there would be greater long-term impact if [donors] were doing projects with the larger population. (Interview, GAC official, Accra, October 10, 2008)

The respondent indicates that programs for key populations tend to be donor-driven and that if global health governance of AIDS is to be results oriented, it should not dilute its resources with these specialized programs. In the process, the official seeks to change the discussion from the human rights focus on marginalized groups to the issue of the efficacy of global AIDS governance. A similar tactic occurred with a Zambian NAC member who sought to redefine which societal groups constitute a key population:

> Continued dependence on donor funding has brought pressure from some AIDS partners to link aid to programs related to sexual preference. . . . But if you look at most of [HIV] infections in Zambia, they are with young people. Out of 82,000 infections which Zambia registers annually, 69,000 plus are among young people between fifteen and twenty-four years old. . . . But then the average funder says they want you to demonstrate that you are addressing key populations, and the global and conventional definition of key populations is men having sex with men, transgenders, bisexuals, LGBT. But in Zambia, our epidemic is largely heterosexual. We can understand that in Europe and America it is a homosexual epidemic. But here, more infections are being registered among young people, among heterosexuals. That group is our key population. So we [on NAC] have called for a redefinition of "key populations." You can't say a key population in America is the same as a key population here in Zambia. (Interview, NAC official, Lusaka, June 13, 2014)

For Zambia, a country with laws against homosexuality and a 12 percent HIV rate, some NAC officials were unwilling to accept policies for men who have sex with men. In a bigger sense, though, both respondents illustrate agency as they seek to use donors' own results-oriented perspective (in Ghana) or donors' own vocabulary (in Zambia) in their arguments. The quotes indicate that while African states have accepted many elements of global health governance on AIDS, they still have the ability to "stand up to powerful structures and even to some extent, change them" through their opposition to some policies (Lonsdale 2000, 7).

The least contested norm for African states is universal access to ART: The number of Africans on ART has expanded from under 100,000 in 2002 to over 10.7 million in 2015. In ten African countries over 80 percent of people who need the medications can access them (UNAIDS 2013, 2015a; WHO, UNICEF, and UNAIDS 2013). In comparison to several other WHO regions, Africa has excelled in providing treatment. According to WHO (2015b), 47 percent of Africans who needed the medications could get them in 2015, a percentage lower than in the Americas region (53 percent) but higher than in the Eastern Mediterranean (11 percent), European (40 percent), and South-East Asia regions (39 percent) and on par with the Western Pacific region (47 percent). African states have improved access by ending user fees at public clinics, addressing problems with supply chain management, and providing more ARVs at rural clinics. However, the fact that more than half of the people who need ART still do not have access shows that while the treatment norm has cascaded, its institutionalization continues to face funding and logistical challenges, particularly in terms of reaching marginalized populations like migrants, men who have sex with men, and people who inject drugs; providing ARVs for children; and preventing clients from being lost to follow-up (UNAIDS 2014d, 2015a).

State Spending on AIDS: Implementation through Resources

Part of state acceptance of global health governance on AIDS is the devotion of resources to the response. To determine African states' level of financial commitment, I used data from the thirty-one Country Progress Reports submitted to UNAIDS by African states in 2014 (or 2012, if 2014 was not available). The reports detail each country's percentage of AIDS spending from government, external sources, and the private sector (see UNAIDS 2014b). The reports show a mixed picture: on one hand, many African states are highly dependent on external resources. On the other hand, many states have increased their contributions to the AIDS response over time. As the Zambia case below illustrates, the outcome is a complicated interplay between dependence and autonomy that illustrates African agency.

In terms of dependence, donors provided on average 73.5 percent of the funding for the region's response, though at the individual state level this percentage varied from 8 percent of total AIDS spending in South Africa to 100 percent of AIDS funding in Somalia and Mali. (South Africa's high commitment to AIDS spending is another indication that it has moved beyond the challenge model evident under Mbeki.) The mean value was 84 percent, indicating a high level of dependence on donors (UNAIDS 2012c, 2014b, 2014f, 2014g). This dependence contrasts with overall health expenditures in Africa, at least two-thirds of which come from domestic sources (*Lancet* 2017, 1985). In the area of provision of ARVs, African states are even more dependent on donors. UNAIDS (2012b, 8) reports that "in 27 countries for which accurate data is available, 87% of expenditures for antiretroviral therapy in sub-Saharan African originate from international sources." Thus, in the aggregate it is difficult to say that African states have devoted their own resources to AIDS.

However, domestic spending by African states for AIDS programs increased 150 percent between 2011 and 2015 (Global Fund 2015b, 38). Thirty-two percent of the states that submitted UNAIDS Country Progress Reports in 2014 (ten states) showed a rise in financial commitment. Friends of the Global Fight (2017) reported that during the 2015–2017 period Global Fund recipient countries in all regions increased their domestic spending on AIDS, TB, and malaria by 52 percent from the 2012–2014 period. Higher spending is situated in the broader context of the above-mentioned Abuja Declaration, though the outcomes of the Abuja Declaration have been mixed. By 2011, twenty-six states had increased government health spending, though only Tanzania had met the Abuja target of 15 percent of government spending for health. Eleven states had reduced spending, and nine had experienced no change (WHO 2011a). Increased AIDS spending is also situated in the context of the African Union *Roadmap on Shared Responsibility and Global Solidarity for AIDS, TB and Malaria in Africa* (African Union 2012). Agreed to in 2012, the roadmap calls for sustainable financial plans for AIDS, TB and malaria programs, increased domestic funding for these health issues, and diversification in funding sources. In terms of AIDS spending specifically, there are positive examples of states that have started to meet these objectives: Botswana, Namibia, and South Africa are transitioning from receiving monetary aid to receiving technical assistance from PEPFAR. Botswana received $52 million from PEPFAR in 2013, down from $84 million in 2011; Namibia's PEPFAR funding declined from $102 million in 2011 to $52 million in 2013 (PEPFAR 2011, 2015a, 2015b). Additionally, as Nigeria's economy grew due to high oil prices during the 2000s, the country took on a greater burden of AIDS funding (from 8 percent in 2010 to over 40 percent in 2012), and PEPFAR decreased its contributions from $488 million in 2011 to $405 million in 2015 (PEPFAR 2011, 2015d).

States illustrated agency as they reacted to donor pressures to increase funding, as the case of Zambia illustrates. Between 2003 and 2014, Zambia experienced an average economic growth rate of 6 percent, fueled by high copper prices and increased trade with China (African Development Bank 2016). The country has a "favorable political climate on AIDS," one with AIDS institutions, civil society inclusion in decision making, and high-level officials who speak about AIDS. But the government's financial commitment to its promises on AIDS has been slow to materialize (interview, AIDS expert, Lusaka, August 20, 2007). A NAC member said:

> We have seen an increase in terms of domestic funding, but it is still within the 10 to 15 percent range, and is still not as it should be. We would want to see 50 percent, or even more than 50 percent coming from domestic resources. That's challenging but [NAC] has been encouraging our government, private sector, stakeholders to look at alternative ways. (Interview, NAC member, Lusaka, June 13, 2014)

The respondent illustrates how NAC officials recognize that the state must increase its contributions. While the official did not detail the "challenges" to reaching this goal, another interviewee pointed to competing government priorities, corruption, and the country's overall high rate of poverty (interview, CCM member, Lusaka, June 12, 2014).

The Zambia case illustrates several points. One is that at least rhetorically, state leaders have a commitment to country ownership and AIDS funding; states do not explicitly demand that donors fund all AIDS activities. Such a rhetorical commitment was partially rooted in the Abuja Declaration and AU Roadmap. Another point is that African actors have used extraversion to maintain donor support by arguing that the AIDS response would falter without continued donor money (Bayart 2000). Several Zambian interviewees said that funding cuts for support groups for people living with HIV would lead to increased HIV rates since these groups educate marginalized populations like youth about HIV and urge HIV testing (focus group discussions, groups of people living with HIV, Mumbwa; April 15, 2011; Kabwe, April 18, 2011). One CCM member said, "In the next four to five years, we will probably see a rise of HIV infections without support for these efforts" (interview, CCM member, Lusaka, June 12, 2014).

Zambian actors also used extraversion when they highlighted the country's success stories, and they reminded external actors that donor money for AIDS had been well spent. In comparison to several African states, Zambia has successfully provided treatment and decreased AIDS deaths. Though it had 4 percent of all Africa's people living with HIV, Zambia had only 2 percent of the continent's AIDS deaths in 2013 (UNAIDS 2014d, 26–27). Many donors agreed with this positive interpretation: "We are in a sense of stabilization with the epidemic and that means we can take a breath . . . We have seen a decline in pediatric infections to practically none . . . and there are a limited number of child-headed households and urban street children due to HIV and AIDS" (interview, multilateral donor official, Lusaka, February 23, 2011). These achievements were echoed at a more personal level in Lusaka AIDS clinics in 2011, where I often encountered Zambian people living with HIV and staff members who spoke of the benefits of ART programs. Government ART programs supported by the Global Fund and PEPFAR allowed people living with HIV to return to work, care for their children, travel, get married, finish school, and even become pregnant (participant observations, three Lusaka AIDS clinics, February–April 2011). Given such successes, it would be difficult politically and ethically for donors to cut funding (see Hunsmann 2015). African actors' ability to use the tool of extraversion meant that even if they were dependent on donor resources, they showed agency in shaping how donors thought about AIDS funding.

In summary, African states have played a role in the design of global health governance through their speech acts at the UN Special Session in 2001, the well-timed and strongly worded Abuja Declaration, and their policy innovations such as routine testing and the public-private partnership in Botswana or the ABC policy in Uganda. African states also illustrate acceptance through participation in the major institutions of global health governance on AIDS and the development of national AIDS strategies. Most assess themselves with a passing grade in terms of political commitment to AIDS (UNAIDS 2014a). They also have sought to promote the norms of inclusive decision-making and universal access to ART, though promotion of nondiscrimination, particularly in terms of key populations, lags. African state hesitancy on policies related to men who have sex with men, people who inject drugs, and other marginalized populations reflects cultural conservatism and criminalization of drug use and homosexual behavior in most African states (see Beyrer and Baral 2011). In terms of financial commitment, even though only about one-fifth of states have taken on a greater financial burden for AIDS, many have adopted the rhetoric of greater monetary responsibility. In the end, African states' acceptance of global health governance of AIDS means that "there is more that has been done on AIDS than any other health issue in Africa" (interview, health NGO official, Kampala, June 20, 2014).

Exceptions to the Rule

While the vast majority of African states accepted most aspects of global health governance on AIDS, two states presented important exceptions to this trend: South Africa under former president Mbeki and The Gambia under former president Yahya Jammeh. Here I outline their challenges. In the next section, I argue that even these cases can be explained by international, state, and societal factors.

In 2007, President Jammeh announced that he had a "mandate" from Allah to cure AIDS (and asthma) using seven herbs listed in the Koran. He said he would personally administer the cure (which included body washes and a drink) at the State House. Over two hundred people living with HIV quit their ART regimens and volunteered to be the president's patients. The president, garbed in long, flowing white robes, administered the treatments to half-naked people living with HIV on state television; patients swallowed (and sometimes vomited) the president's concoction. To validate the efficacy of his cure, the president then asked a Senegalese laboratory to verify that patients' HIV viral loads were undetectable. When the tests indicated this outcome, the president claimed victory. Yet these results most likely occurred because of the individuals' previous ART regimens, a point that the highly respected Senegalese AIDS scientist Souleymane Mboup repeatedly made (Amon 2008; Cassidy and Leach 2009). Instead of gaining health, between 2007 and 2008 at least thirteen of the "cured" individuals died, and AIDS organizations reported others who became ill (Cassidy and Leach 2009). Despite these outcomes, the president continued to claim that his cure worked. In 2013, he opened a homeopathic hospital (*AllAfrica.com*, December 24, 2013), and he welcomed foreign homeopathic healers to practice in the country (*Telegraph*, March 16, 2015). The president's actions had a chilling impact on the country's AIDS efforts. Eight years later, UNAIDS (2015b, 25–26) reported that the country still lagged behind in its commitment to address AIDS. The National AIDS Council had not functioned for many years, the country devoted little money to AIDS (in 2014, 95 percent of AIDS funding came from the Global Fund), and the "active involvement of [government and private] sectors" was "virtually nonexistent."

The South African case has been extensively reported. In 1997, then acting deputy president Mbeki supported the testing and production of Virodene, a medication composed of the toxic solvent dimethylformamide which had been developed by two University of Pretoria scientists (Furlong and Ball 2005; Sidley 1999). When the country's independent Medicines Control Council refused to approve testing of the drug, some council members were replaced. While the drug never received approval, it was tested in South Africa and Tanzania (*Wall Street Journal,* July 19, 2001). When he became president in 1999, Mbeki continued these patterns. He appointed and kept in office as health minister the late Manto Tshabalala-Msimang, who supported alternatives to ART, including nutritional supplements from Matthias Rath (a German doctor) and "the African solution" (a combination of African potato, lemon juice, beetroot, and garlic). Mbeki repeatedly claimed that ART was "toxic," and he blocked distribution of zidovudine (AZT) and nevirapine that effectively prevent HIV transmission from mother to child. He repeatedly questioned the motives of pharmaceutical companies, and he attacked his critics as "sellouts" to Western neocolonial interests (Amon 2008; Power 2003; Epstein 2000; Kapp 2005; Nattrass 2007; Fassin 2007; Patterson 2006).

Mbeki's support for alternative AIDS treatments is situated in his larger questioning of the link between HIV and AIDS. In 2000, he appointed a presidential panel to explore why HIV is often transmitted heterosexually in Africa but is transmitted primarily through homosexual relations and intravenous drug use in the West. Half of the panel members were scientists who espouse AIDS denialism. "Among the most vocal anti-science denial movements," AIDS denialism is an outgrowth of the work of Peter Duesberg, who claims that HIV (and other retroviruses) are harmless. For these scientists, poverty, drug abuse, and/or ART lead to AIDS, not the HIV virus (Kalichman, Eaton, and Cherry 2010, 432). When questioned about the high-level panel, Mbeki asserted that it allowed him to fully understand the science behind HIV; he portrayed himself as a leader who was "just asking questions" (Scheckels 2004, 72). Yet it was clear that denialists swayed his views. In September 2000, Mbeki explained: "[T]he notion that immune deficiency is only acquired from a single virus cannot be sustained. Once you say immune deficiency is acquired from that virus your response will be antiretroviral drugs. But if you accept that there can be a variety of reasons, including poverty and the many diseases that afflict Africans, then you have a more comprehensive treatment response" (*Time Magazine Europe,* September 11, 2000). Mbeki's statement contributed to the "flourishing" of AIDS denialism in South Africa. (On denialism in the United States, see Kalichman, Eaton, and Cherry 2010). The apartheid government's use of biomedical tools against its opponents, as well as the murky boundary be-tween science and politics (Richey 2008), fed this denial and situated it in the context of conspiracy theories about the West meddling in African society (Nat-trass 2012). Mbeki himself promoted such conspiracies, particularly the idea that Western pharmaceutical companies benefit from AIDS.

Mbeki's actions had several long-term effects. First, people, particularly those with low income levels who trusted the Mbeki government, tended to believe him. In a 2009 survey in South Africa, 16 percent of black respondents agreed that sci-entists in the United States invented AIDS to kill black people. In contrast, only 1 percent of nonblack respondents held such views (Nattrass 2012, 45, 52–55). Sec-ond, as a result of this questioning, some South Africans avoided HIV testing and health behaviors to prevent the spread of HIV (Patterson 2006; Chingwedere and Essex 2010). Third, these beliefs led the government to refuse to provide nevirap-ine for prevention of mother-to-child transmission or free access to ART for the thousands who needed it until after 2005. The outcome was devastating. A 2008 study found that the South African government could have prevented 365,000 deaths if it had provided ART and medications for prevention of mother-to-child transmission between 2000 and 2005 ("The Cost of Silence" 2008; *New York Times*, November 25, 2008).

There are three notable aspects of these leaders' challenges. First, both coun-tered the dominant biomedical understanding of AIDS (Youde 2007; Cassidy and Leach 2009; Fassin 2007; Nattrass 2007). Both turned to "African solutions," in-cluding traditional medicine, and they both saw themselves as guardians of Afri-can culture and autonomy. They tapped into a deep fear across the continent about the detrimental effects of technological developments: "The power of science [is] being felt in more intimate ways" (Nattrass 2012, 20). Second, each exhibited inconsistency in his approach to biomedicine. While emphasizing traditional ap-proaches, both embraced the tests, scientific expertise, and jargon of biomedicine. As Rebecca Cassidy and Melissa Leach (2009) point out, Jammeh utilized scientific measurements like HIV viral load and a sophisticated laboratory to demonstrate his cure's efficacy. Mbeki engaged in what he termed an objective investigation of all scientific findings on AIDS. When criticized, he accused the West of "intellec-tual intimidation" akin "to the racist apartheid tyranny we opposed" (Mbeki 2000). Third, their actions impeded global AIDS governance. For example, when the UN representative to The Gambia challenged Jammeh's cure, she was expelled. Two Gambian journalists who wrote about the cure in the state newspaper were fired. Mbeki's actions undermined efforts by the Global Fund and the Clinton Foundation to ramp up early ART programs (Amon 2008; Patterson 2006).

Despite these challenges, the two countries eventually fell into line with other African states. With Mbeki's ouster from the ruling African National Congress (ANC) in 2008, the party quickly moved to reverse his actions. The new health minister, Barbara Hogan, acknowledged the mistakes of the previous government, and the new president, Jacob Zuma, increased funding for ART and HIV prevention (*New York Times*, November 25, 2008). In 2013, UNAIDS Executive Director Michel Sidibé congratulated the country for its positive steps in the AIDS response (*Mail & Guardian*, January 18, 2013).[6] While less pronounced, there are also signs of the move to acceptance in The Gambia. Even though UNAIDS (2015b, 26) reported in 2015 that the country had an "unfavorable social, legal and political environment with regards to key populations," the multilateral agency acknowledged that the country had passed a Strategic Plan for AIDS in 2014 and re-established its National AIDS Council. The 2017 ouster of Jammeh with strong international support, as well as promises of increased foreign aid from Western donors, may bode well for the country's continued acceptance of global AIDS governance (*Reuters*, February 9, 2017).

Explanations for African State Actions

While African states have not fully accepted all aspects of global health governance on AIDS, they have established AIDS institutions and accepted many norms that undergird this governance. One-third have increased AIDS funding, though many more have increased funding for health in general (WHO 2011a). The reasons for this acceptance are complex and present a different situation from what existed during the early challenge period. Acceptance was facilitated by (1) well-developed and well-funded global institutions and relatively coherent norms; (2) democratic governance and neopatrimonial decision-making patterns that urged states to be interested in the benefits and legitimacy that come from global AIDS governance; and (3) an incorporated civil society.

International-Level Factors: Consensus and Resources

As indicated above, by the early 2000s the international community, with the participation of African states, had developed institutions to make, implement, and fund AIDS policies, including UNAIDS, the World Bank MAP, the Global Fund, the WHO 3 by 5 Initiative, and PEPFAR. Unlike during the initial period of global AIDS governance, there was significant funding and high-level political support from major states. Norm contestation was less problematic. This coherence at the international level had three effects. First, because global AIDS governance included resources, it benefited neopatrimonial states, a point I return to below. Second, because of global consensus, there was less space in which African states could challenge international expectations that states should respond to the disease. Denial of AIDS cases and obfuscation against global AIDS policymaking institutions incurred reputational costs, as South Africa discovered with Mbeki's actions. In another example, when Swaziland's king continued to marry young brides, a practice that seemed to support concurrent sexual relations in a country with an HIV rate of roughly 27 percent, he received negative media coverage and criticisms from donors (Patterson 2006). Ignoring AIDS also had become more difficult domestically, as African civil society groups mobilized to push the state to act (see below).

A third effect was that global institutions, norm coherence, and international funding played to African states' aspirational identities. In one sense, the pandemic continued to foster negative views of the continent as a place of suffering and disease. It was this image that Mbeki and Jammeh railed against, viewing the portrayal of AIDS in their countries through highly racialized lenses (for Mbeki) and neocolonial frames (for both of them) (Amon 2008; Fassin 2007; Nattrass 2012). Yet in another sense, the international approach emphasized partnership with African states to alleviate suffering. The Global Fund sought to directly incorporate African state and civil society leaders, since African actors designed and administered their own Global Fund proposals. The emphasis on partnership reflected a gradually changing foreign aid relationship that since the 1990s has put African states "more in the driver's seat" of their own development processes (de Haan 2009, 143–144; Radelet 2010; for a criticism of partnership see Abrahamsen 2004). Donors recognized the need to maintain this partnership, and they astutely praised African state accomplishments on AIDS. In 2013, UNAIDS (2013, 3) reported that "Africa is leading the world in expanding access to antiretroviral therapy . . . by more than doubling the number of people on treatment between 2006 and 2012." And in 2015, UNAIDS (2015a) pointed out that since 2000 the number of HIV infections in Africa had declined by 41 percent and the number of AIDS-related deaths had decreased by 34 percent (see also AMFAR 2015). These statements recognized African leadership and achievements, and they aligned with the characterization of the continent as economically, politically, and socially "rising" or "emerging" (Resnick 2015; Rotberg 2013; *Economist* 2013). It was particularly this type of recognition that the South African government sought after Mbeki's presidency.

While the specific actions of The Gambia and South Africa challenged accepted norms and AIDS institutions, they illustrate how states exhibit agency in the global realm. For both, the emphasis on pan-Africanism against neocolonial forces allowed them to portray themselves as defenders of African societies and populations. Their actions forced the institutions of global AIDS governance to react. Donors and global AIDS activists criticized Mbeki, but in The Gambia they did little beyond initial statements against Jammeh's AIDS cure (Nattrass 2007; International AIDS Society and Society for AIDS in Africa 2007; *United Press International*, March 16, 2007). They feared expulsion or a state crackdown on their programs, actions which would have harmed people living with HIV. Instead of opposing the state, these donors continued their AIDS programs (including ART distribution), as if in a parallel universe with the president's scheme (Cassidy and Leach 2009). These reactions indicated how African states can act as agents, not victims, in the international realm.

State-Level Factors: Democracy and Neopatrimonialism

The above-mentioned international institutions, norms, resources, and opportunities interacted with attributes of the African state to urge acceptance of global health governance on AIDS. Democracy urged policies that "deepened" a country's commitment to AIDS. Neopatrimonialism led states to accept the institutions of global health governance, which, in turn, facilitated the long-term neopatrimonial interests of those states. Over time, states developed a domestic political interest in global AIDS governance.

DEMOCRACY, INCLUSION, AND NONDISCRIMINATION
In general, the relationship between democracy and state AIDS responses is inconclusive. Ashley Fox (2014) finds that public support has correlated with policy adoption on AIDS, indicating some state responsiveness to public opinion. But since public support for AIDS prioritization is generally low (see below), public support for a state's AIDS efforts may be merely a proxy measure for support for the regime (Youde 2010). To examine the relationship between political regime type and state acceptance of global AIDS governance, I use data on regime type from Polity IV (Marshall and Cole 2014, 20–21). Polity IV defines strong democracies as

those with institutionalized processes for open, competitive, and deliberative political participation through elections and with substantial checks and balances on the chief executive. Weak democracies have fewer checks on executive power, some limits on participation, and shortcomings in applying the rule of law. Autocracies have little citizen participation as well as chief executives who are selected according to obtuse criteria and who exercise power with few limits. (Swaziland is a strong autocracy because it has a monarchy.) Because Polity IV does not include Seychelles, São Tomé and Príncipe, and Mauritius, I utilized reports from Freedom House (2016b) to categorize those states. Polity IV classifies Central African Republic and South Sudan with the term "state failure," but because such a designation indicates governance problems, I place these states in the autocracy category. Additionally, while the Polity IV data for some states is somewhat dated—by 2016, for example, Burundi was not classified as a strong democracy—I utilize it because of its focus on elections, power centralization, and rule of law.

Regime type had various effects on state engagement with global health governance on AIDS. According to the National Commitments and Policies Instrument, both democracies and autocracies set up NAC and CCM. Democracies and autocracies also included representation of civil society and people living with HIV on these two institutions, though it was only the autocratic states of Angola, Eritrea, and Uganda that reported no civil society representatives on the NAC, and only Angola and Eritrea reported no representation by people living with HIV on the NAC. The lack of representation on those state AIDS institutions aligns with their repression of media, opposition parties, and other civil society groups (Freedom House 2016b).

In terms of nondiscrimination, fourteen of the sixteen states without mechanisms to prevent discrimination against key populations or people living with HIV were autocracies. Of all autocracies, 70 percent lacked such human rights mechanisms, while only 7 percent of democracies did. (The two democracies were South Africa and São Tomé and Príncipe). As with representation of people living with HIV and civil society organizations, the lack of mechanisms against nondiscrimination reflects broader challenges with human rights protection in those fourteen autocracies. In the case of the two democracies, South Africa already has extensive human rights law and civil society mobilization against human rights violations (Henrard 2002; Johnson 2006); thus, AIDS-specific mechanisms may be viewed as unnecessary. Even during the Mbeki era, South African courts upheld norms of nondiscrimination against people living with HIV, and AIDS institutions included at least some people living with HIV and civil society representatives (Patterson 2006). The other country without mechanisms to prevent discrimination is São Tomé and Príncipe; its relatively small number of people living with HIV (an estimated 1,200 people) affects the prioritization of such decision-making processes (UNAIDS 2015a).

The correlation between democracy and the norm of nondiscrimination was evident in another measure: 83 percent of democracies had policies to incorporate men who have sex with men into the AIDS response, whereas 62 percent of autocracies did. And 68 percent of democracies had policies for people who inject drugs while only 15 percent of autocracies did. The Gambia illustrates this correlation. Human Rights Watch reported in 2015 that the country was one of the most repressive regimes on earth because of extrajudicial killings, torture, and arbitrary arrests (*Telegraph*, December 12, 2015). In the context of AIDS, President Jammeh scapegoated marginalized groups; in 2008, he issued an "ultimatum to homosexuals, drug dealers, thieves and other criminals, to leave The Gambia or face serious consequences." For him, these "bad elements" were corrupting the Muslim country (*Daily Observer*, May 19, 2008). Such comments undermined the norms of human rights embedded in global AIDS governance.

Uganda provides another example of an autocracy that has ignored the rights of key populations. In 2014, the parliament passed legislation with President Museveni's support that made homosexual acts punishable by life in prison and that required people to report homosexual acts to the police. While the law was overturned by the national court, the public action and media coverage surrounding its passage led to increased violence and discrimination against men who have sex with men and inhibited the work of HIV prevention groups working with these men (*Guardian*, February 24, 2014, January 6, 2015). The action directly contradicted the human rights norms embedded in global AIDS governance, and UNAIDS Executive Director Sidibé publicly responded. He reminded Ugandans that the country had played a leadership role in breaking the "conspiracy of silence on AIDS" and in giving voice to people marginalized by AIDS. In short, he said that the legislation would undermine years of good work (*Nation*, February 19, 2014). Uganda paid a price for its act of agency: donors cut funding to the country, and the action exacerbated an already tense relationship with donors over human rights violations, corruption, and unfair elections (*Guardian*, February 24, 2014, January 6, 2015; Wilson Center 2005; Mwenda 2007). Thus, even though adoption of AIDS institutions did not relate to democracy, acceptance of inclusive decision-making and nondiscrimination norms did.

To understand how the nature of the African state itself affected acceptance of global health governance on AIDS, it is crucial to recognize the interplay between the massive amount of global funding for AIDS and state power. As indicated above, African states have been given significant donor funds for AIDS. Nigeria, for example, received $414 million from 2003 until 2015 from the Global Fund and over $3.8 billion between 2004 and 2014 from PEPFAR. During the same period, Kenya got $407 million in Global Fund monies and over $3.9 billion from PEPFAR (PEPFAR 2015c, 2015d; Global Fund 2016b). For low- and lower-middle-income countries, these resources have been essential for promoting HIV prevention and universal ART access. In addition, resources have given African states some autonomy in spending decisions. One Tanzanian explained, "We cannot complain about the donors' priorities on AIDS. . . . Their priorities then free us to do other things, to redirect our work to other topics or concerns. So we will take their money for the issues they are concerned with and then use our resources for our concerns" (interview, government official, Dodoma, July 3, 2015). The speaker demonstrates that one reason African states accept global health governance on AIDS is because the choice enables them to focus on other priorities. This calculation demonstrates agency: In an odd way, these actors' dependence facilitates freedom.

External resources can bolster patronage networks, a crucial aspect of the neopatrimonial state. By enabling leaders to reward followers and buy off challengers, to integrate different societal groups, and to build state and party institutions, patronage can increase regime stability (Boone 1992; Arriola 2009; Lemarchand 1972; Bayart 1993; Huntington 1968). With the economic deterioration of the 1980s and 1990s, African states had fewer patronage resources and thus faced challenges in maintaining power (Clapham 1982). In order to hold governing coalitions together, African incumbents built new patronage institutions that did not undermine the fiscal discipline demanded by neoliberal structural adjustment policies. During the 1990s, many African states established specialized presidential commissions whose members could expropriate resources from society through registration fees or licenses and could interact directly with donors (van de Walle 2001; Englebert 2009). NAC and CCM exemplify this type of institution; they were set up outside the control of the permanent ministries and financed by nonstate resources. As gatekeepers, they control access to external resources for state ministries and civil society groups. Because they tend to be centralized in the president's office, high-level control prevents some of the patronage-grabbing free-for-all that Tim Kelsall (2011) asserts can undermine socioeconomic progress. As such, these centralized, neopatrimonial structures, which are rooted in a long time horizon because "AIDS is a long wave crisis," urge the state to accept global health governance on AIDS (see Barnett 2006, 360). The relationship is reciprocal: neopatrimonial interests urge acceptance of global AIDS structures, and those structures then bring additional benefits to neopatrimonial states.

The NAC and CCM benefit two constituencies: state elites and civil society actors such as religious organizations, groups of people living with HIV, business leaders, and NGOs. The inclusiveness of the NAC and CCM reflected both the multisectoral approach that donors demanded and the state's neopatrimonial goals in rent distribution. Taking on a "governance habitus" (Harman 2009, 357), state elites and their civil society counterparts benefit from rents such as per diems for workshops, payments for travel expenses, and grants to their organizations and agencies (Vian et al. 2012; Smith 2003). Benefits trickle down to communities, with people living with HIV and members of NGOs and FBOs getting foodstuffs and job opportunities (Anderson and Patterson 2017; Patterson 2016; Burchardt 2013). Rents come to be expected: One Ugandan AIDS organization tried to have a workshop with community leaders, but few attended because the organization did not have money to pay for transportation costs or per diems. One representative said: "People just won't come without those things" (interview, AIDS NGO official, Kampala, June 24, 2014).

Rents that are shared sufficiently ensure that no important groups feel excluded and engage in stability-damaging activities (Kelsall 2011, 82). One interviewee observed these AIDS institutions' use of patronage and their attempt to be widely inclusive: "When the Ghana AIDS Commission was established it became a gravy train for all these NGOs and agencies that were set up for [AIDS] . . . because HIV/AIDS is a money winning topic. This happened continent-wide" (interview, international NGO official, Accra, September 23, 2008). In one example, the leaders of a Ghanaian AIDS organization said participation in NAC brought stipends that increased their household incomes (Haven and Patterson 2007). But inclusion brought more than resources: it increased the status and influence of the FBOs, business groups, ministries, and organizations of people living with HIV that were selected for these positions. Prestige then allowed for more community influence and increased ties to donors, who relied on these group leaders to serve as brokers to link their AIDS efforts to the general society (interviews, NAC officials, Lusaka, August 15, 2007, February 17, 2011, and June 13, 2014; GAC official, Accra, October 10, 2008; on the benefits to brokers, see Lewis and Mosse 2006).

Because the NAC and CCM bestow prestige and influence, facilitate connections, and distribute patronage, there is pressure to reward these opportunities to organizations and ministries that might prove the greatest threat to state elites. In short, NAC and CCM positions could be used to incorporate potential opponents. Research on African presidential cabinets illustrates that fewer women tend to be included when politicians must gain support from multiple ethnic constituencies because female politicians (and female voters) are not viewed to be crucial for political survival (Arriola and Johnson 2014). Similarly, the vast majority of CCM and NAC representatives were not from civil society groups, which, as illustrated below, can be weak; instead, they were from state agencies and, because they fund the AIDS response, donor institutions. This limited representation makes it more difficult for civil society groups to get their voice heard; such exclusion occurs because many civil society groups are not threats to the state (Patterson 2006; UNAIDS 2012a, 2014a; Global Fund 2015a). As one example of civil society's limited influence: groups of people living with HIV and small FBOs in Zambia were unable to convince the CCM to include funding for home-based care in the country's 2014 Global Fund application (interview, CCM member, Lusaka, June 12, 2014).

As potential sites of capital accumulation, NAC and CCM, like other state agencies, can experience "intense factional struggles for positions of influence and power" (Beresford 2015, 230). In Zambia, civil society groups competed and engaged in "significant maneuvering" over representation on the CCM and NAC in 2007 (interviews, bilateral donor official, Lusaka, August 14, 2007; FBO official, Lusaka, August 19, 2007). These patterns continued in 2011, when there were tensions as some NAC members sought to "remove some of the NAC representatives" (interview, multilateral donor official, Lusaka, February 23, 2011). The outcome of this jockeying is fluidity in institutional membership, particularly for civil society group members who are easily appointed or demoted. For example, representatives from the ministries of health and finance tend to always be members of these institutions, while a particular FBO, NGO, or group of people living with HIV is not guaranteed such a spot. Some of these smaller organizations lack much bargaining power, a point particularly true of the most marginalized groups in society like youth or men who have sex with men. The constant reshuffling of these less influential groups has the danger of undermining inclusive decision-making and rent dispersal (see Barkan 1994 on the Kenya case).

Given the power of institutional appointments to disperse patronage, state elites have an incentive to create large institutions. Arthur Goldsmith (2000) finds that African states do not employ a higher proportion of the population in bureaucratic jobs than states in other geographic regions, but Leonardo Arriola (2009) discovers that African state leaders who expand cabinet size (as a way to include more groups in patronage distribution) experience greater regime stability. In fact the increase in African cabinet size since the 1980s has correlated with a decline in coups d'état. To investigate if the same stabilizing logic urges state elites to expand AIDS institutions, I use 2014 UNAIDS Country Progress Reports, which provide information on NAC members, as well as information from the Global Fund on CCM composition (UNAIDS 2014b; Global Fund 2015a). In 2014, the average size for both the NAC and the CCM was thirty-four members. Burkina Faso had the largest NAC, with 155 members, while South Sudan had the smallest, with nine members. The largest CCM was in Senegal, with seventy-four members, and the smallest was in South Sudan, with one member. Eighteen countries had CCM with over forty members (UNAIDS 2014b; Global Fund 2015a).

A few points can be made about these institutions. First, there are some political and administrative reasons that these institutions are large. As global health governance on AIDS has become more sophisticated, it has no doubt necessitated the involvement of more ministries and civil society groups to implement policies, manage funds, and monitor results in a multisectoral response. To say that state elites could benefit from such a situation through expanding neopatrimonial coalitions does not discount the logistical and practical reasons to bring more representatives into AIDS governance. These expanded neopatrimonial institutions therefore need not be negative for the AIDS response (Mkandawire 2015). As Alex Beresford (2015, 228) writes, "Informal patronage-based political networks [can] work in parallel with . . . the impersonal political institutions of the state." The ties of reciprocity and dependence that AIDS resources and institutions reinforce can help to ensure low-cost governance and facilitate successes in the AIDS response (Cheeseman 2015). Building political coalitions through large institutions and achieving policy outcomes occurs simultaneously.

Second, one might expect that these bodies would be the largest in states with the highest HIV rates, because of the magnitude and complexity of the epidemic. However, this was not the case for the forty-five states with available data on HIV prevalence and CCM and NAC size. Of the thirty-three states that had HIV rates below 5 percent, 66 percent (twenty-two states) had at least one AIDS institution that was over the region's average size of thirty-four members. In comparison, of the eleven states with HIV rates higher than 5 percent, 55 percent (six states) had at least one institution over the regional average size. When I decreased the HIV rate to 1 percent, the number did not change drastically, with 63 percent of states with this low HIV prevalence still having above-average-sized institutions. Some of the states with the lowest HIV prevalence have the largest NAC and CCM in Africa: Senegal (seventy-four CCM members), Niger (seventy-four NAC members), Mauritania (fifty-three CCM members), and Burkina Faso (155 NAC members).

Third, as William Riker (1962) asserts, state elites seek to build a minimum winning coalition by including only those politicians they need to maintain power. But because of political uncertainty and a desire to reduce their reliance on any one ally, state elites are forced to expand their coalitions. This expansion has been evident over time in the CCM. (Long-term data on NAC membership is not available, so I cannot say the same about NAC.) To be clear, it is not that aid itself has driven the increased size of the CCM (see Arriola 2009); rather, these institutions have grown in importance for resource dispersal. In 2015, the average number of members on a CCM was thirty-four individuals, compared to twenty-seven in 2005. Of forty-seven states for which there was CCM data in 2005 and 2015, twenty-seven (57 percent of states) had increased the number of CCM positions, while thirteen (28 percent of states) had decreased the positions on the CCM. CCM size remained the same in three states (Global Fund 2015a; Patterson 2006, 74–75). As state and nonstate actors have become more aware of AIDS funds, they have pressured states to increase the CCM size. Even community groups want "their share" through CCM membership (focus group discussion, group of people living with HIV, Livingstone, Zambia, June 20, 2011; interview, CCM member, Lusaka, June 12, 2014). Because of the demands for broad membership and because the CCM distribute funds, the CCM in most countries tend to be larger than the NAC. Though the average size for both CCM and NAC in Africa is thirty-four members, in two-thirds of countries the CCM is larger than the NAC. In some cases, the differences are great; for example, the Democratic Republic of Congo has fifty CCM members but only seventeen NAC members.

Fourth, Arriola (2009) finds that cabinet size in democratic countries is smaller than in autocracies because elites in democracies are less concerned about political instability and the incorporation of potential opponents through patronage. In the case of AIDS institutions, the small number of cases makes it impossible to say that a similar pattern holds up to statistical analysis. Democratic states (as classified by Polity IV) were slightly less likely to have either a NAC or CCM with more than the regional average number of members. (The regional average for both institution types was thirty-four.) The average CCM size for African democracies was thirty-seven seats, and it was thirty-five seats for autocracies. However, this difference is not statistically significant.

Fifth, Kelsall (2011) argues that even though neopatrimonial institutions with centralized control over resources do not undermine development, they can still experience problems. One is inefficiency, a by-product of their inclusivity. One Ghanaian respondent echoed this point when complaining about GAC:

> A challenge on GAC is that it takes a while to approve a decision. It must go through different committees. You approve, disapprove, approve with conditions. This can take time. Then there are some people with ego trips . . . people who put their priorities above the larger mission of the organization. (Interview, GAC official, Accra, October 1, 2008; see Haven and Patterson 2007)

Thus, GAC's large number of members creates an inefficient decision-making process in which personalities play a crucial role. The neopatrimonial decision to use the AIDS institution as a patronage tool enables individuals (or the groups or ministries they represent) to highjack the agenda in search of particularized benefits. In a broader sense, this outcome reflects the fact that centralized neopatrimonial institutions face decentralizing pressures when more members are incorporated.

In addition to inefficiency, these neopatrimonial institutions can encourage corruption, though Kelsall (2011, 80) claims that corruption is "more predictable and less harmful" in centralized neopatrimonial regimes. This is because leaders have an incentive to police corrupt actions that undermine long-term access to resources (Kelsall 2011, 80). An examination of Global Fund audit and inspection reports published between 2013 and early 2016 shows both corruption's presence and its relatively limited scope among African states. These reports reaffirm the perception of one donor official: "Allocation of resources can be blurry in the government arena" (interview, bilateral donor official, Lusaka, August 14, 2007). On one hand, of the thirty-seven incidents of reported misuse of funds globally, twenty (or 54 percent) came from African states. This number is proportionally higher than the 43 percent of total Global Fund resources that African entities have received (Global Fund 2015b, 45). For example, Nigeria's National Malaria Control Program staff members submitted fictitious expenses for airline tickets and vehicles (Global Fund 2016c). Auditors in Niger found conflict of interest among CCM members and contractors in the competitive bidding process (Global Fund 2016c). And the Zambia National AIDS Network (ZNAN, a major grant recipient) provided no documentation for grants to community organizations, including the

Maureen Mwanawasa Foundation, a project linked to the country's former first lady (*IRIN News*, March 14, 2011). On the other hand, as of 2016, only fourteen of Africa's forty-nine states had experienced these corruption issues with Global Fund grants. While discovering corruption is difficult, one might also assume that African states have sought to check some of corruption's excesses in AIDS institutions. Indeed, when corruption has occurred, such as in the Zambia case, many governments have quickly moved to address it, even allowing multilateral donors to take over grant administration (on Zambia and Malawi, see Anderson and Patterson 2017; on Kenya, see Dionne 2017).

These dual-edged findings do not deny that when corruption occurs, it has a pernicious effect on the AIDS response. Corrupt procurement processes for ARVs, for example, create delays in delivery and shortages of these life-saving drugs. And countries with higher levels of corruption have shown smaller declines in AIDS deaths because of these inefficiencies in ART dispersal (Friedman 2015). Fictitious NGOs, as were established by Kenya's National AIDS Control Council in the early 2000s, steal money that could be used for AIDS orphans or HIV testing (Transparency International 2006). In the Zambian situation, community groups that relied on ZNAN to pay AIDS educators' stipends and transportation costs were devastated when ZNAN's fraudulent practices led to its demise (Anderson and Patterson 2017). Yet, while corruption in Africa's health sector is a pervasive problem, research on its long-term impact on overall population health remains inconclusive (Moatti and Moatti 2011).

The neopatrimonial explanation presented here elucidates why African states have, for the most part, accepted global health governance on AIDS, but it also sheds light on the South African and Gambian challenges. These neopatrimonial states' search for resources led to their activities. In South Africa, the ANC and the President's Office allegedly received funds and stock shares from the company producing Virodene (Amon 2008), and rumors spread that Matthias Rath paid some ANC officials for the right to distribute his vitamin cures in the country (Geffen 2010, 130). In The Gambia, by promoting his cure as "a mandate from Allah," and by declaring The Gambia to be an Islamic Republic in 2015 (*Telegraph*, December 12, 2015), Jammeh could advance his ties to Muslim countries and gain more foreign aid from the Middle East, a particular concern after the EU cut its aid to the country in 2014 (*Reuters*, December 10, 2014). The cure also provided symbolic and spiritual legitimacy, as well as a media distraction, for his efforts to control donors' AIDS resources. At about the time of the cure's announcement, Jammeh placed the autonomous National AIDS Secretariat—an institution that received most Global Fund monies—under presidential control through the Ministry of Health (Cassidy and Leach 2009).[7] In both countries, the state centralized power over AIDS decisions: ANC officials reportedly feared that they would be sidelined if they spoke against Mbeki's ideas, while leaders (including Nelson Mandela) who did so were publicly attacked (*New York Times*, November 25, 2008). Jammeh's widespread use of repression curtailed any criticisms. These leaders did not create inclusive AIDS institutions to foster buy-in for policies to the detriment of the AIDS response.

In summary, democracy played a marginal role in African state acceptance of global health governance on AIDS. Both democracies and autocracies established AIDS institutions, though autocracies were less likely to support human rights and representation for key populations. Neopatrimonialism urged African states to accept global health governance, and the very institutions of that global AIDS governance then facilitated states' long-term neopatrimonial ambitions. The growth in size in these institutions over time illustrates their role in generating continued acceptance of global AIDS governance. Neopatrimonialism also urged South Africa (under Mbeki) and The Gambia (under Jammeh) to seek resources through alternative AIDS approaches, but because those means lacked inclusion, they crumbled. As the next section illustrates, state-level AIDS institutions have been crucial for the incorporation of civil society.

The Societal Level: Incorporation and Acquiescence

As illustrated above, many civil society groups were initially disengaged from AIDS advocacy. But by the late 1990s, groups of people living with HIV began to challenge African states and the international community to develop AIDS institutions, provide funding, and protect human rights (Smith and Siplon 2006; Haven and Patterson 2007; interviews, advocates for people living with HIV, Lusaka, Accra, Kampala, August 20, 2007, October 14, 2008, November 18, 2008, July 8, 2010, and March 7, 2011; AIDS NGO official, Dar es Salaam, July 6, 2015). Other civil society groups, particularly FBOs, which provide 40 percent of health-care services in Africa, joined in these challenges (Patterson 2011). For example, the Christian Health Association of Ghana urged the state to adopt an HIV education program in the early 2000s; the organization was influential because as a health-care provider, it could give evidence of the effects of AIDS on Ghanaians (Patterson 2011; interview, health FBO official, Accra, November 10, 2008). Many groups of people living with HIV, NGOs, and FBOs continue to hold government accountable for implementation of AIDS nondiscrimination laws and ART programs. In another example, TAC works with the South African police to make sure that perpetrators of sexual violence are arrested, and it has conducted drug audits at local clinics to ensure ART access (informal discussion, TAC activist, Guguletu, South Africa, August 7, 2014).

As global health governance on AIDS has become embedded in institutions and supported by donor funds, civil society groups have been increasingly incorporated into AIDS institutions instead of pressuring the state from the outside. The state has given groups of people living with HIV, faith-based health-care providers, and other civil society groups a place on NAC and CCM. For example, the Inter-Religious Council of Uganda (IRCU) had representation on and funding from NAC (interview, FBO health director, Kampala, June 19, 2014), while the Churches Health Association of Zambia (CHAZ) has been a principal recipient of Global Fund grants since the CCM's establishment in 2003. As of 2017, representatives of the Muslim Council, Christian Council, Catholic Secretariat, Pentecostal Council, Council for the Independent Churches, and the Association of Traditional Healers had seats on the Ghana AIDS Commission (interviews, CHAZ official, Lusaka, August 16, 2007; GAC official, Accra, October 10, 2008; FBO official, Kampala, June 27, 2014; Christian Council of Ghana official, Accra, March 17, 2017).

This incorporation has occurred for several reasons. First, the multisectoral response has necessitated bringing in civil society actors, including groups of people living with HIV and NGO service providers. Second, groups of people living with HIV have been easy to incorporate (and then, when it is not expedient, to exclude), because many lack capacity. One respondent said: "They don't have offices, structures, or policies. There are three or four people who just say 'we are an NGO'" (interview, GAC official, Accra, October 8, 2008). Many of their members come from lower socioeconomic status and thus often lack "real organizational skills, education, human capacity, and leadership skills" (interview, multilateral donor official, Accra, October 8, 2008). Middle- and upper-class people living with HIV have avoided these groups because they have focused on distributing resources such as food and income-generating projects, which middle- and upper-class individuals do not need (see Patterson 2015; Burchardt 2013). One middle-class person living with HIV in Zambia also explained how the AIDS stigma prevented participation in AIDS mobilization:

If people disclose [their status], there will be stigma in the workplace and discrimination. . . . They are afraid of what the next person might do or what they might say. In my case, when my brother-in-law heard I was infected . . .

he stopped his children from visiting my home, afraid his children will get infected. . . . I have a son who is eight years old who is infected and they do not invite him to their home. . . . Now if this is among family, imagine in a workplace. This keeps people from joining support groups, but the professionals are the people who are really suffering silently and need support. (Interview, leader of group of people living with HIV, Lusaka, May 10, 2011)

Even after a generation of AIDS, stigma continues to make AIDS a private issue. In such a context, it is difficult for AIDS groups to effectively challenge the state.

Third, incorporation can be part of a strategy to divide or minimize groups that already have marginal political power. The relatively low economic status of most members of organizations for people living with HIV leads these groups to compete with one another for material benefits from donors or the state (see Kalofonos 2010). For example, one Zambian organization for people living with HIV allegedly tried to "steal the members" of another group in order to bolster its clout with donors (interview, bilateral donor official, Lusaka, August 15, 2007). In Ghana, one women's group of people living with HIV accused another group, whose leaders were all men, of preventing them from working in some villages. The leader of the women's group said, "We hear stories that [the group led by men] has even told the women that if they want to have resources from this PLHIV group they have to sleep with the men" (interview, leader of group of people living with HIV, Accra, October 10, 2008). This competition over resources undermines solidarity among people living with HIV, making it easier for the state to ignore smaller organizations of people living with HIV and to incorporate the bigger AIDS service organizations. Large groups like TASO in Uganda gain resources, while community-level organizations only occasionally benefit (interview, leader of group of people living with HIV, Kampala, June 19, 2014; see also Patterson 2015; Anderson 2015, 144; Boesten 2011).

Fourth, incorporation benefits the state, for it bolsters state legitimacy and increases its knowledge about civil society. One large group of people living with HIV in Tanzania illustrated: "We work closely with the national AIDS control program and they want to work with us because we are in the care and treatment centers. Thus, we know what the problems are" (interview, AIDS NGO official, Dar es Salaam, July 6, 2015). The quote illustrates what James Scott (1998, 2) terms the state's desire to make everything "legible," that is, to know society's attributes, including about the clinic visits and ART adherence of people living with HIV, so that it can more effectively control society. In addition, the state can coordinate and organize these groups, activities that enhance state power and legitimacy and that ultimately lead the state to want to accept global AIDS governance.

Both Ghana and Tanzania provide examples of this civil society incorporation. As illustrated above, in 2008 groups of people living with HIV in Ghana intensely competed for members and resources. They asked GAC officials to arbitrate, heightening the role of the state as a neutral, apolitical entity that, like a parent, guides civil society's actions. Giving the state this allegedly apolitical role enhances a governance hierarchy, in which civil society must rely on the state (interview, leader of group of people living with HIV, Accra, October 10, 2008; on "apolitical" development see Ferguson 1994). In Tanzania, the state moved beyond mediating to organizing civil society. One leader for an organization of people living with HIV explained:

We [the AIDS group] started with support from the National AIDS Council because there were many small support group networks for people with HIV; there were networks of youth, teachers, disabled, etc., but they were all doing different things. So the idea was to put them all together under one council. There were a lot of donors then, and they were calling for a network, so it would be easier for them to work in a systematic way with the groups. They needed some group at the apex for all the people living with HIV. (Interview, AIDS NGO official, Dar es Salaam, July 6, 2015)

The respondent illustrates how organizing people living with HIV fit within the larger structures and expectations of global AIDS governance, since donors needed a network through which to provide benefits. By organizing people living with HIV, the state helps civil society to access resources and thus, gains legitimacy. Broader donor structures make this role for the state possible.

As an outcome of incorporation and the state's mediating and organizing activities, many civil society organizations have limited effect on AIDS policymaking, particularly in comparison to their successes in pushing for access to ART in the early to mid-2000s. Increasingly, civil society groups advise on technical issues, giving groups such as FBO service providers more clout than AIDS activists (Patterson 2015). In Ghana, for example, AIDS NGOs and people living with HIV just "come to the [GAC] meetings, sign the attendance sheets, but they will not really voice their opinions. For many of these groups, their participation is just a way of getting resources" (interview, multilateral donor official, Accra, October 8, 2008). These groups also have been relatively muted in their criticisms of state policies. For example, many donors thought that the IRCU did not speak strongly enough against Uganda's 2014 antihomosexuality legislation. In return, donors cut funding for the organization, which in turn ended grants to smaller FBOs (interviews, FBO officials, Kampala, June 19, 2014, and June 25, 2014). In Zambia, CHAZ officials have been quick to praise the state for "devoting a lot of attention" to AIDS in its "quite strong" response, while people living with HIV, some donors, and health experts have been circumspect in their assessments (interviews, CHAZ official, Lusaka, August 16, 2007; multilateral donor official, Lusaka, February 23, 2011; AIDS expert, Lusaka, August 20, 2007; leader of group of people living with HIV, Lusaka, August 19, 2007).

Weak civil society groups find it necessary to acquiesce to state power; if they do not, they could lose benefits or recognition, as one Zambian group of people living with HIV learned:

> Three years ago [2004] at a World AIDS Day rally the president promised in front of a crowd that he would provide some office space for our group. We then tried to follow up through the normal channels, but nothing. So, the next year at the World AIDS Day event I reminded him of his promise in front of a crowd. We then got the offices, but the president hasn't attended a World AIDS Day celebration since then. And some say it was because I embarrassed him and his government on AIDS. (Interview, leader of group of people living with HIV, Lusaka, August 19, 2007)

The speaker shows how the state acted as a patron by providing the office. But the group then did not play its role in the clientelist hierarchy. By challenging the president publicly, the group leader undermined the state's image as a benevolent patron. The fact that people realized the cost for this defiance (i.e., no high-level participation in World AIDS Day events) showed that groups of people living with HIV understood their weakness in this hierarchy.

The relationship between the state and civil society can also explain the challenges to global AIDS governance that Mbeki and Jammeh presented. Mbeki's flirting with AIDS denialism can be viewed in light of his larger struggle with civil society in the post-apartheid era. Mbeki's years in exile during the anti-apartheid struggle made him less supportive of grassroots mobilization and more inclined to top-down decision-making than Presidents Mandela or Zuma. He gave civil society groups little say in AIDS policymaking (Patterson 2006; Butler 2005). Yet because of their experiences in the anti-apartheid struggle, as well as their linkages to global AIDS activists, civil society groups mounted a successful challenge to the Mbeki government. Through savvy use of the media, human rights and moral framing, direct action, and broad coalition building, the TAC pushed the South African government to provide free medication for prevention of mother-to-child transmission and free ARV access to all South Africans who qualified (Mbali 2013; Johnson 2006; Robins 2004). This pressure moved South Africa from challenge to acceptance of global AIDS governance. In The Gambia, the president's challenge was part of his design to maintain legitimacy and authoritarian control. He sought greater recognition for his rule through ties to important civil society groups, particularly Muslim clerics and traditional healers. These societal leaders pushed the state to act, while Jammeh repressed human rights groups or development organizations that might have urged his acceptance of global AIDS governance (Cassidy and Leach 2009). In both countries tensions between the state and civil society led leaders to challenge global health governance and to marginalize, not incorporate, important civil society actors on AIDS.

In summary, the overall weakness of African civil society (see Englebert and Dunn 2013; Branch and Mampilly 2015; Rothchild and Chazan 1988), and particularly groups of people living with HIV, has enabled their incorporation into the AIDS response. Though these groups opposed the state and urged acceptance of global health governance on AIDS early in the new millennium, once states had accepted global health governance, many civil society groups lost some influence. (This is true even in South Africa, where TAC has faced financial and organizational challenges in recent years. See *SABC News*, October 2, 2014). AIDS institutions like NAC and CCM provided opportunities for the state to organize, reward, and, in some cases, sideline some AIDS organizations. AIDS institutions created ways to disperse patronage to society and foster the inclusion necessary to stabilize politics. Civil society's acquiescence enabled the state to accept global health governance and ultimately to benefit from it.

Conclusion: The Benefits and Dangers of Acceptance?

African state acceptance of global health governance on AIDS has developed over time. During the 1980s and 1990s, many states challenged global health governance because of the lack of international institutions and resources, divisions among donors about AIDS, the ways that portrayals of the disease challenged African state aspirations, and the disengagement of civil society. With the new millennium, many of these dynamics changed. Global health governance was supported by resources and institutions, and it was rooted in human rights norms about participation, nondiscrimination, and access to ART. African states developed AIDS structures which enabled them to reward ministries and civil society groups with patronage and prestige. While civil society groups presented challenges to the state in the early 2000s, once AIDS institutions became entrenched, groups jockeyed for funding and positions. States expanded AIDS structures to include civil society, both to foster representation and to incorporate potential opponents. This political benefit led officials to continue to accept global health governance on AIDS. In the exceptional cases of South Africa and The Gambia, international factors such as reputational concerns, the search for short-term neopatrimonial benefits, and tensions with or repression of civil society drove AIDS actions.

Acceptance has increased states' legitimacy on AIDS. In a survey conducted in thirty-four countries, 69 percent of respondents said their governments were doing a fairly good job or a very good job in combatting AIDS. This number contrasted with the 41 percent who gave high marks to government for providing water and sanitation and the 57 percent who gave government high rankings for improving basic health services (Asunka 2013). The four countries with the highest rankings (Botswana with 94 percent, Swaziland with 92 percent, Burundi with 88 percent, and Namibia with 87 percent) also had high rankings for political commitment in the 2014 National Commitments and Policies Instrument (UNAIDS 2014a). Additionally, public support for state AIDS efforts has increased over time (Fox 2014). As AIDS institutions have become entrenched, the multisectoral approach has generated support from many civil society actors and ministries (interview, multilateral donor official, Kampala, June 30, 2014). Global AIDS governance with its funding and institutional structures has enabled African states to build legitimacy and take credit for AIDS services, particular when citizens see state officials visiting AIDS projects, speaking as NAC officials, or collaborating with donors (Sacks 2012, 7). Mick Moore (1998) asserts that states build legitimacy through service delivery and that dependence on foreign aid prevents them from building capacity to deliver services well. However, in the case of AIDS, donor money enabled the state to build institutions to deliver services. Beyond the provision of neopatrimonial resources, global AIDS governance gives African states ways they can demonstrate their ability to govern.

African state acceptance of global AIDS governance has reinforced that global health governance. The successes on treatment and prevention that have come via African state acceptance have given global AIDS institutions and funding programs a raison d'être. Pointing to successes and Africa's commitment to end AIDS has enabled donors to continue to generate funds and develop programs. For example, in 2012, Michel Sidibé said that Africa is poised to transcend the outdated donor-recipient paradigm and to chart its own course in the AIDS response (UNAIDS 2012d). And during the 2016 International AIDS Conference held in Durban, South Africa, many speakers praised African countries for their progress on universal access to ART and their continued commitment to the disease (*SABC*

News, July 22, 2016). The outcome is a dialectical process: strong global health governance through institutions, norms, and resources fosters state commitments, which then help to justify global health governance.

Because, as this chapter shows, global health governance is not static, acceptance presents dangers for a continued commitment to global health governance of AIDS and ultimately, to the millions of people living with or affected by the disease. As states have gained legitimacy on AIDS, public perceptions that AIDS is a problem have declined. In Zambia, for example, o percent of survey respondents in 2013 said that the government should prioritize AIDS (Afrobarometer 2013; see also Fox 2014). Across society, many people have come to view AIDS as "routine" (interviews, AIDS expert, Lusaka, February 14, 2011; AIDS NGO officials, Kampala, June 24, 2015, and Dar es Salaam, July 6, 2015; physician, Accra, May 9, 2017; Anderson and Patterson 2017). In addition, success can foster donor fatigue, as populations in donor states no longer view the issue to be a problem and thus do not urge those donor states to contribute funds (informal conversation, bilateral donor official, Lusaka, April 14, 2009; Kaiser Family Foundation 2015a; *Science Speaks*, July 19, 2015). In fact, global spending on AIDS declined 13 percent in 2015 (Kaiser Family Foundation and UNAIDS 2016).

As AIDS institutions have become entrenched in a political calculation of African state survival, the norms of inclusion, nondiscrimination, and treatment access that undergird global health governance on AIDS show signs of being undermined. As the state has sought to maintain the status quo and protect its political arrangements, it has excluded some key populations whose involvement matters for the success of the global AIDS response. For example, a Tanzanian AIDS advocate explained the complicated problems that youth living with HIV face:

> Young people who are HIV positive . . . want to start having relationships, but how? They need to know the positives and negatives of relationships, how to protect themselves, the issues of STIs [sexually transmitted infections], new infections, etc. . . . And then there are those who are illiterate and they are afraid to disclose, because they know there is stigma if they do. (Interview, AIDS NGO official, Dar es Salaam, July 6, 2015)

This respondent's concerns are evident in epidemiological data: 25 percent of new HIV infections in Africa are among young women (UNAIDS 2014d). Yet because young women, as well as people who inject drugs, men who have sex with men, migrants, and isolated rural inhabitants, are not easily incorporated into neopatrimonial AIDS institutions, they have remained somewhat forgotten (interview, AIDS NGO official, Kitwe, Zambia, May 19, 2011; see *SABC News*, July 22, 2016). And if pushed to include these groups, the state can become resentful. One GAC official said about donors' focus on key populations in Ghana:

> We are being punished for being successful with our low prevalence. They [donors] think we don't need money, so they only put money into the high-risk groups. But, if 90 percent of your population is HIV negative, why not support keeping them negative? Instead, these donors put all of their money into the other 10 percent. (Interview, GAC official, Accra, October 10, 2008)

As the official indicates, acceptance can lead states to foster policies that benefit the majority, even though successfully combating AIDS requires states to respond to the virus within all subpopulations.

The entrenchment of AIDS institutions could mean states do not address the inequalities that persist in AIDS services. In 2013, 87 percent of people living with HIV in Botswana who needed ART could obtain it, while only 47 percent of people living with HIV in Ghana could (UNAIDS 2014c, 22; UNAIDS 2014e, 68). HIV testing is crucial for treatment access, since almost 90 percent of Africans who test positive for HIV then access treatment (UNAIDS 2014h). Yet the median national rate for HIV testing for twenty-nine surveyed countries was 28.8 percent for women and 17.2 percent for men in 2013 (Staveteig et al. 2013). To fully institutionalize the norm of universal access, HIV testing must increase. Paradoxically, African state acceptance of global AIDS governance, and civil society's incorporation into that governance, makes achieving this goal more difficult because actors have come to accept and benefit from the status quo.

African states focus on AIDS because it fosters patronage networks, helps the state to reward supporters, enables the state to build up its aspirational identity, increases the state's power over civil society, and builds the state's legitimacy. As the next two chapters indicate, not every health concern generates this same political calculus. The result is that some health issues that cause disability, morbidity, and mortality for people who are not living with HIV receive less attention. The lack of political incentives undermines the right to health for all people.

chapter 3

International Confusion, Local Demands

Challenging Global Health Governance during the 2014–2015 Ebola Outbreak

It [Ebola] was terrible, terrible, very, very painful. I lost my wife, my children, my mother-in-law, sister-in-law. It started in July [2014] with my mother-in-law. She got sick. My pregnant wife cared for her. No one knew. No one knew. It was terrible. . . . And then my wife got sick. She miscarried. She was bleeding, bleeding everywhere. I cared for her, just as she cared for my mother-in-law. But she died. Then it was me.

(Interview, Ebola survivor, Monrovia, May 17, 2016)

In a passionate but halting voice the young Liberian described his horrific experience with the Ebola Virus Disease (EVD or "Ebola"), which decimated his family and his livelihood. Two years later, he still struggled to rebuild his life. The disease, which hit Guinea, Sierra Leone, and Liberia during 2014 and 2015, resulted in over 28,000 confirmed, reported, and suspected cases and over 11,000 deaths (WHO 2016e). Research indicates that the outbreak was more deadly than prior outbreaks because a genetic mutation allowed the virus to more easily infect human cells (*New York Times*, November 3, 2016); at the same time, the virus probably infected more individuals than previously thought, with some people never experiencing symptoms (Richardson et al. 2016). In June 2016, the WHO declared the region Ebola-free (WHO 2016c), after isolated cases occurred in Guinea and Liberia in 2016. Even though by 2016 the international community had spent over $7 billion on the outbreak (*Financial Times*, May 23, 2016), the Ebola response has been considered a failure of global health governance (WHO 2015c; Busby, Grépin, and Youde 2016; Moon et al. 2015; WHO 2016d; UN 2016). Within that failure, though, were unique opportunities for African states to challenge global health governance. At the regional level, more than half of African states ignored the WHO recommendation against restrictions on travelers from affected states. One of these affected states— Liberia—challenged both the design and implementation of global health governance, ultimately gaining credit for its response (WHO 2015f).

Liberia provides an important example of how one state relates to global health governance. Like Guinea and Sierra Leone, it has high rates of poverty and underdevelopment: Of the 189 countries listed in the United Nations Development Programme's Human Development Index, Liberia is ranked 177, Sierra Leone, 181, and Guinea, 182 (UNDP 2015, 210). Freedom House (2016b) classifies all three as "partly free" political systems, characterized by corruption, minimal protection of civil rights, and weak rule of law. All have experienced civil war, ethnic conflict, and/or internal population displacement because of violence: Liberia during the 1989–2003 civil war, Sierra Leone during the 1991–2002 war, and Guinea as a result of invasions by Liberian and Sierra Leonean belligerents.[1]

Guinea and Sierra Leone also exhibited some elements of challenge to global health governance on Ebola. Guinea challenged the narrative around the response, particularly with its refusal to report early cases. Fearing that its citizens would be blocked from attending the annual Muslim pilgrimage to Mecca, the government downplayed cases. It insisted on only reporting confirmed cases and deaths, not suspicious or probable cases, a practice that distorted the picture of the epidemic and hindered designing an adequate global response (*Associated Press*, March 20, 2015). More broadly, Guinea was criticized for its slow engagement with the issue and its lack of collaboration with external partners (Morrison and Streifel 2015). Its challenges included the use of violence by some citizens against health-care workers, actions not seen in the other two states (*Washington Post*, September 19, 2014). Sierra Leone, as the final country to experience cases, had less opportunity to challenge the narrative; it was hard for it to deny cases. Rather, it created obstacles during the implementation of global heath governance programs, particularly through corruption and rent-seeking behavior. "Ghost workers" on Ebola project payrolls and the looting and selling for food intended for quarantined communities are two examples (*Guardian*, November 5, 2014). Funds were "siphoned off and misappropriated by a range of actors" (Anderson and Beresford 2016).

While Sierra Leone and Guinea demonstrated some challenges to global health governance, Liberia's efforts were more systematic. The country sought to shape the narrative and design of the response as well as to control its implementation. The country has some unique characteristics that facilitated its challenge. Unlike Guinea and Sierra Leone, it was never officially a colony and thus often does not feel obliged to follow the lead of a former colonial power (Young 2009). And even though it has the smallest population of the three states, Liberia experienced 4,806 Ebola deaths, compared to 2,536 in Guinea and 3,955 in Sierra Leone. Its Ebola fatality rate of 45 percent was between Guinea's (66 percent) and Sierra Leone's

(30 percent). Higher survival rates in Liberia and Sierra Leone resulted from greater attention from donors and the state and from less resistance to biomedicine than in Guinea (Benko 2016; Ammann 2014). The country's historical autonomy and the magnitude of the Ebola outbreak pushed it to challenge global health governance.

However, Liberia's ability to challenge global health governance meant that it had to overcome, or more accurately manipulate, several factors that could have limited its efforts. First, though its relationship with the United States has waxed and waned since 1821 when members of the American Colonization Society claimed land in what was to become Liberia, US political and economic actors have a strong presence in the country (Dunn 2009; Liebenow 1987). Second, Liberia is the most aid dependent of all three countries, receiving 44.3 percent of its gross national income from official development assistance in 2013, compared to 9.1 percent for Guinea and 18.9 percent for Sierra Leone (World Bank 2015b). Third, Liberia hosted a UN peacekeeping mission—the United Nations Mission in Liberia (UNMIL)—during the outbreak, though the mission had limited involvement in the Ebola response (Davies and Rushton 2016). Fourth, Liberia has over 1,500 Ebola survivors, many of whom will require continued food assistance, health care, and dependent support (WHO 2016e; interviews, humanitarian relief agency official and international NGO official, Monrovia, May 18, 2016, and May 19, 2016). The US-Liberia relationship, Liberia's aid dependence, the presence of peacekeepers, and the large number of survivors could have limited the country's challenge to global health governance, particularly if state officials had feared losing important donor assistance. Instead, some of these factors became themes around which Liberia challenged global health governance.

This chapter argues that three sets of inter-related factors made it possible for African states—both the unaffected states that implemented travel restrictions and the Ebola-affected state of Liberia—to challenge global health governance. At the international level, there were no clear norms for addressing infectious disease outbreaks; norm enforcement institutions lacked power; outbreak response programs were weak; funding (at least initially) was limited; and the frames of neglect and crisis not only were contradictory but also undermined the aspirational identities of African states as safe, modern, and "emerging" global economic, cultural, and political players (Rotberg 2013). At the state level of analysis, elections, concerns about tourism revenue, and geographic location pushed states to challenge global health governance through implementation of travel restrictions. However, because the issue was only a short-term crisis and because the adoption of restrictions had little to no impact on externally derived donor resources, neopatrimonialism played no role in these decisions. For Liberia, the country's partial democratic transition, as well as its historically high levels of corruption through competitive patronage networks, led it to challenge global health governance. At the societal level, the general sentiment of fear shaped states' views on travel restrictions. In Liberia, civil society's history of distrust and opposition to the state pressured the state to act, particularly since civil society responses were situated in traditional and religious power centers.

To make this argument, the chapter first provides a short background on the outbreak. It then details the weak, unfunded, and contradictory nature of global health governance on Ebola. The third section investigates how weak international health institutions, contested norms, and democratic concerns led unaffected African states to challenge global health governance by restricting travelers from affected states. The fourth section details Liberia's unique challenge in global health diplomacy and policy implementation: it first framed the outbreak in terms of neglect and crisis to gain international attention and resources and then sought to control policy implementation through its Incident Management System. The fifth section asserts that this challenge resulted because of the weak and contested nature of global health norms and institutions, Liberia's limited democracy, its rule through competitive neopatrimonial networks, and civil society opposition. The conclusion illustrates the often temporary effects of challenges to global health governance.

The Ebola Outbreak in West Africa

Ebola is a hemorrhagic disease with a mortality rate of roughly 40 percent; it is spread through direct contact with the bodily fluids of an infected person. The virus can cause the sudden onset of fever and fatigue, muscle pain, headache, and sore throat, which can be followed by vomiting, diarrhea, rash, and in some cases internal and external bleeding. Early support with rehydration and antibiotics can improve survival rates. Surveillance, contact tracing, social distancing (e.g., no handshaking), quarantine of victims in Ebola Treatment Units (ETUs), community mobilization, safe burial of bodies, training for health-care workers, and distribution of personal protective equipment (PPE) like face shields, rubber gloves, boots, and impermeable gowns are crucial to contain the virus (WHO 2016c). Ebola is not a new disease (humans first encountered it in 1976 in what was then called Zaire), but the 2014–2015 outbreak was different because of its magnitude, because it was the first Ebola outbreak in West Africa, and because of its spread in urban areas (WHO 2016b).[2]

The West African outbreak began on December 26, 2013, with the death of a two-year-old child near Guéckédou, a Guinean community located near the borders of Liberia and Sierra Leone. On March 21, 2014, samples confirmed the disease to be Ebola, at which point the government of Guinea notified the WHO, which then announced the outbreak (Baize et al. 2014). On March 30, 2014, Liberia reported its first two Ebola cases in the populous, ethnically diverse, highly impoverished, and war-torn Lofa County, which borders Guinea and Sierra Leone (Peacebuilder 2011; Fearon, Humphreys, and Weinstein 2007, 2; Moran 2006; Bøås 2009). Cases then spread south to Firestone Rubber Factory and Plantation, as one hospital official described:

A good number of the workforce at Firestone comes from the very area where Ebola was first. There is the Kissi tribe . . . and a lot of them have relatives here. The socioeconomic status of their tribesmen in the company is far better than their situation in the countryside. . . . It is known in Liberia that Firestone has . . . a hospital that provides health care free of charge. So my reasoning was that the relatives who got sick [in Lofa] would run to their relatives here. And then we ourselves would be at risk. . . . [Very soon] we got information that there was a suspected case from Lofa, a patient who had escaped the health team and was headed toward Firestone. (Interview, hospital official, Harbel, May 16, 2016)

The quote illustrates how migration, urban-rural linkages, and family connections enabled the virus to spread. In fact, hundreds of people cross the three affected states' borders each day to visit family, seek employment, and/or engage in trade (Alexander et al. 2015, 12).

In addition, distrust of state officials (see below) and the long war in Liberia contributed to structural inequalities that complicated the outbreak response (Benton and Dionne 2015a, 2015b; Mackey 2016). The war led to the massive emigration of health-care professionals. More than a decade after the war's end, Liberia had only fifty physicians for its four million people (Epstein 2014). And postwar neoliberal economic policies also weakened health-care systems (Jones 2014; Benton and Dionne 2015a; Pfeiffer and Chapman 2010; Kim et al. 2002). To receive loans from the IMF, Liberia had to keep its budget deficit under 3 percent of GDP, leading officials to limit long-term investments in public health infrastructure and personnel training and to cap staff salaries (Rowden 2014). Private providers were urged to enter the market, and NGOs and FBOs became increasingly crucial providers of health-care services (Pfeiffer and Chapman 2010). Even though Liberia had rebuilt many of the 550 health-care centers that the war had destroyed, state spending on health care was low. Of the $179 million spent on health in 2009, only about $19 million was from the state. Donors provided at least $122 million, and households, the rest (Downie 2012, 6). Additionally, donor health spending supported donors' priorities. Between 2002 and 2013, donors provided $1.7 billion in aid to Liberia, Sierra Leone, and Guinea; a substantial amount of that money went for vertical health programs to address AIDS or TB; only $20 million went to train doctors and nurses, and only $24 million was for health-care facility repairs. Many grants were intended for large international NGOs, not local FBOs or NGOs (Harman 2015; Benton 2015). Overall, there was underinvestment in health-care systems, with all three countries having some of the lowest levels of health-care expenditure per capita in the world (ODI 2015).

As a result, health-care systems in the affected states were not prepared for Ebola. The virus spread in hospitals and clinics because health-care workers lacked knowledge and training. They were at least twenty-one times more likely to be infected by Ebola than people who were not health-care workers, with almost two hundred Liberian health-care workers—over 8 percent of all physicians, nurses, and midwives—dying (Al Jazeera, June 25, 2015; Evans, Goldstein, and Popova 2015). Out of fear of infection, citizens avoided hospitals; in turn, some health-care workers were traumatized and afraid. One emergency room nurse said, "People really saw the hospitals as a threat. . . . If you go to the hospital you never know who you are going to meet there. They [patients] were afraid of us and we were afraid of them" (interview, hospital nursing assistant, Kakata, May 16, 2016). After health-care staff were given training and PPE, transmissions subsided. One study found that the rate of Ebola transmission to health-care workers declined from a range of 5–35 percent before training to a range of 0–5 percent after training (Benko 2016).

Global Health Governance on Ebola

Several themes characterize global health governance on Ebola, all of which created openings for African state challenges. These include an initially inadequate, slow response from donors; delayed involvement by weak international institutions; a lack of accepted norms to undergird the response; and contested framing of the issue.

First, the response of multilateral and bilateral donors was inadequate for the first eight months of the outbreak. During early 2014, the WHO downplayed concerns about Ebola because it viewed the outbreak to be similar to previous ones in the Democratic Republic of Congo and Uganda (*Associated Press*, May 20, 2015). WHO officials assumed that if they adopted similar responses, the epidemic would fizzle out. By May 2014, WHO officials misinterpreted a drop in reported cases to signal the end of the epidemic. Ebola received little attention at the World Health Assembly meeting in May 2014, where no specific reports or resolutions related to Ebola were presented (WHO 2014j).

In early July 2014, the WHO convened a panel of regional health experts and deployed additional experts to the WHO Regional Office for Africa (AFRO) in Brazzaville (WHO 2014k). Some experts at AFRO recommended the declaration of a Public Health Emergency of International Concern (PHEIC), an action that illustrates African officials' agency and their attempt to shape the design of global health governance. However, these efforts were unsuccessful. The WHO Secretariat feared the PHEIC would damage relations with the affected countries because it would have a negative impact on trade, tourism, and foreign investment (Garrett 2015b; *Associated Press*, March 20, 2015). On August 8, 2014, eight months after the first case appeared in Guinea, the WHO declared a PHEIC. By then, over one thousand people had died (*Associated Press*, May 20, 2015). As part of the PHEIC, the WHO Secretariat advised against travel or trade restrictions against Ebola-affected countries (WHO 2014e). (I analyze state reactions to this recommendation below.) The organization missed the opportunity to address Ebola sooner (Specter 2015), since a PHEIC allows the WHO Secretariat to coordinate global surveillance, raise funds, mobilize manpower, and promote research for vaccines and therapeutics.

Bilateral donors also did little until September 2014 *(Reuters,* December 17, 2014). The US Centers for Disease Control and Prevention (CDC) deployed a team of scientists and public health officials to Guinea in January 2014 and Liberia in March 2014. But by April, CDC officials thought the epidemic was almost over, and CDC reduced its staff. The lack of a "robust and coordinated response" among bilateral and multilateral donor health agencies, as well as tensions between CDC and the WHO, meant the CDC lacked substantial information to accurately assess and respond to the situation (*New York Times*, December 30, 2014; *Washington Post*, October 4, 2014). The United States allocated no special funds to the response until President Barack Obama asked Congress for $6 billion in October 2014 to support CDC activities and the deployment of 3,000 US troops to Liberia to build ETUs, to transport supplies, and to help with logistics (Garrett 2015b; *Washington Post*, November 5, 2014; CDC 2015c). For some Liberians, the United States' slow reaction was inexplicable: "[Liberians] thought that the US government really didn't care for Liberia because they knew that the US government had everything to prevent the virus and they did not do it" (interview, Liberian community leader, Tennessee, March 14, 2016). Underlying this response was the idea that the international community had a normative obligation to respond but was stingy with its resources. Another Liberian interviewee showed his frustration with these slow actions on Ebola:

> You have to ask, "How did we get to this level of deaths without international attention?" The first case in West Africa was December 2013 in Guinea . . . but there was not much attention to this case, we didn't know anything about this until we heard about the five cases in Liberia in March [2014]. So what was happening between December and March with WHO? Why were they not responding? And the only international body that is around to respond to health issues is WHO. . . . That is their major responsibility. . . . They knew that we have weak health systems because we had suffered in the war. We needed resources, human resources, financial resources, capacity and these things came too late. (Interview, hospital official, Harbel, May 16, 2016)

The response not only illustrates the interviewee's incredulity and frustration but also shows a common assumption that the WHO had the capacity, autonomy, and political support to be proactive on Ebola. Also, similar to the above respondent, this individual believed that the international community had a normative obligation to act. As shown below, the reality was that institutional weakness and normative confusion prevailed.

A second theme was that weak international institutions and limited funding hampered the response. The WHO faces the classic principal-agent problem, in which the principal (in this case, states) establishes an agent (in this case, the WHO) to provide public goods that the principal cannot or will not provide (Moe 1984). But fearing that the agent will develop its own agenda, the principal often seeks to rein it in through resource control and structural limitations (Gailmard 2014). Since the organization's establishment in 1948, the WHO's ability to promote infectious disease control has depended on domestic political considerations in major states, the nature of geopolitics, and the disease to be addressed (Kamradt-Scott 2015). The WHO Secretariat is beholden to all member states, who may not all agree on its objectives. (In 2015, WHO Director-General Margaret Chan complained that she had "194 bosses," one from each WHO member state. See Kupferschmidt 2015.) In order to prevent the WHO from becoming too powerful, member states created a decentralized structure with six autonomous regional offices.

Additionally, member states control WHO resources, which have declined since the 1980s. Between 2011 and 2013, donations to the organization's regular budget were cut 50 percent (*Reuters*, December 17, 2014; WHO 2014d, 2015h). Roughly 75 percent of the WHO's contributions are given as extrabudgetary funds for specific donor-approved programs, not for the WHO regular budget (Youde 2012).

These structural problems shaped the WHO response in several ways.[3] The decentralized structure enabled AFRO to control the Ebola information that the WHO Secretariat received, and it allowed the Secretariat to initially downplay Ebola (Moon et al. 2015; WHO 2014a, 2015c, 2015d). Budget cuts meant that the Global Outbreak Alert and Response Network (GOARN), a technical network of public and private actors that participates in infectious disease outbreak responses (see Mackenzie et al. 2014), was severely underfunded in 2014 just as Ebola and the Middle East Respiratory Syndrome (MERS) emerged. In 2014, the WHO cut 130 positions in the program; these staff members could have potentially detected Ebola earlier or helped affected states to act sooner (Garrett 2015b; WHO 2015h). Perhaps protective of its leadership role in global health, WHO officials ignored NGO warnings about the crisis, even though the International Health Regulations (IHR) give nonstate actors a role in identifying infectious disease outbreaks (Youde 2012). The WHO downplayed pleas from Médicins Sans Frontières (MSF) about the extent of the epidemic (Garrett 2015b), even though MSF is "a highly respected organization with years of experience providing health care in hard places" (interview, international humanitarian NGO official, Monrovia, May 19, 2016). The WHO's weakness was evident when the UN Security Council passed Resolution 2177 in October 2014 (see below), an action that created the UN Mission for Ebola Emergency Response (UNMEER) to coordinate a response (UNSC 2014). The WHO was then left to play a merely technical advisory role in the UNMEER structure.

Even after the WHO increased its efforts in August 2014, the lack of resources and political legitimacy affected its ability to act (Kamradt-Scott, Harman, Wenham, and Smith 2015). An NGO worker in Monrovia explained an encounter with WHO personnel:

Sometimes the people [WHO] sent to help put us more at risk [of infection]. . . . They would say, "We need to go into the unit [ETU]" but then they got into the unit and it became clear right away that they'd never been in a unit. They'd never gone through protocols of what to do and not to do. And they came in and they put all of us at such a huge risk. One day when the "Ebola experts" came, they started to doff—to take off the PPE—and there is a specific way, because that's one of the most dangerous times [for infection]. And they just started taking everything off. I was thinking to myself, "We are in trouble." We were spraying them [with bleach] like crazy. It was incredibly stressful. As time went on, though, they did get better. (Interview, international humanitarian NGO official, Monrovia, May 19, 2016)

The anecdote shows that WHO personnel were unprepared, perhaps as a result of lack of resources and staff cuts at the organization (Kamradt-Scott, Harman, Wenham, and Smith 2015). Ebola demanded quick learning, sometimes for people who had little real-world experience with infectious disease management. The incident (and others like it) reconfirmed the perspective that WHO was not really up for the Ebola task. Most crucially for this chapter's argument, the WHO's lack of preparation and its low capacity created spaces in which other actors with expertise, information, and supplies could maneuver. In the above anecdote, that other actor is an official with a humanitarian NGO (who frantically tries to save everyone from infection by spraying bleach). African states also acted in the gap created by the WHO's weakness.

A third theme of global health governance on Ebola is the lack of accepted, coherent norms to undergird action. The right to health could have pushed early actions, but questions about who is obligated to provide health care in humanitarian crises, what health care should be provided, and how to ensure nondiscrimination, freedom of movement, and health-care access undermined the norm's application to the Ebola case (Davies 2010; Youde 2008; Chapman 2012; Mann 1999; UNHRC 2014). Similarly, the humanitarian norm of providing aid to people in crises could have pushed action, but the disease was not even uniformly understood to be a humanitarian crisis. In fact, the United Nations Office of the Coordination of Humanitarian Affairs was only one of many players involved (Percival and Kreutzer 2016). Notions about providing charity to innocent victims could have mobilized early action, but they did not (Kapstein and Busby 2013; Siplon 2013; Keck and Sikkink 1998). This was despite the fact that the media often portrayed West Africans to be innocent, deserving victims in stories about female caregivers, sick children, and dedicated health-care workers who died doing their jobs (Harman 2016b; Inter-Agency Standing Committee 2015). Indeed, my assistant and I analyzed the almost 180 stories published on the topic in three major newspapers—the *New York Times*, the *Washington Post*, and the *Guardian*—between January 1, 2014, and August 15, 2014. The analysis revealed that almost one-third of stories included photos of Ebola-affected children, visuals that emphasized a charity norm. Yet human rights, humanitarian, and charity norms were undermined by the norm of state sovereignty (see Finnemore 2003 on norm contestation). States exercised the right to protect their own strategic and material interests, and they believed that assisting the three Ebola-affected states, which lack hard power because of their low-income status and weak military capabilities, did little to advance those interests. The norm of sovereignty also allowed nonaffected states to challenge the IHR, an international agreement. Thus, competing and/or weak norms characterized global health governance on Ebola.

The final aspect of global health governance on Ebola was competition among issue frames. The first frame was what João Nunes (2016) terms the "narrative of neglect," while the second was the crisis frame. (See chapter 1 on frames.) Though it undergirded much of the Ebola response, the neglect frame dominated the first eight months of the outbreak, leading to the aforementioned disregard, apathy, inaction, and action with incompetence. Sick populations were ignored, and Ebola was virtually invisible (Nunes 2016, 545). Framing Ebola as a "nonissue" resonated with commonly held perceptions of Africa, which until 2014 was the only continent to experience human deaths from Ebola. Neglect fit with Western beliefs about the "primitive" nature of the continent (Jones 2014; Wilkinson and Leach 2014), the view that Africa has been unable to foster health and development (Englebert 2009; Leonard and Straus 2003), and the perception that infectious diseases are the dominant cause of morbidity and mortality in Africa (see chapter 4). As such, Ebola was yet another "African tragedy."

As Nunes (2016, 549) points out, when the WHO declared Ebola to be a PHEIC, "[it] was doing more than just describing a problem—it was inscribing Ebola as a particular kind of problem." Ebola was a *crisis*, a frame that emphasized how infectious diseases, including new or re-emerging pathogens, spread uncontrollably through global trade and travel and threaten a state's security (Price-Smith 2009). Such outbreaks are perceived to originate in poor countries, where the distant "other" people live (Wald 2008; Wilkinson and Leach 2014). Ebola's high mortality rate, its sometimes grotesque symptoms, its transmission through caregiving activities, and what the media portrayed to be its rapid spread throughout West Africa fueled fear, particularly since therapeutics and a vaccine were nonexistent (Price-Smith and Porreca 2016). Even though several aspects of this frame were inaccurate—the virus requires contact for transmission; state failure because of any disease is extremely rare; well-developed health-care systems could contain Ebola (McInnes 2016, 382)—the crisis frame seemed credible because it aligned with the perception that "disease threats originate in the Global South and require international law to prevent their spread to affluent regions" (Gostin 2014, 179).

Ebola became a threat to Western, postindustrial countries like the United States. Before August 2014, this aspect of the crisis frame—Ebola's direct threat to the West—was not evident in media stories. Joanne Liu, president of MSF, remarked that the absence of this frame led to little global attention to Ebola during the first eight months of the outbreak (MSF 2014).

By fall 2014, several events made Ebola salient to Western audiences and elevated the "Ebola is a threat to the West" frame. First, Patrick Sawyer, a Liberian-American, traveled via plane to Lagos, Nigeria on July 20, 2014 and infected several Nigerian health-care workers, leading to twenty cases and eight deaths (*BBC News*, August 4, 2014; Kamradt-Scott 2016). The event seemed to indicate how the virus could spread through air travel. Second, on August 2, 2014, Kent Brantly and Nancy Writebol, a doctor and a nurse who worked with the international FBO Samaritan's Purse in Monrovia, were infected with Ebola and returned to Emory University Hospital in Atlanta for treatment. Third, on September 2, 2014, Joanne Liu told the United Nations that the world was "losing the battle" with the "transnational threat," phrases that stressed the uncontrollable, global spread of the pathogen (MSF 2014). Fourth, in late August, the WHO predicted there would be at least 20,000 cases in the affected countries by November 2014 (*New York Times*, August 28, 2014). The CDC then forecast that without action there would be over one million Ebola cases by February 2015 (Meltzer et al. 2014). These statements seemed to signal that the outbreak would destroy societies. Fifth, on October 9, 2014, the World Bank predicted that West Africa's GDP could lose $2.2–$7.4 billion in 2014 and $1.6–$25 billion in 2015 (World Bank 2014a), a statement that showed the economic cost of the outbreak. Sixth, in mid-October 2014, Liberian Thomas Eric Duncan travelled to the United States. His Ebola infection was misdiagnosed in a Dallas hospital, he infected two nurses, and he ultimately died from Ebola. The situation seemed to emphasize the pernicious effects of globalization and the ill-prepared nature of health-care systems for new pathogens (*Time*, October 25, 2014).

Just as the neglect frame led to inaction, the crisis framework, particularly with its focus on Ebola's danger to the West, catalyzed state activities. On September 18, 2014, the UN Security Council recognized the magnitude of the outbreak and unanimously passed Resolution 2177 which set up UNMEER, making Ebola only the second health issue after AIDS that the Security Council had addressed (McInnes and Rushton 2010). UNMEER was the first UN mission established for the sole purpose of addressing a health crisis, a precedent that some UN Security Council members privately questioned for fear that it equated Africa with insecurity (interview, UN Security Council delegate, New York, October 5, 2015; phone interview, African UN representative, October 15, 2015). The resolution also directly termed Ebola a "threat to international peace and security," a label not used for AIDS (Rushton 2016). At the bilateral level, the United States sent troops to Liberia, and the British sent troops to Sierra Leone. For the United States, these actions reflected concern about the disease's spread, the historic relationship with Liberia, and geostrategic calculations since China had ramped up its Ebola response (Kamradt-Scott, Harman, Wenham, and Smith 2015; interview, government official, Monrovia, May 18, 2016).

The tension between the neglect and crisis frames was evident in the media "spectacle" (McInnes 2016). As an example of neglect: Between January 1, 2014, and June 1, 2014, our analysis revealed fewer than fifteen stories on the West African outbreak in the *Washington Post*, the *New York Times*, and the *Guardian*; a LexisNexis search for newspaper articles using the term "Ebola" during the same time period uncovered fewer than twenty stories. During this early period, media coverage emphasized that the disease was spread through cultural practices like eating bush meat, touching corpses before burial, reliance on traditional healers over biomedicine, and belief in witchcraft. These messages drove fear and seemed to blame West Africans for their suffering and death (WHO 2015d; Alexander et al. 2015; Jones 2014; interview, government official, Monrovia, May 18, 2016; Abeysinghe 2016).

After August 2014, media stories exhibited the "Ebola as a threat to the West" crisis motif. Of thirty-nine stories published in August 2014 in the above-mentioned three newspapers, eighteen focused on Americans and five described experimental drugs for Ebola. These stories made Ebola a Western problem, wrapping it up in US domestic politics: "Party and electoral politics was the predominant frame through which Ebola management was cast" (Abeysinghe 2016, 457). Indeed, US media coverage of Ebola dropped precipitously after the midterm elections in early November 2014 (Media Matters 2014). But this was not before the Republican-majority Congress criticized the CDC and President Obama named an "Ebola czar." The public's attention to Ebola coverage further advanced the crisis narrative: By October 2014, 67 percent of Americans said they were following media coverage of the diagnosis of an Ebola case in the United States (Saad 2014). As a result, 63 percent of Americans said that they were somewhat or very afraid that the country would experience a large number of Ebola cases, while 45 percent were somewhat or very worried that someone in their family would get Ebola (Hamel, Firth, and Brodie 2014). In a Gallup poll in November 2014, Ebola ranked third among Americans' top health-care concerns (with 17 percent of respondents prioritizing the disease), after health-care costs (19 percent) and health-care access (18 percent) (Saad 2014).

The crisis frame "masked the underlying continuance of deep-seated neglect" of the larger political, economic, and social structures such as corruption, weak health-care systems, donors' misguided health priorities, and poverty that had enabled the disease to quickly spread (Nunes 2016, 543). In addition, stories only included very general discussions of Africans, thus continuing to ignore the people harmed by the disease or to treat them as "exotic and racialized" (Nunes 2016, 543; see Seltzer et al. 2015 on social media and Ebola). For example, of the thirty-nine above-mentioned stories, six described African practices such as traditional healers, Pentecostal healing services, and communal burials as drivers of the outbreak. Only two stories focused on African doctors or health-care workers, portraying them as more than faceless victims of Ebola.

As the next two sections illustrate, these four aspects of the response—its slow start, its institutional disorganization, the lack of accepted norms to drive action, and the tension between neglect and crisis framing—created spaces in which nonaffected states and Liberia could act. I now turn to the reasons that nonaffected states challenged global health governance on Ebola, particularly the IHR.

African Challenges to Global Health Governance on Ebola: Travel Restrictions

This section investigates how nonaffected African states challenged WHO recommendations on travel restrictions, an action which indicates these states' role in the implementation (not the design) of global health governance. As part of the process of declaring a PHEIC, the WHO can recommend trade and/or travel restrictions (Davies, Kamradt-Scott, and Rushton 2015; Youde 2012; WHO 2005). In August 2014, WHO advised against such restrictions for Ebola-affected countries, fearing they would isolate the already impoverished states (WHO 2014e). Instead, the WHO encouraged "states with Ebola transmission to conduct exit screening of people at airports, ports, and major land crossings" in order to check "for unexplained febrile illness consistent with potential Ebola infection" (WHO 2014e). In Resolution 2177, the Security Council implicitly criticized many African states when it called on member states to drop their travel restrictions against visitors from the three affected countries. The fact that African states with restrictions ignored this criticism demonstrates their agency. The resolution also urged transportation carriers to continue flights, based on the WHO's finding that the risk of transmission through air travel was low (WHO 2014g).

Over 30 percent of states globally disregarded these statements and implemented travel restrictions and/or screening requirements (Ryhmer and Speare 2016). These include screening body temperature upon entry, requiring an "Ebola free" health certificate, quarantining visitors, and forbidding entry for anyone from an affected state. The United States, for example, required individuals coming from the three affected countries to enter through New York, Atlanta, Newark, Washington, DC, or Chicago and to be screened upon entry (*Guardian*, October 21, 2014). The WHO received over five hundred complaints about restrictive trade and travel barriers related to Ebola, and it reported that forty-seven states had imposed excessive measures (WHO 2015a, 41; Rhymer and Speare [2016] identified fifty-eight states). When states impose barriers, they also send a signal to private actors to alter their behavior (Lee and McKibbin 2004). Mining and agricultural companies, as well as major airlines such as British Airways, Delta Airlines, and Air Emirates, left the Ebola-affected countries (*Economist*, August 16, 2014). One NGO official told a terrifying story of furtively flying to Accra from Monrovia, hoping to be allowed on a flight to Europe (interview, international humanitarian NGO official, Monrovia, May 19, 2016). Many Liberians have family in the United States, and the airlines' exit led to panic: "I barely got out before Delta cut its flights" (informal conversation, Liberian professional, Monrovia, May 15, 2016).[4] Liberians praised Brussels Air and Royal Air Maroc for continuing flights and providing them with a lifeline (informal conversation, Liberians with family in United States, Harbel, May 22, 2016; see *Time*, October 10, 2014).[5]

African states were more likely than states in other regions to impose Ebola-related travel restrictions (Worsnop 2016b). Data compiled from the risk management agency SOS International (2015), Catherine Worsnop (2016b), and C. Poletto et al. (2014) reveal that thirty-two of forty-nine states in sub-Saharan Africa enacted some type of screening or entry restrictions on passengers from affected countries (see also *Free Republic Post*, October 8, 2014).[6] This number includes states in the Southern African Development Community (SADC), which announced a common policy of monitoring travelers from Ebola-affected countries for twenty-one days (*News 24*, September 9, 2014). Some SADC states, such as Namibia, Zambia, and Botswana, also developed their own policies.

Both the weakness of global health governance and domestic political considerations led to these restrictions. In order to encourage states to report outbreaks, the IHR allows the WHO to publicly name states that impose excessive trade and travel barriers (WHO 2005, Article 43.3; Davies, Kamradt-Scott, and Rushton 2015). States are aware of the reputational costs for their actions as well as the potential loss of aid, trade, and cooperation on other issues when they do not comply with international agreements (Keohane 1984; Goodliffe and Hawkins 2009). Thus, WHO statements could potentially shape state behavior. However, the WHO did not "name and shame" states that imposed barriers. Instead of serving as a "norm custodian" to enforce international cooperation (Harman 2016a), the WHO also issued confusing statements about screening travelers. After the WHO initially said that states should not implement any entry screening, it then said that any screening needed to comply with the IHR's policies on nondiscrimination and human rights protection. When some states adopted screening, the WHO then urged states "implementing such measures to share their experiences and lessons learned" (WHO 2014f). These inconsistencies gave states room in which to maneuver.

Limited by structures and funding concerns, the WHO could not easily name and shame states for travel restrictions, particularly after its biggest donor, the United States, set up screening procedures. Additionally, after the WHO's failures to act early on Ebola, it lacked credibility. Imposing barriers demonstrated African agency in the international system, and the norm of sovereignty enabled these states to make these decisions regardless of the WHO's recommendations (Brown 2012, 2013). The sovereignty norm competed with weaker norms about international cooperation through the IHR, and while travel limitations could have undermined the norm of humanitarian assistance, a point the WHO tried to make when it said restrictions would hamper the movement of health-care workers, this argument did not sway many states.

Domestic politics, particularly in combination with geographic location, also drove the decision to implement restrictions. Table 3.1 lists states with restrictions as a percentage of all African states with particular characteristics. (A complete list of states with Ebola-related restrictions is provided in appendix A.) The table indicates that of the four states that share borders with the affected states—Senegal, Mali, Côte d'Ivoire, and Guinea Bissau—75 percent (all of the four except Mali) placed restrictions on travelers. In addition, of the twelve states in the Economic Community of West African States (ECOWAS) that were not heavily affected states, 66 percent (or eight states) enacted restrictions. Location seemed to matter, as state officials feared the virus would spread across borders as it had between the three affected states.

The effect of regime type—democracy or autocracy—on implementation of restrictions was less clear cut. On one hand, one might expect that democracies, particularly those with upcoming elections, would face public pressure to enact limitations (as the US case above illustrated). Indeed, Worsnop (2016b) finds that at the global level, states with some democratic qualities and low health spending were more likely to impose barriers. (I examine health spending below.) On the other hand, states with a commitment to rule of law, a characteristic of a strong democracy, might be more likely to comply with international agreements, a pattern Worsnop (2016a) finds in terms of reporting outbreaks to the WHO.

I examine African states with democratic characteristics, using the classifications provided by Polity IV in order to align my study with the work of Worsnop (2016b) (see Marshall and Cole 2014, 20–21; see chapter 2 on Polity IV definitions.) As Table 3.1 shows, of Africa's thirty weak and strong democracies, 66 percent (twenty states) imposed restrictions. This is the same percentage as the ECOWAS members with restrictions, a finding that seems to indicate that democracies are not necessarily more willing to follow the rule of law embedded in international agreements (Worsnop 2016a). But 63 percent of the continent's nineteen autocracies (twelve states) also imposed restrictions; democracies and autocracies were equally concerned about the spread of the outbreak. Of the region's seventeen strong democracies, eleven (or 65 percent) imposed restrictions. This number increases to 73 percent when the two Ebola-affected states of Liberia and Sierra Leone are excluded. An upcoming election also correlated with a state's noncompliance with the WHO recommendations: thirteen of the twenty-one states (62 percent) that the National Democratic Institute (2016) reported as holding a general or presidential election in 2014 or 2015 imposed barriers. In the context of the Ebola outbreak, democracy did not lead states to comply with the WHO's travel recommendations. Instead, the free press, competition in elections, and demands for executive accountability that democracy includes pushed some states to impose restrictions, even states such as Botswana, Namibia, and South Africa that are located thousands of miles from the disease outbreak. In fact, proximity to the outbreak seemed to have no discernible impact for democratic states: of the five strong democracies in ECOWAS that were not Ebola-affected (Senegal, Cape Verde, Ghana, Niger, and Benin), only three imposed restrictions.

Because Ebola was a short-run crisis, neopatrimonial states' concern over long-term resource acquisition was not a driver of restrictions. But what about other economic considerations? Limited capacity might urge states to implement restrictions out of fear that the state could not respond to an outbreak if one did occur (Gray 2014; Chayes and Chayes 1998; Tallberg 2002). At the global level, weak domestic health-care capacity (as measured by health expenditure as a percentage of

TABLE 3.1 African States with Ebola-Related Travel Restrictions

State type	Total number of states	Number with Ebola-related restrictions	Percentage with Ebola-related restrictions
All African democracies	30	20	66
All strong democracies	17	11	65
All autocracies	19	12	63
States with elections in 2014 or 2015	21	13	62
ECOWAS members	12*	8	66
Border states	4	3	75
Health spending less than 3% of GDP	31	20	64
States with above-average number of tourists	13	12	92

Source: Compiled by author from World Bank (2014c); Marshall and Cole (2014); National Democratic Institute (2016); UNWTO (2013); SOS International (2015); Worsnop (2016b); ECOWAS (2016); and Poletto et al. (2014).

   * The number of ECOWAS members does not include the three affected states.

GDP) made a state more likely to implement restrictions (Worsnop 2016b). In Africa, of the thirty-one states that spent less than 3 percent of their GDP on health in 2014, twenty (or 64 percent) imposed restrictions. I use 3 percent of GDP as a simple benchmark because it is the average spending for the forty-eight sub-Saharan states for which the World Bank (2014c) has data. (It does not have data for Somalia.) States with Ebola restrictions spent on average 3 percent of GDP on health, compared to states without restrictions which spent an average of 2.8 percent of GDP on health. The difference between these two percentages is not statistically significant, and the finding does not support the argument that states with low capacity supported travel restrictions. Because some of the region's middle-income states with greater health spending and health-care capacity imposed restrictions (e.g., South Africa, Gabon, Botswana, and Namibia), the argument about capacity has little explanatory value.

Another economic consideration revolves around lost revenue: States might impose restrictions on people from affected states because they fear losing money from trade or tourism (Worsnop 2016a). In fact, of the thirteen African states that hosted more tourists than the continental average in 2010, 92 percent (twelve states) imposed restrictions. (The state without restrictions was Uganda.)[7] The fear of losing tourism revenue was real, particularly because Western populations have limited knowledge about African geography and thus might equate travel to South

Africa or Kenya with risk of Ebola infection in Liberia (Lundy and Negash 2013). The *Wall Street Journal* (August 19, 2014) reported that tour companies in South Africa and Kenya had lost large contracts with foreign travel agents (see also phone interview, South African government official, October 13, 2015). When Kenya announced that it was blocking people from the affected states (unless they were Kenyan citizens or aid workers), tourism agencies were relieved.

In all likelihood, fear of lost tourism income pressured strong democracies, especially those with upcoming elections, to implement restrictions. Indeed, all four strong democracies with both elections in 2014 or 2015 and greater than average numbers of tourists—Botswana, Namibia, South Africa, and Zambia—imposed some barriers. These democratic states were responding to public concerns. In addition, these states' aspirational identities played a role, since South Africa, Namibia, and Botswana have sought to present positive views of Africa to the world: they support democracy, support health and education, maintain regimes that are less corrupt than others in Africa, and play a leadership role in IGOs. Crisis and neglect frames that portrayed Ebola as an outbreak linked to ignorance, tradition, and backwardness challenged these states' efforts.

Namibia illustrates some of these dynamics. As a strong democracy with a growing tourism industry, Namibia held presidential elections in November 2014, when the number of Ebola cases was high. While there was little doubt that the incumbent South West Africa People's Organization Party (SWAPO) would retain power (*BBC News*, December 1, 2014), opposition political leaders and the media did raise questions about the state's actions on Ebola. On October 1, 2014, the presidential candidate for the opposition Democratic Turnhalle Alliance, McHenry Venaani, called for a ban on travelers from Ebola-affected countries (DTA 2014). And in almost thirty articles published between March 2014 and January 2015, the *New Era* raised concerns about Ebola. One central theme was the loss of revenue from foreign firms and travelers.[8] According to one government official, the public became very afraid. Adopting travel restrictions was a relatively easy way to respond to public fear and the potential loss of state revenue. Yet it is ironic that nonaffected states like Namibia ignored norms of cooperation under the IHR while also supporting norms of humanitarian assistance, as when the African Union sent a team of physicians and nurses to fight the epidemic "in a sign of solidarity to our fellow Africans" (interview, Namibian government official, New York, October 6, 2015; African Union 2015).

In summary, roughly half of African states imposed travel barriers on people from the affected states, challenging the WHO's recommendations and, more broadly, global cooperation under the IHR. This challenge was possible because of the institutional and funding weakness of the WHO and its inability to enforce the IHR. Norms of sovereignty competed with norms of cooperation and humanitarian intervention, with sovereignty empowering African states to act. African states' aspirational identities also motivated action. For example, Rwanda's identity as a developmental state that demands that donors follow its guidelines led it to require travelers from the United States and Spain (two high-income countries with Ebola cases) to report their medical conditions for twenty-one days (US Embassy Rwanda 2014; see Matfess 2015 on Rwandan aspirations). In terms of state-level variables, most democracies with upcoming elections implemented restrictions, particularly if they relied on significant tourism revenue. But it was not true that states with limited capacity were more likely to impose restrictions. Finally, possibly because of the short-term, crisis nature of the outbreak, civil society organizations did not mobilize to drive policy decisions. In the end, aspirational identities urged states to exhibit agency in a low-cost way through travel restrictions.

Challenges from an Ebola-Affected State: The Case of Liberia

Liberia exhibited challenges in both the design and implementation phases of global health governance on Ebola. In terms of design, it shaped the disease narrative through its slow response, its emphasis on the neglect and crisis frames, and its utilization of the unique US-Liberia relationship. These means enabled it to promote its views in global health diplomacy and to gain global attention and resources. Here I provide background on these actions, while the next section analyzes the international, state, and societal factors that drove these activities.

First, Liberia was criticized for foot dragging. It was slow to report cases to the WHO; it claimed that Ebola was defeated in May 2014, when there was a temporary lull in cases; officials did not speak openly about the epidemic until July 2014; it did not close the border with Guinea in March 2014; and it did not quarantine Lofa County (interviews, health-care workers, Margibi, Montserrado, and Bong Counties, May 16, 2016, May 20, 2016, and May 22, 2016; Moran and Hoffman 2014). One respondent said that it was only after health-care workers, NGO officials, and donors presented data to the president's cabinet in July 2014 that the "government finally got it" (interview, international humanitarian NGO official, Monrovia, May 19, 2016). And when the president declared a state of emergency only a few days before the WHO's PHEIC declaration, some found the action to be a little too late (*BBC News*, August 6, 2014; interview, hospital senior nurse,

Kakata, May 16, 2016). In reaction, Liberian officials said it took time to develop a culturally appropriate response (interviews, government officials, Monrovia, May 18, 2016, and May 21, 2016). This slow response led to a global delay, but it also enabled Liberian officials to dictate the pace of actions in global health governance.

A second way that Liberia challenged the design of global health governance was when it emphasized the neglect and crisis frames in order to gain global attention and resources. In the process, officials forced global health governance to change from inaction to action. In these efforts, Liberian officials used the media spectacle to their advantage: "Interviews with [international] journalists . . . presented the opportunity to get information out and to call for international help" (interviews, government officials, Monrovia, May 19, 2016, and May 21, 2016). President Ellen Johnson Sirleaf's "Letter to the World," broadcast on *BBC News* on October 19, 2014, provides one example.[9] In it, she highlighted the frame of neglect: "The international reaction to this crisis was initially inconsistent and lacking in clear direction or urgency." She also used the crisis frame, stressing the magnitude of the pandemic ("millions of West Africans"), the outbreak's transnational character ("the disease respects no borders"), and its social and economic destruction (the "effect on the economy or within communities is already reverberating throughout the region and across the world").[10] The infection of the two American health-care workers in Monrovia helped to reinforce these points and particularly the idea that the crisis was a threat to the West. One respondent said that the event "signaled to comfortable Americans" that "this disease is going to follow you . . . it is not a national event but an international one" (interview, government official, Monrovia, May 18, 2016; See *Washington Post*, August 2, 2014). Neglect and crisis necessitated "a commitment from every nation that has the capacity to help—whether that is with emergency funds, medical supplies or clinical expertise" (*BBC News*, October 19, 2014).

Performances such as the letter utilized both diversionary nationalism and extraversion. In the former, the state "diverts the blame for development failure onto others, particularly the West" (Englebert 2009, 199), as President Sirleaf did when she said the initial international reaction was "lacking in clear direction" and "urgency" but did not mention her own government's foot dragging. Intended for national audiences, such nationalism can legitimate state power and justify state actions, since the state's role is presumably to protect its people. In terms of extraversion (see chapter 1), the president emphasized how as a "fragile state" recovering from war, Liberia was unprepared for the outbreak, and she began the letter by highlighting the deaths of children and dedicated health-care workers (*BBC News*,

October 19, 2014). Extraversion seemed to sway an international audience. Liberian officials said the letter was a "crucial stepping stone" and a "catalyst" for generating global support; ultimately, it "saved the sub-region" (interviews, government officials, Monrovia, May 18, 2016, May 19, 2016, and May 21, 2016).

A third way that Liberia challenged the narrative and design of global health governance on Ebola was by capitalizing on its special relationship with the United States in order to place the outbreak on the Security Council's agenda. According to one Security Council representative, West African states, and particularly Liberia, approached the United States about writing the resolution, urging the US delegation to frame the issue as a security concern (interview, UN Security Council delegate, New York, October 5, 2015; Hamel, Firth, and Brodie 2014). High-level Liberian officials had "very cordial relationships" with the then US ambassador to Liberia Deborah Malac and the US Assistant Secretary of State for the Bureau of African Affairs Linda Thomas-Greenfield, who had been the US ambassador to Liberia from 2008 until 2012 (Thomas-Greenfield 2016). According to one respondent, the US officials deeply understood that the disease posed a significant threat to donor investments in the subregion and to the US Global Health Security Agenda—an initiative begun in 2014 to improve infectious disease control, particularly in low- and middle-income countries. Liberian officials repeatedly articulated these dangers as well as the transnational nature of the disease. What John Kingdon (1995) terms the "policy window" opened with the aforementioned infection of the two American health-care workers, leading the United States to push for passage of Resolution 2177 (interviews, government officials, Monrovia, May 18, 2016, and May 21, 2016; CDC 2015b). While this action partly reflected the Security Council's need to improve its image in the face of its failures on Ukraine and Syria, as well as its desire to protect its investments in UNMIL (Rushton 2016), the passage of Revolution 2177 did lead to increases in monetary resources and personnel for the Ebola response.

Liberia's challenge was also evident in the implementation of the Ebola response, particularly when state officials insisted that Liberians, not international actors, direct the response. One respondent explained:

The president put her foot down that ownership for decision making . . . was going to be done by the government, not by any international organization. . . . This meant that sometimes advisors were adversarial toward the international community. . . . In the end, I think they [the international community] realized that we were not going to be kicked around. (Interview, government official, Monrovia, May 18, 2016)

The quote illustrates both how sovereignty enabled the state to devise its own institutions (Brown 2012, 2013) and how the president played a central role in policymaking. As a result, Liberians headed all levels of the Incident Management System, such as case management and social mobilization, while officials from UNICEF, the WHO, and the World Food Programme served as technical advisors. This meant that it was the government instead of donors that ordered unpopular policies like the quarantine of some communities and the cremation of Ebola-infected bodies (see below).

There are several reasons these actions in global health diplomacy and policy implementation can be interpreted as challenges to global health governance. First, these actions contrasted with governance patterns in Sierra Leone, where donors played a larger role in the response: At one point, the WHO coordinated country activities with UNMEER (Kamradt-Scott, Harman, Wenham, and Smith 2015). Second, these actions contrast with prior management of international efforts in the country. For several years, UNMIL had directed security initiatives; thus, the state's insistence on overseeing the Ebola response indicated a relatively new level of autonomy. Also the US military usually oversees its foreign operations, but in this case, the Ministry of Health and the Incident Management System coordinated these efforts. Third, as the above quote indicates, tensions between Liberians and donors also seemed to indicate that international actors would have preferred to play a larger role in directing the response. Liberians complained about donor-driven health messages, exclusion from initial decision making, and the use of unsupported data to make decisions (interviews, government officials, Monrovia, May 18, 2016, and May 21, 2016). Donors cited "serious logistics problems," poor management by Health Minister Walter Gwenigale (he was replaced abruptly in mid-November 2014), inefficient meetings with the Incident Management System, and a lack of accurate data to drive the response (*New York Times*, November 19, 2014; interviews, international NGO official and international humanitarian NGO official, Monrovia, May 19, 2016).

An example illustrates these tensions while also suggesting donors' desire to direct the response. International partners met early in October in the UNMEER headquarters in Accra, Ghana, but excluded Liberian representatives. After the international advisors presented the plan that resulted from the meeting, Liberian officials questioned several of its underlying assumptions, particularly the September 2014 WHO prediction that if nothing was done to fight Ebola, there would be 20,000 deaths by November (WHO 2014h). In reality, by late July 2014, the Liberian government had closed schools, required nonessential government staff to stay home from work, quarantined hard-hit communities, developed public health messages, and established the Incident Management System. In short, government had already "done something." Donors' desire to control the response created a backlash, as state officials then challenged the UNMEER plan (interviews, government officials, Monrovia, May 18, 2016, and May 21, 2016; *BBC News*, July 30, 2014; *NBC News*, August 6, 2014).

In summary, Liberia presented challenges to global health governance through its slow response to the disease, its emphasis on the neglect and crisis frames, and its manipulation of its relationship with the United States to gain resources and attention. Media performances and private advocacy, facilitated by connections with US officials and global journalists, became the means by which this global health diplomacy occurred. Through its emphasis on the neglect and crisis frames, and the uncertainty that accompanied the Ebola outbreak, Liberia was "really able to get the world to listen" (interview, multilateral donor official, New York, October 1, 2015). And once Liberians had the world's attention, they challenged usual donor patterns by insisting that they control the management of the response. The next section illustrates the reasons why Liberia took this approach.

Explaining the Liberian Response

Liberia exhibited agency in its response, showing that "donors have less bargaining power than recipients assume and recipients have more power than they use" (Whitfield 2009, 16). Multiple factors combined to make this outcome possible. At the international level, weak global institutions and frames that challenged the country's aspirational identity catalyzed state action. At the state level of analysis, the country's weak democracy and its decentralized forms of neopatrimonial governance that focused on short-term benefits mattered, while a civil society that used a variety of individual and collective means to directly and indirectly oppose the state pushed Liberia to challenge global health governance.

International-Level Factors: Weak Global Action and Aspirational Hope

The limited capacity of the WHO to enforce the IHR created space for Liberia's actions. As an international treaty, the IHR requires that states report outbreaks of specific diseases (e.g., cholera, yellow fever, and viral hemorrhagic fevers like Lassa and Ebola), outbreaks of unknown origin, and unusual or unexpected outbreaks that could have serious public health effects. States also must develop core capacities in surveillance, outbreak response, personnel capacity, and laboratories in order to detect, control, and ultimately report such outbreaks (Davies, Kamradt-Scott, and Rushton 2015; Youde 2012; WHO 2005). Yet most low-income countries have not met these IHR requirements. In 2012, all African states missed the deadline for attaining the minimum IHR core capacities (Kasolo et al. 2013), and in 2014 many African states were either unable to provide data on compliance or did not meet the target of 75 to 100 percent progress in core capacity areas (Harman 2016a; WHO 2014i). The lack of compliance reflected some African states' suspicion that the IHR (and "pandemic preparedness" in general) was merely a tool for combatting pathogens in the Global South that might travel to high-income countries, not a means for building health-care systems (Nguyen 2014; Youde 2011, 2012). When these states did not comply, they utilized the norm of sovereignty to contest international cooperation in disease control.

Noncompliance also reflected states' lack of resources to develop these capacities and donors' unwillingness to provide needed funds for this objective. Thus, even if a norm of compliance with the IHR was emerging, many low- and lower-middle-income countries lacked the ability to institutionalize that norm (Davies, Kamradt-Scott, and Rushton 2015). And even if the WHO had engaged in naming and shaming for states that did not comply, such labels would carry little reputational cost, because donors recognized that low- and lower-middle-income countries could not afford to comply. Yet, as discussed above, faced with structural, resource, and political challenges in playing the role of enforcer, the WHO was unlikely to force compliance. As a result, Liberia could be slow in its initial Ebola response and then demand to control the effort.

Another international-level consideration was that the neglect and crisis frames undercut the aspirational identity of Liberia, shaping its actions. The country has come to view itself as moving beyond the trauma and destruction of war. In her BBC letter, President Sirleaf spoke about how Liberia's "future was looking bright" and the country was "bouncing back." She said, "After thirty years of brutal civil and political unrest, Liberia was a nation reborn" (BBC News, October 19, 2014). These views of progress contrasted with media images that portrayed Ebola-affected countries as mired in misery, destruction, and disease. And when Liberian officials were excluded from decision-making, this seemed to indicate disrespect for the progress the country had made (interview, government official, Monrovia, May 18, 2016).

News stories and public health messages that blamed cultural practices such as touching during caregiving, shaking hands, using traditional medicine, and isolating sick community members also undermined Liberia's aspirational identity (Richardson et al. 2015; Jones 2014). As a result, "The primary reason [the Liberian government needed to control the response] was that there were a lot of assumptions made by the international organizations that lacked contextualized knowledge. . . . Ebola was not one of those outbreaks that you could understand without understanding the culture" (interview, government official, Monrovia, May 18, 2016). In order for Liberia to reach what John Ruggie (1998) terms an "aspirational hope," Liberia used its sovereignty to address the response on its own timeline, with autonomy, and through the manipulation of the very neglect and crisis frames that contradicted its own aspirations.

The State Level: Exclusive Democracy, Decentralized Neopatrimonial Networks

Two aspects of the Liberian state—its weak democracy and its decentralized and winner-take-all form of neopatrimonialism—led it to challenge global health governance. In reality, these factors are intertwined, since neopatrimonial practices undermined the trust, state accountability, and citizen participation needed for democracy. For the sake of parsimony, I dissect these two factors. In the case of the country's weak democracy, the high level of citizen distrust for the state and the country's problematic elections led the state to challenge global health governance. Additionally, its decentralized neopatrimonial structures that foster elite competition and that have enabled corruption necessitated that the state control the Ebola response and seek international resources.

EXCLUSIONARY DEMOCRACY

Freedom House (2016b) reports that while Liberia has made improvements in rule of law, judicial independence, and press freedoms, democracy is still hampered by corruption, intimidation of journalists and civil society leaders, harassment of ethnic minorities, and executive over-reach. These are symptoms of Liberia's exclusionary politics and the war which pitted people of different religious and ethnic backgrounds against one another (interview, international humanitarian NGO official, Monrovia, May 19, 2016; Bøås 2005). Liberia has at least fifteen major ethnic groups, each with a specific language and culture; 86 percent of its population is Christian, and 11 percent is Muslim (Alexander et al. 2015; Peacebuilder 2011). Historically, these groups have jockeyed for political control, making politics a zero-sum game and fostering distrust between citizens and the state.

From its establishment until the 1980 coup d'état, Liberia was ruled by an Americo-Liberian elite who used nation-building projects, national identity promotion, repression, cooptation, and patronage to hold on to power (Ellis 1999). After Samuel Doe staged the 1980 coup, his increasingly corrupt regime gave positions to ethnic Krahns and aligned with northern Mandingo business leaders (Williams 2016, 74–84; Liebenow 1987, 192; Ellis 1999, 65). In a context of increasing poverty and desperation, Charles Taylor's National Patriotic Front of Liberia (NPFL) invaded the country in 1989; popular among ethnic Lorma in Lofa County and Kpelle in Nimba and Bong Counties, it targeted Krahn and Mandingo.[11] In response, the Mandingo-dominated United Liberation Movement for Democracy in Liberia (ULIMO) invaded Lofa County from Guinea in 1991. Because of long-standing distrust between the Mandingo and the Lorma (Bøås 2009; Ellis 1999, 38–39), ULIMO targeted Lorma. Retaliation against the Mandingo followed (IRIN 1999).[12] After a hiatus between 1997 and 1999, the war began again when Liberians United for Reconciliation and Democracy (LURD), a loose coalition with Krahn and Mandingo leadership, and the Movement for Democracy in Liberia (MODEL), a group of refugees from Côte d'Ivoire and Ghana, challenged then-president Taylor. With pressure from international donors and Liberian civil society (Westendorf 2016; Reticker 2008), MODEL, LURD, and Taylor agreed in 2003 to the removal of Taylor, a coalition government for two years, national elections in 2005, and the establishment of UNMIL, a UN peacekeeping mission with over 14,000 military personnel and the mandate to foster stability and recovery (Paes 2005; Bøås 2005).

The war increased societal distrust. A 2007 survey showed that one-fourth of people in Lofa County felt tensions related to wealth, religion, ethnicity, and age. Even though most inhabitants trusted kin, coethnics, and people from their town, only 37 percent trusted district officials, and only 28 percent trusted state officials in Monrovia (Fearon, Humphreys, and Weinstein 2007, 3, 40). This distrust had implications for the Ebola response. It is probably no coincidence that counties with the highest number of Ebola cases (Montserrado, Bong, Lofa, and Nimba) were the most war-torn and have high levels of ethnic diversity (Peacebuilder 2011; WHO 2016a). Their histories of division meant people had low trust for one another and for government's messages about Ebola. This fact led the government to adopt the most basic slogan about the disease (which was plastered on billboards and bumper stickers): "Ebola Is Real." Distrust of government also meant that people did not go to health-care centers or believe health-care workers. One respondent who worked on the Ebola response in Lofa County commented: "It was really hard to get anyone to listen to us" (interview, international humanitarian

NGO official, Monrovia, May 19, 2016). And distrust meant the state had to demonstrate resolve and results: "The president became overcome with the desire to show action" (interview, government official, Monrovia, May 18, 2016). Such pressure led the state to challenge global health governance by insisting that Liberian officials control the response and by seeking global attention and external resources through diplomatic and media performances.

Liberia's electoral experiences in 2011 and 2014 also colored the state's Ebola response. The 2011 presidential election was marred by violence and low voter turnout that "exposed deep divisions" based on ethnic and wartime alliances (Carter Center 2011; see also Bøås and Utas 2014). Some people asserted that the state initially ignored Ebola because the first cases were in counties and neighborhoods that had not supported Sirleaf in 2011 (interviews, health-care workers, Margibi, Montserrado, and Bong Counties, May 16, 2016, May 20, 2016, and May 22, 2016). In four of the six most Ebola-affected counties—Bong, Margibi, Nimba, and Montserrado—a majority of voters had not supported Sirleaf on the first-round ballot in 2011 (NEC 2011). In 2014, the government was perceived to have manipulated the Ebola response for its political advantage. In that year's senatorial elections, Robert Sirleaf (the president's son) competed to represent Montserrado County against George Weah, a former world soccer star who is popular among urban youth and who ran for president in 2005 and vice president in 2011 (*New York Times*, December 20, 2014). Sirleaf lost decisively, but events around the campaign became heated. As Weah's campaign began to hold well-attended public rallies, the president banned street parades, rallies, and demonstrations ostensibly because of the danger of Ebola (Government of Liberia 2014). The opposition parties were not above similar actions when they "tried to exploit the [Ebola] situation . . . by arousing disadvantaged groups" and by establishing charity organizations to distribute food to Ebola-affected communities (interview, government official, Monrovia, May 18, 2016; see also *New York Times*, October 30, 2014; *Financial Times*, April 8, 2016; Epstein 2014; *Guardian*, December 28, 2014; *Liberian Observer*, October 15, 2014). Because the government was accused of politicizing Ebola, the state needed to show strength in the Ebola response through autonomous decision-making and use of the media and international arenas to gain attention and resources.

NEOPATRIMONIAL NETWORKS

The state's desire to access neopatrimonial resources was one, though not the only, driver of its challenge to global health governance. The zero-sum nature of Liberian politics, the country's history of violence, and its fluid political alliances have led to governance through networks (Ellis 1999; Moran 2006; Utas 2008). Rather than foster long-term development, these rent-seeking networks create a resource-searching free-for-all, with "Big Men" heading networks that utilize reciprocity, patronage resources, and personal loyalty. Networks are "instrumentalized for roughly any socioeconomic or social-political action" (Utas 2008, 4). As informal, behind-the-scenes nodes of power and decision-making, they often overlap with societal structures such as chieftaincy, religious groups, and secret societies. Network members play multiple roles. For example, politicians are also business leaders, church parishioners, founders of NGOs, relatives of people in the diaspora, and/or members of secret societies. Each node in the network is a place where resources are gained and then passed along to other network members. As "endless," mutable, and fluid, networks facilitate great variation in the "flow of goods and favors," and they are the site of real power in Liberia (Utas 2008, 6).

Widespread corruption has been the result of this type of neopatrimonial governance, with public goods like education and health care distributed through private networks and gatekeepers who control access to these services, creating a "shadow state" that perpetuates structural violence against most citizens (Utas 2008; Moran 2006; Ellis 1999; on the shadow state, see Reno 2000; on gatekeeper politics, see Beresford 2015). As one respondent said, "Let's be candid . . . corruption is widespread in this country" (interview, government official, Monrovia, May 18, 2016). Transparency International (2013) found that 75 percent of surveyed Liberians had paid a bribe in the education sector, and 77 percent had paid a bribe to a police officer. Overwhelming majorities thought that civil servants (67 percent), national legislators (96 percent), the police (97 percent), political parties (71 percent), and the judiciary (89 percent) were corrupt.[13] Fifty-two percent said that corruption increased between 2011 and 2013, while only 2 percent said it declined.

The pattern of rent grabbing through networks and the history of corruption affected state actions on Ebola in three ways. First, they meant the neopatrimonial state needed to strongly challenge the international community to act in order to access resources and gain political clout. This accounted for the state's use of extra-version, its manipulation of the "Ebola as threat to the West" frame, and its use of the country's special relationship with the United States. Second, the state had to fight widespread distrust of its actions on Ebola (and other issues) through a strong response. Here timing and context matter. Ebola emerged in the aftermath of a high-level corruption scandal. In 2010, then minister of agriculture Chris Toe was accused of stealing donor funds intended to fight an army worm infestation. He resigned and was never convicted, but in 2013, the Supreme Court ordered *Front-*

PageAfrica, the newspaper that had investigated the story, to pay fines for libel against the minister (*AllAfrica.com*, September 3, 2013; *VOA News*, August 26, 2013). The scandal led citizens to distrust the state's messages about Ebola. One interviewee said: "When Ebola arose, there was a general belief that the government was just making it up in order to get donor money" (interview, church official, Monrovia, May 17, 2016; Jerving 2014; *Reuters*, February 10, 2015).[14] Strong state actions in global health governance were essential to repair such trust.

Third, informal patterns of neopatrimonial rule through networks necessitated that Liberian officials, not international actors, control Ebola decisions. Unaware of or without links to network players, UNMEER, international NGO, and bilateral donor officials could not exert real power in the Ebola response. It was Liberians who were rooted in such governance layers and network ties, not outsiders. Additionally, the fluid nature of Liberian networks made it possible to set up a new structure— the Incident Management System—to make and implement Ebola decisions. Since networks revolve around individuals, the president could "use her bully pulpit" to plead the country's case internationally in order to gain resources and attention (interview, government official, Monrovia, May 18, 2016). However, Ebola governance through networks also led to the above-mentioned donor criticisms, as external actors sought greater efficiency and clearer power structures than networks provide.

The outcome of the state's challenge was that international resources poured in, making the disease a "windfall event [that] was particularly conducive to rent seeking behavior" (Anderson and Beresford 2016). There was an abundance of opportunities for network members embedded in these social hierarchies to benefit. To reward many competing factions and shore up state legitimacy, the state distributed resources widely, as two health-care officials explained. One nurse was given $125 to attend a one-day training, during which "we ate four times." She said with incredulity, "They were just stuffing us with food. It was obscene. Why do we need to eat four times in one day?" A clinic administrator then described her training with high-level government officials at a very exclusive hotel. After talking in detail about the food, alcohol, music, and dancing, the administrator said, "But it was terrible! This was a very serious disease and for people to be dancing and having a party was just not right!" (informal conversation, two health-care workers, Harbel, May 22, 2016) The conversation illustrated the almost farcical nature of rent distribution within these decentralized networks. One respondent complained that overinflated bids to donors and large contracts meant "some people just used Ebola to make money" (informal conversation, Liberian professional, Monrovia, May 22,

2016), while another interviewee said about the large number of new homes being built outside of Monrovia: "That is all Ebola money" (interview, international humanitarian NGO official, Monrovia, May 19, 2016). Charges of outright corruption led to the closing of the Liberian branch of the Red Cross (*Reuters*, March 10, 2016). Rule through networks facilitate this short-term rent dispersal, though did little to institutionalize a long-term and concerted effort to promote public health (interviews, international NGO official and international humanitarian NGO official, Monrovia, May 19, 2016).

While neopatrimonial governance drove state challenges to generate resources for rents, it is important to recognize that not everyone gained materially. Networks competed in a decentralized free-for-all, one in which many health-care workers, ambulance drivers, and Ebola survivors gained few benefits (interviews, hospital nursing assistant, Kakata, May 16, 2016; Ebola survivor, Monrovia, May 17, 2016; government official, Monrovia, May 18, 2016; priest, Gbargna, May 20, 2016; pastor, Gbargna, May 21, 2016). This competition partly resulted from the fact that Ebola was a short-term crisis that gave state elites no incentive to construct institutions that centralized control over resources. The disease itself did not push the state to have a long time horizon, one that might limit resource grabbing or foster an inclusive strategy to bring civil society groups into policymaking and rent management. On this point, Liberia's Incident Management System contrasts with the National AIDS Commissions that managed AIDS resources and increased buy-in for AIDS efforts. As this chapter's conclusion argues, without such centralized and inclusive institutions, the improvement of health services that is needed to address public health crises is undermined (see Kelsall 2011).

In summary, the country's weak democracy undermined citizens' trust in state Ebola messages, a distrust which divisive elections exacerbated. Within the 2014 election, the state and opposition parties manipulated Ebola for their political advantage, a dynamic that pushed the state to demand autonomy in Ebola decision-making and to act internationally in order to claim credit. Governance through networks of clients that expected benefits required that the state control the response and use extraversion to gain resources. To build trust, shore up networks, and with an eye to the 2017 elections (when President Sirleaf cannot compete), the president promoted Liberian unity and the country's aspirational identity when she asserted that the Ebola response had created a "window of opportunity that can be used to come together as a people" (Government of Liberia 2015, 22). In the end, donors and many citizens credited the government with an effective response, though its impact on the country's long-term advancement in health and development remains to be seen (*Reuters*, March 10, 2016).

The Societal Level: Informal and Formal Mobilization in Opposition to the State

Societal reactions to Ebola took many forms, some which directly opposed the state and others which, by taking over the state's tasks, indirectly opposed the state. These actions included diffuse and relatively disorganized activities like denial, rumors, and protests, both individual and collective. Society also engaged in formally organized activities, such as service delivery and advocacy. Unlike in the case of AIDS or, to an extent, NCDs, Liberian mobilization was not linked to international civil society groups. There was no global Ebola movement, for example, to provide local groups with resources, advocacy advice, or training. When these assets emerged, they tended to come through international NGOs and FBOs that engaged in service delivery. Additionally, unlike with the AIDS response, the membership of the epistemic community of Ebola experts was relatively small and technically focused; biomedicine was also accused of ignoring the cultural drivers of the epidemic (Richardson et al. 2015; *National Public Radio*, September 28, 2014).[15] The epistemic community did little to engage with societal activities, sometimes even "looking down on" traditional and religious actors involved with the response (interview, international NGO official, Monrovia, May 19, 2016). Thus, transnational linkages did not bolster the power or influence of Liberian civil society. These informal and formal actions highlighted the power and legitimacy of civil society and the relative weakness of the state. As such, they pushed the state to respond in ways that challenged global health governance.

THE INFORMAL ACTIONS OF DENIAL, RUMORS, AND PROTEST
Denial of the disease's existence led people to avoid health-care centers and to transport dead bodies for community burials (*Reuters*, December 15, 2014). Denials resulted because of limited information on the disease, fear, and distrust of state leaders and health-care workers. One health-care worker described how such denial led to what seemed to be irrational behavior for one patient:

When [the patient] was brought to the clinic the workers saw that he had red around his mouth. So they ask him, "Have you been to the latrine [to vomit]?" And he said, "No, I have been drinking a tonic." He didn't admit [he was throwing up blood]. Then he walked outside to throw up again. And there was just blood. He couldn't use his shirt to wipe his mouth because the blood would have shown. So he took a handful of grass and wiped his mouth. Then he came back in. And the nurses, they looked at him, and said to one another, "This guy is throwing up blood." They asked him, and he denied it. He went out again . . . to [another hospital]. But then he came back and died.

(Interview, hospital official, Kakata, May 16, 2016)

The story illustrates the extreme form that denial could take, as the patient frantically tried to hide his symptoms and then escape the situation. In the process, denial endangered many other patients and health-care workers—at this particular hospital, thirteen of seventeen Ebola-infected workers died. The vignette also showed how the state's inability to convince society about Ebola's danger made it more likely for society to respond through its own means.

Denial could also feed rumors, which took several forms. One, which was published in Liberia's *Daily Observer* (September 9, 2014), suggested that Ebola was a genetically modified organism manufactured by Western pharmaceutical companies or the US Department of Defense and tested by the CDC on West African subjects (see also *New York Times*, October 18, 2015; interview, Liberian community leader, Tennessee, March 14, 2016). This rumor reflected popular suspicion that what Elwood Dunn terms an historic "mutuality of interests" between the United States and Liberia really meant that the United States was meddling in Liberian affairs (Dunn 2009, 185; see also Huband 1998; Ciment 2013; Ellis 1999, 50–52, 68; Liebenow 1987; Moran 2006; Epstein 2014; Global Witness 2015; Frontline 2014). (The rumor also echoes aspects of the AIDS conspiracy, showing how such global theories can morph to fit particular contexts. See Nattrass 2012) A second rumor theme portrayed Ebola as a curse from witches or a punishment from God because of "the sins of the nation" (Bolten 2014; interviews, hospital official, Kakata, May 16, 2016; church relief agency official, Monrovia, May 18, 2016). Because the vast majority of Liberians are highly religious, these rumors aligned with popular understandings of life, death, power, and the occult (Ellis 1999; Moran 2006, 7; Pew Forum 2010). They also fit within a larger dynamic in which religion has served as a counterbalance to the state, with religion (and its intermediaries like pastors, priests, imams, and shamans) perceived to access spiritual power for good or ill.

While denial and rumors opposed the state's official biomedical approach to Ebola and hampered the response by causing people to avoid health-care centers or to engage in unsafe burials, these forms of "creative resistance" also enabled marginalized people to indirectly shape the state's actions (Scott 1990; see also Anderson and Patterson 2017). As "directed, meaningful, intentional and self-reflective social or political action" (Chabal 2014, xv), rumors and denial illustrate what John Lonsdale (2000) calls "agency in tight corners." Even in contexts of poverty, dependence, and disease, local people could act to affect the Ebola response. In terms of the state's engagement with global health governance, rumors and denial gave the state space and time in which to develop its own Ebola-control plan and structures. But to respond to society's denial and rumors, state officials had to use their knowledge of culture, and they had to direct that response (Jerving 2014; interviews, church relief agency official, Monrovia, May 18, 2016; international NGO official, Monrovia, May 19, 2016; government official, Monrovia, May 21, 2016).

Another informal societal reaction that opposed the state was protest, particularly against quarantine. On August 20, 2014, the president announced a quarantine of West Point, a seaside slum neighborhood of between 60,000 and 120,000 people just north of Monrovia (*New Democrat*, May 17, 2016).[16] The policy indicated the state's control of the response: Though civil society leaders and international public health experts did not support the policy, it was "urged by the security forces," who enforced the policy ostensibly to prevent the spread of the virus (interview, church official, Monrovia, May 17, 2016; see also *Inquirer*, August 27, 2014; *Yahoo News*, September 7, 2014). The quarantine caused food and water shortages, and citizens complained that they would die of hunger, not Ebola. West Point citizens both disengaged from state control and opposed that control. Since roughly half of residents work outside West Point, many searched for creative ways to escape the barriers, including swimming to Monrovia (West Point is a peninsula) or bribing security officials to allow them to enter and exit. In the face of mounting frustrations, though, residents began to actively oppose the state. Crowds stormed an ETU, setting patients free and destroying equipment, and after the community's commissioner was evacuated by police, riots began. The security forces fired on protesters, ultimately killing a fifteen-year-old boy (*New York Times*, August 29, 2014; *Guardian*, August 21, 2014). Soon after, the president lifted the quarantine (*Financial Times*, April 8, 2016).

The incident negatively affected trust of the state, the state's image abroad, and its overall legitimacy, particularly because West Point has a history of opposing state power. Founded by Kru and Bassa fishermen, the neighborhood recently has been inhabited by northern Lorma and Kissi, many of whom were former war combatants who flocked there from Lofa, Nimba, and Bong Counties (Bøås and Hatløy 2008). This population dynamic facilitated the spread of Ebola between Monrovia and those areas. In postconflict Monrovian society, alliances are fluid, and individuals are "subjected to arbitrary, uncertain, and unpredictable forms of discipline" including state and criminal violence (Hoffman 2007, 405–406; see also Westendorf 2016; Medie 2013). The West Point *gronnah* (a colloquial term for "grown up child" and one which implies street thugs, drug users, and homeless people) often acts outside the lines of authority, frightening Liberian elites who fear instability (*New Democrat*, May 17, 2016). This historical fear conditioned the president's actions on the Ebola quarantine. But when faced with opposition, lost authority, and embarrassment, the state had to illustrate its control of the Ebola response (and, more broadly, of the West Point society), and it needed to show the Liberian population that it could mobilize resources for the response. Challenging global health governance through autonomous decision-making and the use of the neglect and crisis frames facilitated these goals.

FORMAL RESPONSES OF COMMUNITY MOBILIZATION AND ADVOCACY

Society also acted in more organized ways through civil society groups, frequently without the aid of donors or the state (informal conversation, Liberian priest, Tennessee, December 5, 2015; *Al Jazeera*, November 5, 2015; Huster 2016). Some of these actions replaced state efforts, while others opposed state activities. While the media often highlighted negative social mobilization, such as communities that destroyed health-care centers and stigmatized Ebola victims (*US News and World Report*, April 27, 2014; *Reuters*, July 30, 2014, December 15, 2014), several examples illustrate that Ebola-related activities varied greatly. First, when a pastor in Bong County heard about the Ebola cases in Lofa, he sought to educate his congregation about Ebola transmission; he was convinced (rightly) that his city of Gbargna would eventually face the disease, and he wanted to be prepared (interview, pastor, Gbarnga, May 21, 2016). Second, in April 2014, the major Liberian churches established a weekly prayer service to "pray the [Ebola] devil back to hell . . . though this was three months before the donors and government even realized we were in hell" (interview, church official, Monrovia, May 17, 2016).[17] Though it was a symbolic action, the prayer service became a site for organizing tangible responses, sharing information, and publicly shaming state officials for their slow actions. In a third example, young people in Dolo's Town established an Ebola Task Force to educate people about the virus, care for the sick, and transport people to hospitals "before government or NGOs or anyone came into this community" (interview, Ebola Task Force member, Dolo's Town, May 17, 2016). After the West Point riots, the *gronnahs* organized a similar response (*New Democrat*, May 17, 2016; see also Mogelson 2015).

Many factors fostered mobilization. "Love of the community and country" drove some participants to act (interview, Ebola Task Force member, Dolo's Town, May 17, 2016), while a basic desire to survive urged others. One person explained: "If we all got afraid and ran away, we were not going to solve the problem. . . . We ourselves may have then died" (interview, psychosocial team member, Gbargna, May 21, 2016). For some participants, "It was a matter of life and death; there wasn't a choice" (interviews, psychosocial team members, Gbargna, May 20, 2016, and May 21, 2016). Cultural practices also informed the work. One Liberian employee at an international NGO explained: "When people here receive a stranger [a person not from the community], they have to go and let the chief know. Then everyone in the community knows that there is a stranger, and so, if anything goes wrong . . . then they know they need to ask some questions." The respondent then described how during the Ebola outbreak chiefs set up a system in Grand Gedeh County so they could know if a "stranger" had crossed from Nimba County and was "within one hundred kilometers." The interviewee summed up: "And even though we may condemn these traditional people, these structures helped. Because if you talk about contact tracing or surveillance, they already had that in place" (interview, international NGO official, Monrovia, May 19, 2016). It was necessary to recognize and incorporate these traditional practices and leaders into the response, something Liberian officials, not international donor officials, were most qualified to do.

In addition to its roots in compassion, patriotism, survival instincts, and cultural practices, social mobilization was made logistically possible through civil society organizations, including the chieftaincy structure and religious groups. Liberia has roughly 250 senior chiefs and over five hundred clan chiefs, while churches range from mainline Protestant to new Pentecostal to syncretist (Liebenow 1987, 42–43, 81–82). One chief near the Guinea border deployed the youth in her district to sleep in the forest ("with all its snakes and wild animals") in order to prevent anyone from crossing the unofficial border and sneaking into her village. If someone crossed illegally, the youth took the person to the police (interview, international NGO official, Monrovia, May 19, 2016). The Bong County Churches Association established a psychosocial team to educate people about Ebola. Partnering with local Muslim leaders, it filled a void when seven healthcare workers at a local hospital died (interview, pastor, Gbargna, May 21, 2016). And an imam in Cape Mount County developed a roll call system for his community. Each morning, one person from every household had to report on the health of household members. If they reported that someone was ill, then the person was taken to the hospital (interview, international NGO official, Monrovia, May 19, 2016).

Because they tend to be trusted, religious and traditional leaders have been relatively effective in encouraging community mobilization in Africa (Patterson and Kuperus 2016; Gifford 2009; Dorman 2002; McCauley 2012; Patterson 2011). Because of their perceived link to spiritual power and their moral authority, religious organizations have the potential to oppose the state. While Gus Liebenow (1987, 81) reports that the mainline churches tended to support the state before 1980, Stephen Ellis (1999) shows how religious groups exhibited a certain level of autonomy during the war, allowing them at crucial periods like the 2003 peace process to challenge the state (Gberie 2008; Ellis 1995; Reticker 2008). In the context of Ebola, these groups potentially had even more power than usual because citizens distrusted the state and lacked accurate information on the outbreak. This power could be used to oppose the state and/or to take on the state's tasks. Illustrating the latter role, one pastor described how a group of religious leaders interacted with a village in which many people had died. Despite repeated visits from state health-care workers, the villagers "just could not believe it was Ebola." He said:

> There had seen someone earlier who had died . . . and they believed that the person had been bewitched. So [the villagers] engaged in a traditional burial with cleansing and herbs. All those who were involved died. But then even those who weren't at the burial began to die . . . So we pastors said, "You want to tell us that everyone in this town died from witchcraft? . . . And it is not only in this town that people are dying from this sickness." So the villagers started to see. But they listened because it was religious leaders who showed concern and started to act. . . . As a result, the people agreed to call the Ebola emergency phone line . . . when their relatives were ill. And you know what? Then the sickness stopped. (Interview, psychosocial team member, Gbargna, May 21, 2016)

The delivery of a clear message by trusted leaders facilitated the end of the community's outbreak. But the example demonstrates a bigger lesson: civil society often mobilizes without state assistance and because of state limitations. Civil society's ability to act when the state could not led state officials to both marvel at these nonstate efforts and, at times, to shrink with embarrassment about the state's weakness (interviews, government officials, Monrovia, May 18, 2016, and May 21, 2016). Civil society's activities pressured state officials not only to control the response but also to show this control in international arenas. In short, to augment its power in the state–civil society dynamic, the state needed to illustrate that it was in charge.

In some cases, autonomous civil society groups advocated against state policies. As early as June 2014, representatives of the Interfaith Religious Council and the Liberian Council of Churches met with the president to push for a response (interview, church official, Monrovia, May 17, 2016). In October 2014, traditional chiefs lobbied to be incorporated into the Incident Management System (interview, international NGO official, Monrovia, May 19, 2016). Advocacy was particularly important in shaping the state's policy on burial and cremation. When the number of victims in Monrovia escalated, government health-care workers buried the bodies on swampy land outside the city. When it rained, some bodies floated in the street (*Reuters*, August 4, 2014). Facing community anger and a public health crisis, officials with the Incident Management System quickly decided to cremate the bodies. The policy went against traditional practices and ignored family members' desire to have a place where they could visit their dead relatives. In short, the decision "did not go down well" (interview, church relief agency official, Monrovia, May 18, 2016). People resisted by hiding their relatives with Ebola or moving bodies (interview, government official, Monrovia, May 18, 2016; *Time*, October 7, 2014). In response, the Liberian Council of Churches and the Traditional Council of Liberia lobbied to change the policy. State officials agreed that if the chiefs found land for a cemetery, cremations would stop. The chiefs quickly found the land (interview, international NGO official, Monrovia, May 19, 2016). The example showed the pressure that civil society could put on the state and why the state then needed to show agency in global health governance.

Three broad lessons about societal mobilization emerge. First, organized and unorganized societal actions pressured the state to challenge global health governance. While denial and rumors created space in which the state could initially drag its proverbial feet on Ebola, over time societal responses required state action, particularly because this "was the first time in our country in peacetime to see these high numbers of deaths" (interview, government official, Monrovia, May 18, 2016). After civil society groups began to mobilize, protest, and advocate, the state had to react. Faced with a strong society composed of traditional and religious power brokers, the relatively weak Liberian state had to respond in order to maintain power (Migdal 1988). Civil society opposition meant that Liberians—not international donors—needed to direct the response because policies needed to be culturally sensitive and to respond to civil society demands (interview, international NGO official, Monrovia, May 19, 2016). As state officials learned with the cremation fiasco, when they were not sensitive to cultural norms and did not consult civil society leaders, these leaders reacted negatively (interview, government official, Monrovia, May 18, 2016).

Second, in the face of civil society actions, the state needed to show it was searching for resources. The use of extraversion enabled Liberian officials to say they were pushing an apathetic international community to help. Involvement with the Security Council's resolution showed Liberian society that the state was responsive to the population's actions. Third, the crisis nature of the issue and the informal nature of civil society's response meant that societal actors had few claims to make on the state once the crisis ended. As a result, some participants like the "burial boys" or members of community Ebola Task Forces were forgotten (see *New York Times*, December 9, 2015; *FrontPageAfrica*, April 8, 2016, on unpaid workers). They had not been brought into inclusive centralized institutions, which, as with the AIDS response (see chapter 2), could distribute rents and contribute to state legitimacy. Only time will tell if the confidence that the Liberian society gained through its activities during the Ebola tragedy will have long-term consequences for the state–civil society relationship and Liberian politics (interviews, government officials and international NGO official, Monrovia, May 18, 2016, May 19, 2016, and May 21, 2016).

Conclusion: Challenge Is Never Absolute

Several African states challenged global health governance during the 2014–2015 Ebola outbreak in West Africa. This occurred when over half of African states defied the WHO recommendations on travel restrictions for people from Ebola-affected states. The WHO was unable to enforce the IHR for multiple reasons: its own structural, political, and funding limits; contested norms; and African states' need to show democratic responsiveness (particularly for West African states, states with upcoming elections, and states with large tourism industries). Ebola also undermined African states' aspirational identities, leading them to distance themselves from the disease and its victims. As the Namibia case illustrated, ruling parties—even those in noncompetitive elections—faced pressure from the public, media, business elites, and opposition party candidates to enact travel barriers. Challenges also came from Liberia, a state that suffered more Ebola deaths than any other. Liberia shaped the disease narrative with its slow initial reaction, its manipulation of the neglect and crisis frames, and its use of the US-Liberia relationship. The state then challenged implementation of global health policies by devising its own management structures. As with nonaffected states that implemented travel restrictions, Liberia had room to maneuver because of weak international cooperation on disease outbreaks and its own aspirational identities as a postwar state. Weak democracy and neopatrimonial networks necessitated state control over decisions and the use of extraversion to gain resources. Societal activities pressured the state to act by embarrassing officials, highlighting societal distrust, and demonstrating the state's overall weakness.

African states were able to take advantage of unique political opportunities that Ebola presented—the immediacy of the outbreak, the media spectacle, the weakness of global health institutions and norms, and Ebola's spread to the West—to challenge global health governance. But events after the outbreak illustrate that challenge is difficult to sustain. Even though the affected states lobbied donors to provide resources for health system strengthening (Sirleaf 2014), donors seemed more eager to establish a global health emergency workforce and to improve poor countries' disease surveillance systems (*Guardian*, May 18, 2015, February 13, 2015; Kupferschmidt 2015). In April 2015, the CDC and African Union announced the development of an African CDC to "prevent, detect and respond to any disease outbreak" (Yasmin 2016a; CDC 2015a), and the United States allocated most health funds in Liberia for "build[ing] capacity to identify and contain future EVD cases" and for training individuals in epidemiological reporting systems (USAID 2016). In May 2016, the World Bank announced the development of a $500 million Pandemic Emergency Financial Facility, a fund to help low-income countries fight outbreaks of infectious diseases (*Financial Times*, May 23, 2016). Despite donors' efforts to build programs for pandemic preparedness, a 2017 World Bank report showed that less than one-fourth of the 162 states surveyed were ready for the next outbreak. Donors also seemed to move on to the next crisis, causing concern for Liberian health-care workers. In 2016, the Obama Administration shifted $500 million from the Ebola response to Zika (*STAT News*, June 1, 2016; *The Hill*, February 3, 2016). In mid-2016, a Liberian health-care worker explained the potential impact of these changes:

> If the [donor] partners withdraw, we are asking the Ministry [of Health], "Where would we continue to get PPE? Those suits cost $150 to $250. Where would we continue to get gloves? Where would we continue to get the face shield or aprons?" So [the government] now says we need to do risk assessment before [using PPE] with each patient. So if I see a patient and she has respiratory problems, then I say, "Do I need a face mask? Yes, but maybe not an apron." Or another patient, "Do I need gloves?" So we have put the ball

back to the health worker, which means you have to be very sharp when you are working . . . prioritize quickly in terms of supplies. (Interview, hospital senior nurse, Kakata, May 16, 2016)

The respondent shows that despite Liberia's astute use of the crisis frame, health-care services still suffer from a deep neglect that forces health-care workers to potentially take on unnecessary risks. Distrust of the state remains, as the suspicion underlying this worker's questioning indicates. Neglect also emerges from vertical programs that result from crisis framing. In contrast to AIDS's privileged position (see chapter 2), attention to Ebola meant that AIDS was demoted. In this particular hospital, boxes of gloves lined nurses' stations, but the laboratory had no reagents for completing CD4 tests for people living with HIV (participant observations, public hospital, Kakata, May 16, 2016). Neglect reflects a state that governs through short-sighted, decentralized networks, societies that distrust and oppose the state, and weak, underfunded global health institutions that lack roots in coherent norms. Ultimately, neglect has the potential to create new crises and new opportunities for African states to challenge global health governance.

chapter 4

What Is the Problem?

Ambivalence about Global Health Governance of NCDs

There is so much loss . . . [people] not working, loss of limbs, blindness, economic destitution, depression, death.

(Interview, advocate on NCDs, Dodoma, July 2, 2015)

Over half of the rural population has no clue how harmful tobacco is.

(Interview, tobacco control advocate, Lusaka, June 13, 2014)

There's a lot of ignorance amongst the medical personnel regarding the signs and symptoms of cancer. So, by the time you are finally diagnosed, even if you go in good time, there are so many cases of misdiagnoses. [A friend] died of cancer of the colon, which had spread to the bone. They said he had arthritis until it was too late.

(Interview, advocate on NCDs, Lusaka, June 12, 2014)

We have seen these NCDs arising in our country for many years. But there are few political statements on how the global community is dealing with this.

(Phone interview, South African government official, October 13, 2015)

These respondents illustrate the high costs of noncommunicable diseases (NCDs), the need to educate citizens and medical personnel about these diseases, and national and global inaction on this health issue. This chapter tackles these themes. As described in chapter 1, NCDs are diseases that do not result from an infectious agent, that are often chronic, and that usually do not have a complete cure. They include mental health illnesses, musculoskeletal diseases, unintended injuries, chronic neurological disorders, cancers, cardiovascular diseases, diabetes, and chronic respiratory diseases (e.g., asthma and chronic obstructive pulmonary disease). Cancers, diabetes, cardiovascular diseases, and chronic respiratory diseases make up the vast majority of cases. As the top cause of death globally, cardiovascular diseases (heart attacks and stroke) led to 17 million deaths worldwide in 2013. Cancer was second, with 7.6 million deaths. Chronic respiratory diseases caused 4.2 million deaths, and diabetes, 1.3 million deaths (Sturchio and Galambos 2014, 6). It is estimated that by 2020, NCDs will account for 80 percent of the global burden of disease (Boutayeb and Boutayeb 2005).

As an issue relatively new to the global health governance agenda, NCDs provide an opportunity to analyze the response of weak states on an emerging health issue. This chapter argues that African states' position on NCDs has been ambivalent: While a few states have adopted structures and policies to fight NCDs, most have not. Those policies and institutions that do exist often are poorly implemented. The ambivalence emerges because of weak international institutions, limited global funding, and competing issue frames that make norm coherence problematic. These attributes of global health governance on NCDs interact with state-level factors: Democracy has not led to demands for action, while a disengaged civil society, as indicated by the lack of mobilization on the issue and low citizen knowledge of or interest in these diseases, creates no urgency for states to act. The result is that state leaders hedge their bets, remaining ambivalent on the issue but aware that in the future, global interest in and funding for these health concerns, as well as civil society mobilization, could increase.

The chapter first examines the global crisis of NCDs, particularly as it affects the Global South. It then highlights global health governance on NCDs, illustrating its nascent institutions, contentious norms, competing frames, and lack of funding. The third section investigates African states' ambivalence in two phases of global health governance: (1) shaping the narrative around the global responses to NCDs and (2) implementing WHO-recommended strategies and funding mechanisms. The fourth section uses the three levels of analysis to analyze this ambivalence. It argues that weak global structures and contending frames have created spaces for African states to engage in performances of compliance and extraversion while doing little on the issue. State characteristics such as democracy or neopatrimonial governance show no discernible pattern of influence on policy adoption, though in particular country cases they matter. Despite some international advocacy on NCDs, African civil society has been relatively disengaged from the issue, with few African groups and limited societal interest. The chapter concludes that the weakness of global health governance on NCDs leads to highly contextualized explanations for weak states' involvement with these health problems.

African States and the Global Crisis of NCDs

In 2012, NCDs caused 68 percent of global deaths, an increase from 63 percent in 2008. Eighty percent of those deaths occur in the Global South (Editorial Board 2011; WHO 2015j). The impact of NCDs on Africa is hard to measure because of low levels of reporting and paltry surveillance data, but scholars agree that Africa's cases of NCDs will increase by 25 percent between 2014 and 2025 (White et al. 2012; Parkin et al. 2008; Sturchio and Galambos 2014, 1). In high-income countries, the number of premature deaths (or deaths of people under the age of sixty) due to NCDs has declined since 2005, while this number has steadily increased in low- and lower-middle–income countries; over 80 percent of Africans who die from NCDs are under sixty years old (Daniels, Donilon, and Bollyky 2014). Reflecting inequalities in income and access to health care, NCDs that are preventable and treatable in high-income countries, such as cervical cancer, cardiovascular disease, liver cancer, and diabetes, have high mortality rates in poor countries. Only 5 percent of cancer patients in Africa, for example, have access to chemotherapy (*Lancet* 2013). At least 30 percent of these deaths in low- and middle-income countries are avoidable (Sturchio and Galambos 2014, 6). In addition to premature death, NCDs contribute to increased morbidity and disability, cutting productive years from individuals' lives and increasing costs to families for long-term health care (Harvard School of Public Health and World Economic Forum 2011). NCDs require greater management than most infectious diseases, thus demanding health-care capacity and access to pharmaceuticals. Each year, developing countries collectively lose roughly 4 percent of their GDP (or $500 billion) due to NCDs (UNGA 2013).

The WHO highlights four factors that increase the risk of suffering from one or more NCDs: tobacco use; diets high in salt, sugar and fat; physical inactivity; and alcohol use. Exposure to these factors has been exacerbated by globalization, urbanization, and the rise of incomes in low- and middle-income countries. Trade liberalization opened markets in poor countries to Western tobacco companies, who were eager for new customers since tobacco use in the West has declined as a result of taxes, public smoking bans, and public awareness of health risks. Major tobacco companies now control large shares of markets in low- and middle-income countries. For example, British American Tobacco controls 93 percent of the South African tobacco market (Warner and MacKay 2006), and Japan Tobacco International controls 97 percent of the market share in Tanzania. And while Japan Tobacco owns 75 percent of the Tanzanian Cigarette Company (MacKenzie, Eckhardt, and Prastyani 2017), the company kept the Tanzanian brand name in order to retain local buyers (interview, tobacco control advocate, Dar es Salaam, July 4, 2015).

As a result of these actions, as well as aggressive marketing by tobacco companies, the number of smokers has increased in low- and middle-income countries, because of weak (or nonexistent) tobacco regulations, a lack of awareness of the health effects of tobacco use, and a general belief among people globally that infectious diseases will kill people in the Global South before cancer or heart disease will (Drope 2011; interview, physician, Accra, May 9, 2017). One Tanzanian health worker said, "Among the general population, people don't see it as a problem. Even here in the clinic, people will just light up and no one bothers to tell them to stop" (interview, physician, Dar es Salaam, July 8, 2015). The doctor's comment helps explain how nearly 80 percent of the 6.3 million deaths from smoking in 2010 occurred in low- and middle-income countries (*Guardian*, November 20, 2013). A lack of country-specific studies that demonstrate how tobacco use causes morbidity and mortality also hampers the formation and implementation of tobacco control laws, with policymakers sometimes asking: "If smoking is so dangerous, why am I not sick?" (phone interview, Rwandan tobacco control advocate, May 3, 2017; see also interview, expert on NCDs, Accra, May 4, 2017). Youth have been particularly impacted; in Zambia, for example, 25 percent of students (both boys and girls) report using tobacco products (University of Zambia, Ministry of Health, and University of Waterloo 2014). In Ghana, despite overall low rates of smoking (8.9 percent of males and 0.3 percent of females use tobacco products regularly), youth report that cigarettes often seem "appealing" and "attractive"; some also use "shisha" ("hookah" or the water pipe) during social gatherings (focus group discussion, university students, Accra, April 26, 2017; Owusu-Dabo et al. 2009).

Additionally, trade liberalization has increased people's exposure to processed food that is high in fat, salt, and sugar. Transnational food companies engage in marketing activities that change traditional eating habits; in urban areas the "relentless advertising and ubiquity of outlets" for such food, and the fact that urban individuals have little (if any) space for growing healthy food, have created demand for these products. Unhealthy, processed foods have become cheap, while healthier foods often are more expensive and require more time for shopping, storing, and preparation. Increasingly consumed not just by elites, processed products are "conduits of Westernisation" (Barraclough 2009, 106–107). Susan Bridle-Fitzpatrick (2015) finds that "food swamps," or geographic areas where people have excessive exposure to unhealthy foods and drinks, undermine Mexico's antiobesity efforts. In Accra, an increasing number of low-income workers now purchase packaged and premade food with high salt content from market sellers (interview, physician, Accra, May 9, 2017; personal observations of health-related behaviors, Accra, January–May 2017). These processes of globalization have changed the global diet, which during the last fifty years has become more homogeneous with increased consumption of wheat, corn, dairy products, and meat (*Los Angeles Times*, March 3, 2014).

The rise of urban populations has created crowded conditions that increase vulnerability to chronic respiratory diseases, limit opportunities for exercise, and expose more people to processed food, alcohol, and tobacco. (Over 90 percent of urban growth is currently happening in the developing world; see World Bank 2015c). One Ugandan interviewee said, "If you look around this city, there is no place to walk; we get no exercise. We just drive or sit in traffic. And lack of physical activity is a risk factor for NCDs" (interview, advocate on NCDs, Kampala, June 26, 2014). A Ghanaian physician who oversees a clinic for diabetes and hypertension patients commented that successfully persuading patients to increase their physical activity was the hardest aspect of preventing and managing NCDs (interview, physician, Accra, May 9, 2017).

As many individuals in low- and middle-income countries experience greater exposure to risk factors, they also find affordable, efficient primary health care difficult to access. As chapter 3 showed in relation to West African states' preparedness for the Ebola outbreak, neoliberal structural adjustment policies that started in the 1980s led to the erosion of health-care facilities, shortages in health-care personnel, and greater suspicion of the health-care system by the population (Kawachi and Wamala 2007; Wilkinson and Leach 2014). Even with the end of user fees in many countries by the mid-2000s, uptake in services has been slow (Meessen et al. 2011). These problems with health-care systems have made it more difficult to diagnose various NCDs early in their progression and to provide the continual monitoring many patients need. One Tanzanian respondent described the situation:

> We see five hundred to six hundred patients each day in outpatient, many with hypertension or diabetes. But there is no time to educate the patients about risks . . . alcohol use, cheap processed foods. . . . Many don't even know they have these diseases. . . . And the high cost of drugs for diabetes control and hypertension makes it impossible to treat them. Every day we see stroke victims as a result . . . there is no support for these patients. (Interview, physician, Dodoma, July 2, 2015)

Working on the frontlines of health care in a midsize city in Tanzania, the speaker outlines overwhelming challenges that range from lack of knowledge to costly medications. The respondent's comment about "no support" for these patients also alludes to donors' focus on vertical health programs for AIDS, TB, and malaria, not programs to combat NCDs or to strengthen health systems (Giles-Vernick and Webb 2013; interviews, NGO health-care system administrator, Accra, April 18, 2017; bilateral donor official, Accra, May 18, 2017). As chapter 2 indicated, this emphasis led to new institutions such as National AIDS Commissions and funding mechanisms like the Global Fund. But vertical programs marginalized other diseases, reinforced the idea that Africa's major health challenge was communicable diseases, and promoted the belief that disease-specific programs are the most cost-effective way to achieve measurable results (Crane 2013; Shiffman 2008). Often omitted in health care has been health education (e.g., on tobacco use or nutrition), early identification of chronic health conditions (e.g., hypertension), and consistent monitoring and treatment for these chronic health problems (on hypertension in Africa, see Kayima et al. 2013). As the next two sections illustrate, the lack of willingness to engage the "big health picture," with all its complexity and structural causes, is evident at both the international and national levels (interview, multilateral donor, Kampala, June 30, 2014).

Global Health Governance on NCDs

Weak institutions, contested frames that problematize normative expectations for state behavior, and meager funding characterize global health governance on NCDs. With the rise of AIDS onto the global health agenda in the new millennium, NCDs have gained little traction, despite the fact that the WHO first mentioned them as a health challenge in *The Global Burden of Disease* in 1996 (Editorial Board 2011; Murray and Lopez 1996). In 2000, the WHO director-general issued a call for a global strategy on prevention and control of NCDs to the World Health Assembly, but it took eight years before the WHO issued its 2008–2013 Global Action Plan (Editorial Board 2011). This section details the general weakness of this global health governance.

Slow Institutional Development

The design of institutions to address NCDs has been centered in the United Nations and the WHO, though it was countries in the Caribbean Community (CARICOM), after realizing the high burden of NCDs on their populations in the early 2000s, which pushed for international actions. In 2007, these states passed the Declaration of Port-of-Spain, which called for national commissions on NCDs, stronger implementation of the Framework Convention on Tobacco Control (FCTC), and national policies on physical activity and food labeling (CARICOM 2007). CARICOM members (particularly Barbados) became a driving force for the UN High-Level Meeting of the General Assembly on the Prevention and Control of Noncommunicable Diseases held in 2011 (interview, multilateral donor official, New York, October 1, 2015; phone interview, South African government official, October 13, 2015). Given that this was only the second UN special session held to discuss a health issue (the first was the 2001 meeting on AIDS), global health officials and activists hoped the 2011 meeting would galvanize media and state attention and mobilize resources. Before the meeting, the Lancet NCD Action Group, the NCD Alliance, and public health experts called for specific outcomes such as leadership commitment, action on tobacco, prevention targets on the marketing of processed foods, and access to affordable medical technologies and generic medications (Editorial Board 2011; Beaglehole and Lancet Action Group 2011a, 2011b). They advocated for UN member states to set measurable goals that focused on key diseases and risk factors.

The outcome of the meeting was the unanimous endorsement of the Political Declaration of the High-Level Meeting of the General Assembly on the Prevention and Control of Noncommunicable Diseases (the "Political Declaration"). The document called attention to the crisis of NCDs, noted prior regional efforts to address these diseases, recognized the high cost of these diseases, called for government and societal action to reduce risk factors for NCDs, urged states to adopt specific policies to combat NCDs, and placed the issue squarely under the jurisdiction of the WHO (UNGA 2011e). But the Political Declaration's initial effect on institutional development was somewhat meager. It set no specific targets or timelines, leaving that task to WHO bureaucrats, ministers of health, and activists. The difficulty in target setting partly reflected the challenge of gathering data about NCDs in the Global South, but it also indicated significant foot dragging on the part of some member states (*Devex News*, June 3, 2016).

After the 2011 meeting, member states engaged in a contentious process of policy formation and institution building that required two additional years of bargaining (Sturchio and Galambos 2014, 13). In 2013, the World Health Assembly unanimously endorsed the resulting WHO Global Action Plan for the Prevention and Control of Noncommunicable Diseases 2013–2020, which set nine voluntary targets to be achieved by 2020 (WHO 2013). The targets are not disease specific; instead they focus on risk factors and health systems or primary health care. They have been criticized for concentrating on individual behavior (such as physical inactivity and salt intake) and for ignoring the structural inequalities and vulnerabilities such as undernutrition that many African populations face (see Nulu 2016). The targets are:

1. A 25% relative reduction in overall mortality from cardiovascular diseases, cancer, diabetes, or chronic respiratory diseases;
2. At least a 10% relative reduction in harmful use of alcohol, as appropriate, within the national context;
3. A 10% relative reduction in prevalence of insufficient physical activity;
4. A 30% relative reduction in mean population intake of salt/sodium;
5. A 30% relative reduction in prevalence of current tobacco use in persons aged 15+ years;
6. A 25% relative reduction in the prevalence of raised blood pressure or contain the prevalence of raised blood pressure, according to national circumstances;
7. A halt in the rise in diabetes and obesity;
8. At least 50% of eligible people receiving drug therapy and counselling (including glycaemic therapy) to prevent heart attacks and strokes;
9. An 80% availability of the affordable basic technological and essential medicines, including generics, required to treat major noncommunicable diseases in both public and private facilities. (WHO 2013, 5)

To achieve these targets, the WHO established the Global Monitoring Framework, which in turn developed nine indicators to determine states' progress toward meeting the Global Action Plan targets (WHO 2014b). Each individual state measures its response to NCDs using the following indicators:

1. Has an operational unit/branch or department within the Ministry of Health, or equivalent
2. Has an operational multisectoral national policy, strategy or action plan that integrates several NCDs and shared risk factors
3. Has an operational policy, strategy or action plan to reduce the harmful use of alcohol
4. Has an operational policy strategy or action plan to reduce physical inactivity and/or promote physical activity
5. Has an operational policy, strategy or action plan to reduce the burden of tobacco use
6. Has an operational policy, strategy or action plan to reduce unhealthy diets and/or promote healthy diets

7. Has evidence-based national guidelines/protocols/standards for the management of major NCDs through a primary care approach
8. Has an NCD surveillance and monitoring system in place to enable reporting against the nine global NCD targets
9. Has a national, population-based cancer registry. (WHO 2014b)

By 2014, the United Nations had formed additional structures to help states meet their targets: the UN secretary-general established the UN Interagency Task Force on NCDs, and the WHO set up its Global Coordinating Mechanism on NCDs to improve engagement between member states and civil society. The 2014–2015 WHO Programme Budget also included a dedicated line to provide technical assistance to countries as they worked to develop their own plans, targets, and monitoring systems (WHO 2014b, 2014d). To promote these institutions, WHO Director-General Margaret Chan spoke extensively on NCDs (see M. Chan 2014). In addition, one of the six major departments of WHO Geneva specializes in NCDs and mental health.[1] Despite these efforts, it is notable that unlike AIDS, NCDs do not have their own UN program. And because the WHO department addresses the range of health conditions and diseases defined to be NCDs, health issues constantly compete for resources and personnel. The inclusion of NCDs in the Sustainable Development Goals could potentially generate more institutional focus, though in 2017, it was too soon to draw such a conclusion (UICC 2016).

The limited commitment to institutional development at the global level was mirrored at the state level. In 2010, only 32 percent of the WHO's member states had policies with a budget to combat NCDs. While that number increased to 50 percent in 2014, half of states still had no policy or resources to combat various NCDs (UNGA 2014). Many of those in compliance were high-income states that already had such policies, meaning that their adoption of global health governance on NCDs was a low-cost action (WHO 2011b, 2014b). Some of these states also have policies that undermine the prevention of NCDs, particularly in the area of tobacco control. For example, the United States has not ratified the FCTC, even though the scientific evidence shows that tobacco use is the single greatest preventable cause of death in the world and a risk factor for six of the eight leading causes of mortality (WHO 2009). In addition, proposed protocols to the FCTC that would limit illicit trade of tobacco have received little support among almost all WHO member states (Bollyky and Fidler 2015; *Lancet*, March 5, 2016). These obstacles led the WHO to acknowledge that "progress [on NCDs] has been insufficient and uneven" (UNGA 2013, 18).

Competing Issue Frames

The underdevelopment of global-level institutions reflects the fact that NCDs have been framed in multiple ways. And unlike with AIDS, when the human rights and security frames mobilized different constituencies for the same outcome (funding AIDS programs), three distinct frames for NCDs have competed and stressed different policy solutions. Additionally, a variety of groups have espoused different perspectives, including the NCD Alliance, public health experts with the Lancet NCD Action Group, economists, private foundations like the Bloomberg Initiative, and IGOs like the WHO.[2]

The first frame emphasizes human rights and how the hardship and suffering that accompany NCDs undermine the right to health. Activists assert that people should not die premature and "avoidable" deaths from NCDs and that it is inequitable that such deaths primarily occur in low- and middle-income countries (NCD Alliance 2014b; UNGA 2011g; Casswell 2016). Some activists highlight marginalized groups, such as women and children. For example, the Bloomberg Initiative points to the vulnerability of youth to tobacco industry marketing, and the NCD Alliance stresses the stories of children with NCDs on its website. These portrayals illustrate how discourses about the prevention of bodily harm for vulnerable or "innocent" groups are often necessary to facilitate mobilization and eventual norm acceptance, a point illustrated in chapter 2 about AIDS (see Keck and Sikkink 1998). One respondent said as much: "With NCDs you don't necessarily get a very striking sort of imagery, like with some diseases of poverty. I know it is politically incorrect to say, but those images really do wake a lot of people up" (phone interview, global advocate on NCDs, October 9, 2015). Yet, despite these attempts to frame NCDs as a human rights issue, the Global Action Plan 2013–2020 demonstrates a "lack of concrete attention to human rights," with, in contrast to the inclusion of people living with HIV in global AIDS governance, no emphasis on patients' participation or rights (Gruskin, Ferguson, Tarantola, and Beaglehole 2014; NCD Alliance 2014b).

Additionally, the human right to access lifesaving medications (including generic versions of hypertension and diabetes drugs) is noticeably absent from the 2011 Political Declaration, which calls for the private sector "where appropriate" to "contribute to efforts to improve access to and affordability of medicines and technologies in the prevention and control of noncommunicable diseases" (UNGA 2011e, 8; see Smith and Yadav 2014 on access to medications). Even though medications for diabetes and cancer are often costly and inaccessible in low- and middle-income countries, the human right to health and the alleviation of suffering that such medications can bring was downplayed (on suffering, see Livingston 2012). This outcome reflects the fact that during the 2011 negotiations for the Political Declaration, the United States and the European Union (EU) sought to protect the intellectual property rights of Western pharmaceutical companies. In a month of negotiations that involved foreign ministers and trade officials (not health ministers), Brazil and India, countries involved in the production of generics for the global market, challenged the US/EU position. South Africa, speaking for the Africa bloc, also lobbied for medicine access, particularly because of the country's prioritization of diabetes drugs and its need for the vaccine against the human papillomavirus (HPV) to prevent cervical cancer (phone interview, South African government official, October 13, 2015).[3] One observer said: "The whole Political Declaration came down to this one issue—protecting intellectual property rights" (phone interview, global advocate on NCDs, October 9, 2015). As a result of negotiations, only two of the nine targets in the Global Action Plan (numbers 8 and 9) relate to the human right to access medications. This omission is noticeable because global AIDS governance has successfully stressed the human right to universal access to ART (see chapter 2).

A second frame emphasizes economic issues and portrays NCDs as a "major challenge to development," because they contribute to household and national-level poverty, and because poverty in low- and middle-income countries makes it difficult to prevent and control NCDs (Beaglehole and Lancet Action Group 2011a, 2011b). The Sustainable Development Goals linked NCDs with "ending poverty, transforming all lives, and protecting the planet" (Garrett 2015a). The development frame often refers to NCDs using the language of cost-benefit analysis. For example, the World Economic Forum estimated in 2011 that within the next twenty years, NCDs will cost more than $30 trillion in medical care, lost productivity, morbidity, and early mortality in low- and middle-income countries. In 2012, the global burden of smoking-attributable deaths was $1.4 trillion in health-care costs and lost worker productivity, with 40 percent of this cost being borne by developing countries (Goodchild, Nargis, and Tursan d'Espaignet 2017). Preventing such economic losses will require spending less than forty cents per capita annually, or around $2 billion (Harvard School of Public Health and World Economic Forum 2011). This cost-benefit analysis assumes that prevention of NCDs is cheaper than their treatment (NCD Alliance 2015; UNGA 2011e, 5; Glasgow 2012; WHO 2011c). Development officials also have asserted it is not cost effective for donors and governments to ignore NCDs while at the same time treating other communicable diseases: "NCDs undermine the effectiveness of existing US global health investments. . . . It is poor stewardship of scarce US global health resources to spend substantial resources to save an individual from one preventable and treatable disease [HIV and AIDS] while that individual succumbs prematurely to another preventable and treatable disease" (Daniels, Donilon, and Bollyky 2014, 30–31).

Those who frame NCDs as a human rights issue or development concern face a challenge, because NCDs have often been understood to be a private issue or the result of personal health decisions. That is, some NCDs, particularly cardiovascular diseases, diabetes, and some cancers, are perceived to result from individuals' poor food choices, their overuse of alcohol, their tobacco use, and their lack of exercise (Nulu 2016). In this framing, conquering NCDs necessitates empowering individuals with information so that as autonomous decision makers, they can make positive eating, lifestyle, and health choices (Glasgow 2012; *Devex News*, June 3, 2016). This approach makes it difficult to rally the public for policies to address NCDs. For example, surveys show that because most individuals view diabetes and heart disease to be the result of an individual's poor health choices, they are unlikely to support public policies to fight these conditions (Kapstein and Busby 2013). Indeed, in a 2014 survey only 26 percent of Americans said prevention and treatment of heart disease and other chronic diseases should be one of the top priorities in US global health programs. This compares to 57 percent who supported clean water and 53 percent who supported child health and immunizations (Kaiser Family Foundation 2014).

This individual responsibility frame decouples risk from the structural violence embedded in unequal socioeconomic status, trade inequalities, and human rights discrimination (Farmer 2005). Emphasizing individual responsibility makes it unnecessary to regulate the food or alcohol industries for their pricing or marketing strategies that are intended to capture market share and develop brand loyalty (see Hesse 2015 on African beer markets; Hawkins, Holden, Eckhardt, and Lee 2016 on the global alcohol industry), with only the tobacco industry's products being singled out as "incompatible" with public health (World Health Assembly 1986). The food, beverage, and alcohol industries' participation in the 2011 UN High-Level Meeting indicated their role in defining NCDs as the result of individual choices. And the Political Declaration merely urges the food, beverage, and alcohol industries to voluntarily redesign healthier products or to limit advertisements to children (UNGA 2011e).

Tensions among the human rights, development, and individual responsibility frames are apparent, particularly in terms of recommended policy outcomes. If health is a human right, the state has the obligation to ensure that people with NCDs receive access to medicines. But if health is the result of personal decisions, then individuals should solve their own health problems and industries should not be held responsible. If health is viewed in terms of cost-benefit analysis, then when health interventions are not economically viable they can be discarded, even if doing so undermines the right to health. (On the tension between various health frames see McInnes and Lee 2012). These tensions contribute to a lack of norm coherence and murky normative expectations of states. Thus there is no belief that states must address NCDs because their identities and legitimacy in the eyes of other states depend on such behavior (Legro 1997; Florini 1996). States do not label other states as "inappropriate" because of their lack of implementation of the WHO Global Action Plan or, if they are donor states, their lack of development assistance for NCDs. States do not feel the need to explain their inaction on NCDs. This lack of admonishment contrasts with the situation with AIDS, a disease for which global action became a moral and ethical imperative.

Little Funding

Ultimately, if one of the hallmark measures of prioritization of a health condition is funding (see Shiffman and Smith 2007), then NCDs cannot be said to be a priority. The 2011 High-Level Meeting led to no new funding mechanism, unlike the 2001 AIDS meeting which was followed by the establishment of PEPFAR and the Global Fund. Global funding to address NCDs is woefully inadequate. The WHO (2011b, 5) estimates that it will cost $11.4 billion annually to provide all low- and middle-income countries with the best interventions such as tobacco control, access to generic drugs to prevent heart attack and stroke, and preventative education.[4] Most African states lack capacity to adequately address these various diseases, and bilateral donors, who provide most global health aid, have allocated little money for programs on NCDs. In its 2015 budget justification to Congress, for example, USAID requested funds for HIV and AIDS, TB, malaria, child and maternal health, family planning, nutrition, and health system strengthening, but not directly for NCDs (US Department of State 2014). The United States has no programs specifically dedicated to these diseases. Even though US funding for global health increased from $1.3 billion in 2001 to over $8 billion in 2014, only $10 million of this total amount was spent on the prevention of NCDs (Daniels, Donilon, and Bollyky 2014, 25). And of the $31.4 billion for global health allocated by all donors in 2011, only $68 million went for tobacco control, one prevention activity (Bollyky and

Fidler 2015). As another sign of the low priority that NCDs face among donors, the Development Assistance Committee of the Organisation of Economic Co-operation and Development (OECD) has established few measures for the dispersal of aid for NCDs (NCD Alliance 2014b). Indeed, in Ghana, a country where 42 percent of deaths are attributed to NCDs (WHO 2014b), as of early 2017, only the UK Department for International Development (DFID) supported programs on NCDs, and in that case, only for mental health (interviews, NGO health-care system administrator and mental health expert, Accra, April 18, 2017, and May 18, 2017). And even though the WHO was criticized in the wake of the Ebola crisis for focusing too heavily on NCDs (and not outbreak surveillance and control), NCDs received less than 10 percent of the WHO's $3.97 billion budget in 2014 (Daniels, Donilon, and Bollyky 2014). This amount increased from $113 million in 2013 to $192 million in 2015. (The total is $318 million if disabilities, mental health, and violence are included; WHO 2012c, 2014d). Despite these efforts, these numbers do not reflect the fact that NCDs are the biggest cause of mortality, morbidity, and disability globally.

African Participation in the Emerging Governance of NCDs

African states engaged in the emerging governance of NCDs in two phases: global health diplomacy and implementation of policies. To discern involvement in the first phase, I relied on interviews with participants in negotiations surrounding global actions on NCDs, particularly WHO officials, state officials, and global activists. In addition, I examined the thirty-two speeches of African presidents and ministers of health who spoke at the 2011 High-Level Meeting. For any country that had implemented at least five of the nine WHO Global Action Plan indicators in 2013 (see below), I also examined the Ministry of Health website for speeches or documents on NCDs. My goal was to discover the themes that African states stressed as well as their overall interest in this health issue. In speeches, I paid particular attention to the competing narratives of "development," "human rights," "treatment access," and "personal responsibility" as well as concerns about "foreign assistance."

To ascertain state implementation of global health governance on NCDs, I again used interviews with national-level activists and state officials. I then examined the 2014 reports from African states-parties to the WHO FCTC to discover states' implementation of two tobacco control measures: a ban on public smoking and taxes on tobacco products (WHO 2015g). I chose those two policy areas because they tend to face high political opposition and their passage demonstrates state commitment to tobacco control. While these reports can be colored by respondents' own objectives, the fact that many officials provided glaringly uncomplimentary statements about FCTC policy implementation made me reasonably confident in their responses.[5]

I also compiled a database of all African states policy actions on NCDs that related to the above-listed nine indicators of the Global Action Plan. Data come from country reports submitted in 2010 and 2013 to the WHO. In 2010, all African states (forty-eight) submitted reports; in 2013, thirty-nine did. Because not all states completed reports in 2013, and because three of the nine questions in the 2013 survey differed from the 2010 survey, I rely on this data as a secondary source to support interview themes and lessons drawn from the country case studies below. While self-reported assessments are always problematic, the country data on the Global Action Plan are reported in conjunction with WHO officials and, in some cases, civil society representatives. If governments sought to improve their global image on the issue of NCDs, one might expect that these numbers would show higher levels of policy implementation than they do. While governments might have incentive to underreport their actions, the fact that there is little global funding for NCDs gives state officials little incentive to engage in underreporting. (That is, there is little to be gained by claiming high levels of NCDs or a lack of policies to address them.) To determine if states had committed financial resources to this health issue, I searched government websites, reports from activists, responses to the WHO 2013 Global Action Plan surveys, and African leaders' statements at the 2011 High-Level Meeting for information about states' funding for programs to control NCDs. These financial data were limited and difficult to verify.

A Limited Role in Global Health Diplomacy on NCDs

African state efforts to shape global health diplomacy on NCDs were minimal. It was only two months before the 2011 High-Level Meeting that the African Union adopted the Brazzaville Declaration on Noncommunicable Diseases Prevention and Control in the WHO African Region. In contrast to the Abuja Declaration on AIDS (see chapter 2) and CARICOM's proactive efforts, the Brazzaville document was "very general, weak, and with minimal state commitments" (interview, multilateral donor official, New York, October 1, 2015). In short, it illustrated state leaders' ambivalence about these health issues.

The situation was similar during the run-up to the 2011 High-Level Meeting, a period during which behind-the-scenes discussions occur to iron out policy differences. Except for South Africa and, to an extent Senegal, Botswana, and Ghana, African states were absent during these negotiations. The region was also under-represented in the roundtable discussions during the High-Level Meeting: only 10 of the 112 roundtable speakers were from Africa, and only one NGO speaker was African (WHO 2011d). Representation in the roundtables was important because these less formal arenas provide an opportunity for more in-depth discussion and negotiations (Sturchio and Galambos 2014). Africa's minimal role was partly because most African states do not have health attachés at their UN missions, but it was also because "many African leaders just don't see NCDs to be an issue . . . even though the region has a very high prevalence of hypertension" (interview, multilateral donor official, New York, October 1, 2015; see also interview, government official, Dodoma, July 3, 2015). Echoing this sentiment, one African UN representative said: "Some African diplomats questioned why we needed to raise this issue to the level of a High-Level Meeting, when there are other issues that need more time, money, and attention" (interview, African state UN representative, New York, October 6, 2015).

The low saliency of NCDs for many African states was apparent at the podium during the 2011 High-Level Meeting: only six heads of state (four presidents and two prime ministers) spoke at the meeting in contrast to the fifteen heads of state (including ten presidents) who spoke at the 2001 UN Special Session on HIV/AIDS (UNGA 2001). This limited participation by high-level officials cannot be explained by the continent's general under-representation among plenary speakers: 24 percent of speakers (32 of 139) represented African states, and 25 percent of the UN General Assembly is composed of African states. Rather, high-level officials simply chose not to attend. Speeches delivered at the meeting lacked urgency or emotion: No speaker shared stories of family, friends, or citizens lost to NCDs, despite the fact that activists and UN officials had urged them to view the impact of NCDs in a personal light (interview, multilateral donor official, New York, October 1, 2015). The rhetoric contrasted greatly with African leaders' speeches at the 2001 UN Special Session on HIV/AIDS, during which they spoke openly and passionately about people from their countries who were suffering and dying from AIDS (UNGA 2001).[6] After the High-Level Meeting, African states had little role in the negotiations that ultimately led to the WHO Global Action Plan (Sturchio and Galambos 2014, 13).

"No Strategy, No Funding, No Plans": Slow Implementation of Global Health Governance on NCDs

Interviews and the aforementioned dataset illustrate several themes related to African adoption of the policies and institutions aligned with the WHO Global Action Plan indicators. The first observation is government's overall inaction on these diseases. At the 2011 High-Level Meeting, leaders from Cameroon, Namibia, and Gabon even admitted their limited activities (UNGA 2011f, 17). One interviewee said, "Look, they had the High-Level Meeting in 2011 [on NCDs] in New York and here it is 2015, four years later, and we have no action. We have no strategy, no funding, no plans" (interview, advocate on NCDs, Dar es Salaam, July 9, 2015; see also interviews, advocates on NCDs, Lusaka and Kampala, June 12, 2014, and June 26, 2014). The long timeline for policy development after the 2011 meeting contrasts with African states' relatively prompt implementation of AIDS structures and policies after the 2001 Special Session on HIV/AIDS.

Data compiled from country reports to the WHO confirm that African states have been slow to implement global policies on NCDs. By 2013, the majority of countries that had adopted few or none of the nine Global Action Plan indicators outlined in 2013 were African states. Table 4.1 shows that 36 percent of states in the WHO African region that completed the WHO's 2013 survey reported that they had adopted zero items. In comparison, 13 percent of thirty-one reporting states in the Americas region had adopted zero items, and none of the ten reporting states in the South-East Asia region had adopted zero indicators. Additionally, only 21 percent of reporting African states said they had adopted five or more policies, compared to 56 percent of Latin American states and 70 percent of South-East Asian states. (However, for those eight African states—Ghana, Côte d'Ivoire, Eritrea, Mozambique, Togo, Zambia, Guinea, and Madagascar—their reported actions put them on par with middle- and high-income states like Mexico, Poland, Switzerland, Sweden, Luxembourg, and Australia.) No African state reported having adopted eight or nine indicators. In short, Africa lagged behind. (See appendix B for a list of all WHO member states implementing the Global Action Plan indicators.)

Second, inaction partly relates to officials' ignorance about or apathy toward these health conditions. For example, then Senegalese president Abdoulaye Wade said at the 2011 High-Level Meeting that he needed to educate himself more about NCDs (UNGA 2011f, 17). Two other interviewees said that government officials, just like the public, lack much information about these diseases,

TABLE 4.1   Adoption of Policies on NCDs by WHO Region

Region	Reporting states with with 0 policies (%)	Reporting states with 1–5 policies (%)	Reporting states with 5–9 policies (%)
Africa	36	43	21
Americas	13	31	56
South-East Asia	0	30	70

Source: Compiled by author from WHO 2014b.

particularly the risk factors that drive them (interviews, global advocate on NCDs, October 9, 2015; multilateral donor official, New York, October 1, 2015). But for some respondents, it was not just ignorance that led to state inaction. Rather, state officials had not prioritized these health conditions. One interviewee explained: "Many of these people [government officials] know about cancer or diabetes. But if they get sick, they just go to Europe or the States and get help. So public policies are not that important to them" (interviews, advocate on NCDs, Kampala, June 26, 2014; expert on NCDs, Accra, May 4, 2017). Another respondent echoed this view: "The government knows that these NCDs are a problem . . . diabetes, cancer, hypertension . . . but there is no effort to limit them. . . . If these were a priority, we'd do something by now" (interview, advocate on NCDs, Dar es Salaam, July 9, 2015).

Third, even though actions to address NCDs are limited, there has been some improvement in African activities. Government policies are not stagnant. One Tanzanian advocate reported in 2015 that the government was finally putting together a planning committee to work on a strategy, while a Zambian advocate reported that breast cancer testing had become more available in hospitals in the last five years (interviews, advocates on NCDs, Lusaka and Dar es Salaam, June 12, 2014, and July 9, 2015). Casual observations over several years indicate this change: In the mid-2000s, for example, public billboards or newspaper advertisements urging breast cancer testing or physical activity were practically nonexistent on the continent; instead, public health messages revolved around AIDS, childhood immunizations, and malaria. By 2015, public messages on NCDs had started to appear (personal observations of health messages, Zambia, Tanzania, South Africa, Ghana, Liberia, and Uganda, 2007–2017). Table 4.2 illustrates small advances in the development of policies related to alcohol use, physical activity, tobacco control, and nutrition. (The decline in countries with population-wide cancer registries, though, paints a confusing picture. The 2010 survey did not specify *population-wide* registry.) Despite these improvements, in 2013, it was still only about one-third of African states that had these policies, indicating that "this [change] is slow going" and uneven across the continent (phone interview, global advocate on NCDs, October 9, 2015).

Fourth, even for the aforementioned countries that have been relatively active on NCDs, there remains a gap between "policy makers' recognition of a national chronic disease burden and the development and implementation of chronic disease policies and plans" (de-Graft Aikins et al. 2010, 5). Interviewees echoed this point. One said, "The taxes on alcohol and tobacco are very low," actions that could decrease use of these two harmful substances (interview, advocate on NCDs, Dar es Salaam, July 9, 2015). A Ugandan respondent bemoaned the lack of policies on cancer and other NCDs (interview, advocate on NCDs, Uganda, June 19, 2014). And one study on cancer control in Africa found that "the political will to fund national cancer control plans is limited, even though the plans exist and are otherwise well conceived" (Stefan et al. 2013, e189; see also Camacho et al. 2015). The challenges of policy implementation are evident in the 2010 and 2013 WHO surveys, particularly the question about the presence of an "NCD department in the Ministry of Health." (See table 4.2.) Most African states reported having such a department in 2010, but when they were asked about an "operational" department to combat NCDs in the 2013 survey, the number of affirmative answers declined. One activist explained that many states that claimed to have a department for NCDs in 2010 really just had a tobacco control focal point person in the ministry of health. There really was not an operational department for NCDs. In some states, the tobacco control person then de facto became the point person for all NCDs: "Their agenda increased eight fold. So it is one person, and it's not like the budget increased or their capacity increased. Nothing changed except that they are now tasked with dealing with a bunch of disparate but related health issues" (phone interview, global advocate on NCDs, October 9, 2015). Such a situation raises questions about state commitment to provide resources and personnel needed to implement policies.

As table 4.2 indicates, of all policies to combat NCDs, African states have been the most likely to adopt tobacco control efforts. As of 2017, forty-five of the forty-nine African states had signed and ratified the FCTC, with most doing so between 2004 and 2007.[7] Of the states-parties to the FCTC, 67 percent (thirty of forty-five countries) had passed laws that ban smoking in some public spaces, and 49 percent (twenty-two of forty-five countries) had implemented taxes on tobacco products. Taxes are a more recent policy, with most states implementing them between 2012

TABLE 4.2   African States Adopting Policies on NCDs by Year

WHO Action Plan indicator	2010	2013
Has department to address NCDs in ministry of health	42	15
Has multisectoral strategy on NCDs	N/A	6
Has alcohol use policy	1	10
Has physical activity policy	3	12
Has tobacco control policy	7	17
Has nutrition policy	5	14
Has evidence-based national guidelines for managing NCDs through primary care	N/A	7
Has surveillance/monitoring system against the nine global targets for NCDs	N/A	1
Has population-wide cancer registry	9	4

Source: Compiled by author from WHO 2011b, 2014b.

Note: N = 48 in 2010; *N* = 39 in 2013. "N/A" indicates that the question was not asked in the 2010 survey.

and 2014. Few African states have comprehensive tobacco control laws. South Africa and Mauritius are exceptions (Drope 2011; Tumwine 2011). Yet in comparison to the WHO Americas and South-East Asia regions, African states are policy laggards on passing and implementing tobacco control efforts. Of the twenty-nine states-parties to the FCTC in the Americas region in 2015, 86 percent had laws prohibiting smoking in public, and 72 percent had taxes on tobacco products. Of the ten states-parties to the FCTC in the WHO South-East Asia region in 2015, 80 percent had taxes on tobacco, and 100 percent had bans on public smoking (WHO 2014c, 2015g).

Despite support from the Bloomberg Initiative and Gates Foundation to advocate for passage and implementation of tobacco control policies in Africa, states have been relatively slow to respond, particularly in countries like Tanzania and Uganda, where tobacco is grown. In Tanzania, for example, the parliament has been unwilling to pass legislation that taxes tobacco products or requires warning labels that cover at least 30 percent of the product packaging. In fact, when the Tanzanian Cigarette Company (owned by Japan Tobacco International) exports to Rwanda, the Democratic Republic of Congo, and Burundi, it must use larger warning labels on its packaging. The hesitancy to pass strong tobacco control legislation reflects the fact that some Tanzanian legislators own large tobacco farms, that tobacco production has been framed as a "job creator" and "national industry," and that the transnational tobacco companies have intensely lobbied the legislature and ministry of health (interviews, tobacco control advocates, Dar es Salaam,

July 4, 2015, and July 9, 2015; TTCF 2012). Throughout Africa, the global region where smoking prevalence is increasing the fastest, tobacco companies engage in corporate social responsibility activities, such as community development and education projects, environmental education, and even disease prevention programs such as providing funding to AIDS organizations in order to build societal goodwill (Drope 2011; Smith, Thompson, and Lee 2016; McDaniel, Cadman, and Malone 2016). In other countries, tobacco companies offer to write legislation or regulations, they fund African academics to conduct research that advances the companies' interests, and they use rumors to insinuate that tobacco regulators are corrupt. Some respondents also reported that tobacco companies engage in outright corruption, "buying off" legislators to hinder legislation or ministry of health officials to stall implementation (informal conversation, Kenyan health activist, Cape Town, August 8, 2014; interviews, tobacco control advocates, Lusaka, Dar es Salaam, and Accra, June 13, 2014, July 4, 2015, July 9, 2015, and April 6, 2017; phone interviews, transnational tobacco control advocates, April 27, 2017, and May 5, 2017).

Yet just because states have passed legislation does not mean that they have implemented it. In Zambia, tobacco control policy has been relegated to the ministry of health, a "silo" ministry with little political clout, instead of the state adopting a high-level multisectoral approach as it did with AIDS (interview, advocate on NCDs, Zambia, June 13, 2014; see also Alleyne and Nishtar 2014). The ministry's weakness makes it more difficult to implement the law against smoking in public, though reasons for the limited implementation are complicated, as the following speaker shows:

> [We have had this law against smoking in public places since 2007] but we did this survey and 87 percent of people say they still see people smoking in all public places, including in offices . . . People are aware of the smoking ban and [even smokers] say they don't want smoking in public places. . . . So why is it not being implemented? It is a lack of political will and public will. We are very polite people. If you pick up a cigarette and say, "Do you mind if I smoke?" I will just say, "Oh no! It's okay." . . . People are unaware of the real dangers. (Interview, tobacco control advocate, Lusaka, June 13, 2014)

Because the government does not have the capacity to police public places, it must rely heavily on public education and support to limit smoking. Yet to gain that support, the public must be educated and mobilized, a process that demands political will and public monies.

A final point about African state commitment to NCDs is that responses to these diseases receive few financial resources. Historically the continent's health-care systems have focused on communicable diseases, and roughly 80 percent of spending goes for such conditions (de-Graft Aikins et al. 2010). Interviewees confirmed this situation: "There is no money for cancer control" (interview, advocate on NCDs, Lusaka, June 12, 2014); "We are only now [in 2015] starting to draw up a budget for NCDs" (interview, advocate for NCDs, Dar es Salaam, July 9, 2015); and "African countries just have so little money for these problems" (interview, global advocate on NCDs, October 9, 2015).

However, the picture about funding is complicated. During their speeches at the 2011 High-Level Meeting, fifteen African representatives (or 31 percent of all African states) discussed national funding mechanisms, though only the Tanzanian representative mentioned the specific amount of $2.5 million for disease surveillance programs (UNGA 2011a, 2011b, 2011c, 2011d, 2011f, and 2011g; NCD Alliance 2011). In the 2010 WHO country reports, 56 percent of the region (twenty-seven states) reported providing some state funds for treatment and control of NCDs, and 60 percent (twenty-nine states) reported funding prevention programs (WHO 2011b). These claims provided no information on funding amounts or specific prevention and treatment priorities, and the obtuseness or unavailability of most government health budgets prevents clarification. Most likely, as a resource-strapped region where NCDs are not high on the public agenda, most African states have devoted few funds to NCDs. Or, as in the case of Ghana, they have sought to redirect funds from some communicable disease to address NCDs. For example, in its 2011 strategic plan on NCDs, the Ghanaian government proposed to use funds for TB for education on the dangers of smoking and to devote some malaria funding to public education on childhood asthma (Ministry of Health 2011). Despite these proposals, informants in 2017 said there remained little money to address these health conditions (interviews, NGO health-care system administrator and expert on NCDs, Accra, April 18, 2017, and May 4, 2017).

In summary, while the region's participation in global health governance on NCDs varies with the state, overall, Africa lags behind in its adoption of many global policies and structures. However, African states have not challenged global health governance on NCDs. They have not denied the existence of NCDs or explicitly blamed people with these health conditions, as many African states did early in the AIDS pandemic. They have not challenged WHO policy recommendations, as half of African states did with travel restrictions during the Ebola outbreak, or as Liberia did with its efforts to shape the narrative around and response toward the outbreak. Rather, African states seem to be biding their time to see what happens on this health issue at the societal and global levels. As such, they remain ambivalent to, though, as indicated by their participation in the 2011 High-Level Meeting, not always inactive in, the global health governance of NCDs.

Explanations for African State Actions

The international, state, and societal levels of analysis provide reasons for this ambivalence. The underdevelopment of global institutions and funding, coupled with competing frames, did not urge African states to accept governance, though the incoherence and inconsistencies created spaces for what James Scott (1990) terms "performances of compliance" and what Jean-Francois Bayart (2000) calls "extraversion." (See chapter 1 on extraversion.) Additionally, unlike with the early days of AIDS or the Ebola outbreak, neither NCDs nor the lackluster global policies to address them challenged African aspirational identities. At the state level, democratic governance did not push states to adopt policies, because NCDs lack clear constituencies or high public salience (see below). Neopatrimonial goals did not encourage states to develop institutions and policies because there were few resources to be gained. Civil society mobilization has had little impact on state actions because few advocacy groups on NCDs have resources and political traction. The result is that for the vast majority of states, the pattern is ambivalence; even states with policies on NCDs are slow in implementation. Most states hedge their bets for the future, when donors may inject resources into this health challenge and civil society groups may effectively exert pressure. At that point, global health governance will help neopatrimonial states to bolster their ruling networks and links to civil society, patterns that ultimately increase state legitimacy and advance policy outcomes.

The International Level: Unclear Commitments Create Room for Agency

The ambiguity of global health governance on NCDs created space in which African actors could reframe the issue, utilize extraversion, and engage in performances of compliance. All three of these approaches were evident in the speeches given by African leaders at the 2011 High-Level Meeting (UNGA 2011a, 2011b, 2011c, 2011d, 2011f, and 2011g). States sought to reframe the issue in two ways. In the first, several speakers wanted to expand the focus on NCDs from just cancer, cardiovascular disease, diabetes, and chronic respiratory diseases to include sickle cell anemia, motor vehicle accidents, and mental health (UNGA 2011a, 2011b, 2011c, 2011d, 2011f, 2011g; see also Mensah and Mayosi 2013). The second effort prioritized the human right to health and medication access over neoliberal trade agreements. Along with many other low- and middle-income states, African states had a view "sharply at odds with the majority of donors (such as the United States and the EU), [because they] focused on the need to change trade rules to enable LMICs [low- and middle-income countries] to gain improved access to the essential medicines required to treat NCDs" (Sturchio and Galambos 2014, 9). Similar flexibilities in trade agreements had facilitated access to generic ARVs in the global AIDS response.

Many speeches could be viewed as tools of extraversion because they emphasized Africa's poverty and low health-care capacity, as well as wealthy countries' obligation to assist these states (Bayart 2000; Harris and Siplon 2006). The Rwandan delegate reminded donor countries that global cooperation was possible on health: "Let us not forget what happened in this very hall 10 years ago during the 2001 UN Special Session on HIV/AIDS. That meeting fundamentally changed the way that HIV was fought in developing countries" (UNGA 2011c, 11). In the process, state officials sought to frame NCDs as a "social justice and equity issue in the same way HIV/AIDS is an equity issue" (phone interview, global advocate on NCDs, October 9, 2015). Among others, Namibia pointed to the ways that NCDs undermine development ("We are concerned about the impact of these diseases on the lives of our people, the socio-economic development of our country"), and several states played up the misperception that combatting NCDs requires large amounts of money (UNGA 2011f, 14; see Bollyky 2012 on low-cost policies to address NCDs). Twelve African leaders stressed poverty and the need for external assistance: Mozambique's health minister said, "[We] cannot treat these new diseases, which are chronic and extremely costly," while President Robert Mugabe of Zimbabwe said that "developed countries need to make concrete commitments . . . to this scourge" (UNGA 2011g, 4). Several bemoaned the fact that they could not implement policies on these health problems because of a "lack of human, material and financial resources." As a result, as the representative from Central African Republic said, "The international community [needs] to mobilize resources . . . to ensure that we save many lives" (UNGA 2011g, 5). Many African leaders wanted new funding structures that resembled global AIDS institutions. Yet they had to be careful that they did not push the idea of a global fund for NCDs too far, since doing so might lead donors to decrease their AIDS funding, an outcome no

African state official wanted (phone interview, global advocate on NCDs, October 9, 2015).

In addition to being tools for extraversion, the speeches provided an opportunity for performances of compliance, or speech acts in which weaker players go along with hegemonic discourses in order to protect themselves or to gain specific benefits from powerful actors (J. Scott 1990, 108). Eighteen leaders repeated statistics on cancer, diabetes, cardiovascular diseases, and/or tobacco use in their countries; while relatively dull and impersonal, the recitation of data seemed to be aimed at demonstrating to donors these leaders' awareness of and concern for the issue. (Leaders also were performing for home audiences, trying to educate them about these issues.) In these performances, twenty-one African leaders also spoke of their "political commitment to NCDs" or "the political priority of NCDs." These terms have become buzzwords in global health governance, since donors have recognized the need for high-level political attention (or "political will") to address health issues, particularly in contexts like Africa where executives are crucial for policymaking and implementation (Lieberman 2012). One advocate on NCDs from Tanzania summed up African state leaders' engagement in these performances: "These high-level meetings are just a chance for the politicians to talk and get attention. But if you look at what they sign, what they agree to, at the country level, there is nothing. They are just politicizing the issue" (interview, advocate on NCDs, Dar es Salaam, July 9, 2015).

William Brown (2012) asserts that African agentic actions are shaped by "external conditions [with] the possibility for agency." The High-Level Meeting provided a unique global arena ripe for attention grabbing and credit claiming with domestic and donor audiences. For African states, the cost of agency was quite low. Domestic populations had little knowledge about the diseases and, most likely, the UN meeting, so they had no expectations of leaders. And since donors have done little on NCDs, African leaders' performances could not undermine existing aid programs. The forum of the United Nations, with its emphasis on state sovereignty and legal equality of all member states, provided the opportunity for African leaders to speak freely (Brown and Harman 2013; Englebert 2009). And while the interconnected processes of global health governance have weakened African state sovereignty in some areas, such as domestic health-care financing (see Kirton, Cooper, Lisk, and Besada 2014), in the context of NCDs, African states used their sovereignty to urge global action while engaging in very little action themselves. The weakness of global institutions, their lack of funding, and tensions among frames facilitated this ambivalence.

The State Level: Ambivalence in Divergent Contexts

Ambivalence toward global health governance on NCDs is evident both within states—they adopted some but not all policies, or they partially implemented adopted policies—and across the region—some states adopted more policies than other states did. Here I use four country case studies to illustrate ambivalence within states' implementation as well as the complexity of factors that drive action. I use countries that differ in the state-level characteristics of regime type, neopatrimonialism, disease severity, and income level to show how global health governance on NCDs is contextually situated. Each of these countries has accepted a majority of WHO Global Action Plan indicators, but, except for the case of South Africa, all continue to face hurdles in implementation. I then present an aggregate-level analysis that confirms these murky patterns.

I first hypothesize that democracy will correlate with more state actions on NCDs, because leaders in democracies must be responsive to citizens' demands for social welfare (Patterson 2006; Strand 2012; Sen 2001). Democratic states should be more likely to act than autocratic states. This statement assumes, though, that there is an identifiable constituency for policies on NCDs and that people find NCDs to be politically salient. (As illustrated below, these two conditions are not always met.) I distinguish a country's regime type using Polity IV classifications and Freedom House reports (see chapter 2; Marshall and Cole 2014).

Second, I predict that neopatrimonial states will not implement policies on NCDs because such states tend to have weak capacity, shortages in health-care personnel, some level of corruption, and political manipulation of the civil service (van de Walle 2001; Englebert 2009; Beresford 2015; Bates 1981). Because donors give few resources for NCDs, I do not argue that neopatrimonialism will lead states to adopt policies to get external resources, though some of the cases below do illustrate how donor actions condition state interests (Callaghy 1988; Clapham 1996; Bayart 1993; Kelsall 2011). I assume that because of their weak capacity, political manipulation, and mismanagement, neopatrimonial states will be less effective in governance, as indicated by a World Bank (2015d) government effectiveness score that is lower than the regional average of twenty-six (on a scale of 0 to 100, with 100 being most effective).

Third, I maintain that disease severity will lead a country to act on NCDs. As chapter 1 showed, some states began to address AIDS once the magnitude of the pandemic became evident. However, as chapter 2 demonstrated, states with both high and low HIV rates have now accepted global AIDS governance. To measure severity, I look at the percentage of a country's deaths attributed to NCDs (WHO 2011b, 2014b). I hypothesize that countries with rates higher than the regional average of 33 percent will enact policies on NCDs. Disease severity percentages range from a high of 85 percent for Mauritius to a low of 19 percent in Somalia (WHO 2011d, 2014d).

Fourth, because of the perception that addressing NCDs is costly, I argue that countries with higher income levels will be more likely to accept global health governance around these diseases. I classify countries using the World Bank's categories of low-income (GDI/capita of $1,045 or less); lower-middle income (GDI/capita of between $1,046 and $4,125); upper-middle income (GDI/capita of $4,126 to $12,745); and high-income (GDI/capita above $12,745). In 2015, twenty-seven African states were classified as low-income, fourteen were lower-middle income, and seven were upper-middle income (World Bank 2015a). I assume that upper-middle or lower-middle–income level countries will be more likely to act on NCDs than low-income countries.

As the first case study, South Africa supports these hypotheses. Heralded for its actions on NCDs, the country has implemented all Global Action Plan indicators (WHO 2011b). It has a department that works on NCDs in its ministry of health; funding for treatment, prevention, and surveillance of NCDs; systems for reporting on morbidity, mortality, and risk factors associated with NCDs; and policies on physical activity, tobacco use, alcohol use, healthy diet, and the four major NCDs (interview, multilateral donor official, New York, October 1, 2015; phone interview, global advocate on NCDs, October 9, 2015; see also Stefan et al. 2013; Kayima et al. 2013). It has developed a National Health Commission with civil society representation to manage activities on NCDs. And it has begun to integrate its programs on AIDS and its programs on NCDs in order to "maximize synergies" (WHO 2011b; phone interview, South African government official, October 13, 2015). It has been praised for its strong tobacco control legislation as well as its 2017 implementation of a tax on sugary beverages (WHO 2017). The country's activities are situated within a democratic context in which civil society organizations have mobilized to promote social development, health, and human rights (Patterson and Kuperus 2016; Johnson 2006; Lodge 2003). While corruption and neopatrimonialism do exist (Beresford 2015; Lodge 2014), its government effectiveness score is 65.4, well above the regional average (World Bank 2015a). Thus, it has relatively efficient institutions for implementing health policies. It also has an incentive to respond: 43 percent of deaths in South Africa result from NCDs (WHO 2011b). As an upper-middle income country, South Africa has resources to spend on NCDs.

Ghana presents a mixed picture, having adopted five of nine Global Action Plan indicators (WHO 2014a). The country passed tobacco control legislation in 2012 as part of its Public Health Act (though no laws on illicit trade in tobacco) and a national strategy on NCDs (on tobacco trade, see *GhanaWeb*, June 12, 2015). It has operational strategies on alcohol use, tobacco control, physical activity, and nutrition (WHO 2014b). In 2014, Ghana launched a public-private partnership with three pharmaceutical companies (Sanofi Associates, MSD, and Pfizer) to provide needed medications for diabetes and hypertension (*Daily Graphic*, March 27, 2014). A visitor to Ghana can see evidence of the country's efforts, particularly in terms of the promotion of physical activity and tobacco control. Tobacco advertisements are difficult to find, and in urban, elite areas, people engage in exercise and talk about healthy diets (personal observations of health-related behaviors, Accra, January–May 2017). Yet many policy challenges remain. Most care for people with NCDs occurs at the tertiary level, and community-level education about diabetes and cardiovascular diseases is limited. The national health insurance scheme requires out-of-pocket payments for many medications related to NCDs (such as cancer treatment and mental illness), making the health maintenance that many patients with NCDs require unaffordable. The widely praised Community-Based Health Planning and Services program has improved maternal and child health but done little to address NCDs at the local level (Ofori-Asenso and Garcia 2016; interviews, expert on NCDs and mental health expert, Accra, May 4, 2017, and May 18, 2017). And, as mentioned above, government funding remains inadequate for programs to prevent NCDs.

Several factors push Ghana's actions: It is a strong democracy, with highly competitive elections, an independent media, and citizens who increasingly demand accountability (Freedom House 2016a). With 42 percent of the country's deaths attributed to NCDs (WHO 2014b), the country has an incentive to adopt strong policies. Ghana is a lower-middle–income country with some resources for programs on NCDs (World Bank 2015a, 2015d). And it is less neopatrimonial than many states (its effectiveness score is 44.2), a fact that facilitates policy implementation. It also has a growing epistemic community situated at the University of Ghana–Legon that has conducted evidence-based research on multiple NCDs, government policies, and societal attitudes and behaviors related to the prevention, control, and treatment of NCDs (See Agyei-Mensah and de-Graft Aikins 2010; Ofori-Asenso and Garcia 2016; de-Graft Aikins, Anum, and Ogedegbe 2012). Despite these factors, why does Ghana continue to face some hurdles in policy implementation? One clue lies in the fact that donors have focused on malaria, maternal mortality, TB, and AIDS, not NCDs. They have only recently added health-system strengthening to their activities. Ghana, which relies on external funding for its health programs and which since 2003 has experienced a massive increase in the number of donors that work in the health sector, finds it difficult to ignore donors' priorities and to address both communicable and noncommunicable diseases (USAID 2015; Pallas, Nonvignon, Aikins, and Ruger 2015; interview, bilateral donor, Accra, May 18, 2017).

Zambia resembles Ghana in its partial implementation of agreed-upon policies on NCDs, though some of the reasons for this outcome are different. The country has adopted six of nine Global Action Plan indicators. It has a department to address NCDs in the ministry of health, operational plans for alcohol use, tobacco control, physical activity, and nutrition, and guidelines for managing NCDs through the primary health-care system (WHO 2014b). Its 2011–2015 National Health Strategic Plan considered NCDs to be a health priority. Yet, as in Ghana, most care for NCDs occurs at the tertiary level; there is little data on NCDs; and health-care workers have almost no training in the education and monitoring of NCDs. It was only in 2012 that the government began to train community health assistants in the screening of hypertension and diabetes. Similarly, while the country has tobacco control legislation, it needs to strengthen provisions for labeling and increase taxes on tobacco products (University of Zambia, Ministry of Health, and University of Waterloo 2014). Zambia's efforts on NCDs have suffered from a "lack of clarity at the policy level" (Aantjes, Quinlan, and Bunders 2014; see also Oelke et al. 2015).

Several factors have pushed the country to act on NCDs. Zambia is a lower-middle–income country with more resources than many states; it is a partial democracy with competitive elections and some level of governmental accountability (Freedom House 2016c; *AllAfrica.com*, September 18, 2013; Simutanyi 2013). It also is home to one of the most politically powerful nongovernmental health-care organizations in Africa. The Churches Health Association of Zambia (CHAZ) administers almost half of Zambia's health-care services; it has received millions from donors for AIDS, TB, and malaria; and it has substantial influence over government health policies (Patterson 2011; see also informal conversation, international NGO official, Accra, February 4, 2017). Sadly, Zambia also has experienced the deaths from NCDs of several high-level leaders: one sitting president (Levi Mwanawasa) suffered a stroke and died in 2008; one sitting president (Michael Sata) died in 2014 after a heart attack; one former president (Frederick Chiluba) died of a heart attack in 2011; and there were rumors in early 2015 that the current president, Edgar Lungu, had kidney disease (*Telegraph*, January 20, 2015; *Lusaka Times*, December 31, 2014; *AllAfrica.com*, November 23, 2014).[8] Thus, the country's ruling elites are particularly sensitive about NCDs.

Zambia illustrates how leaders can influence policy adoption, particularly in contexts with unclear norms, weak global institutions, little social mobilization (see below), and weak government ministries (Rotberg 2012). As one donor official explained:

> I have found that for the African countries, they may have interest in a health issue for a while, and then they will drop out and disappear on the issue for five or six years. It is really like they have personalized the issue and thus, for that one person who was the spokesperson and for that short time, it is on the agenda. And they will play an important part on it. But then the next thing you know, you are calling the Ministry of Health and find that they have no one who knows anything about the issue, so there is no one there you can mobilize, you can work with. (Interview, multilateral donor official, New York, October 1, 2015)

The speaker highlights the negative effects of leadership-centered decision-making, particularly as an obstacle to policy continuity. But leaders also can urge countries to act when bureaucratic institutions or civil society organizations do not exert such pressures.

While leadership, advocacy by CHAZ, and state capacity drove Zambia's actions on NCDs, two factors created obstacles for full policy implementation. Unlike Ghana and South Africa, where over 40 percent of deaths result from NCDs, in Zambia this number is 23 percent (WHO 2014b). AIDS remains a top cause of mortality, with 14 percent of Zambians between fifteen and forty-nine years old living with HIV (WHO 2015i). Zambia's neopatrimonial state has benefited from donor AIDS programs that have given almost $1 billion to the country since 2003. The entrenched nature of AIDS programs—and the neopatrimonial benefits they bring to a state with a World Bank governance effectiveness score of 38.28—discourages action on NCDs (World Bank 2015d; on corruption in Zambia's donor programs, see Patterson 2015; Anderson and Patterson 2017). Because of "limited interest by donor agencies" in incorporating NCDs into Zambia's AIDS efforts, and because of Zambia's long-standing positive relationship with donors (Barnes, Brown, and Harman 2015), the state fears the loss of donor funds if it acts on NCDs (Aantjes, Quinland, and Bunders 2014). Donors themselves seem to be only interested in NCDs such as cervical cancer that are linked to AIDS (CDC 2015d). Even CHAZ has benefited immensely from donor-funded AIDS programs, a fact that tempers its advocacy for policies on NCDs (Patterson 2011). As one donor official stated, leaders become content with the patronage resources that AIDS generates and do not wish to jeopardize those programs for activities on NCDs (interview, multilateral donor official, Kampala, June 30, 2014).

The final country I examine is Eritrea. The country has adopted six of nine Global Action Plan indicators.[9] It has an operational department to address NCDs in the ministry of health, a national strategy on NCDs, and operational plans to combat alcohol use, tobacco use, physical inactivity, and nutrition (WHO 2014b). It provides free medications and diagnostic tests for NCDs through its primary health-care system. But the country is not a state-party to the FCTC, and even though its national tobacco control plan limits advertising and levies moderate taxes on tobacco products, the country also has weak laws to limit smoking in public places (WHO 2015k). Health-care centers often lack medications for diabetes, stroke prevention, and hypertension, and there is a shortage of personnel needed to treat NCDs (Mendis et al. 2012; Dalal et al. 2011).

Several state-level factors prevent Eritrea from doing more on NCDs. First, Eritrea is a low-income country with limited resources to act on NCDs. Second, it lacks any semblance of democratic accountability and responsiveness. As a highly repressive state, the country has not held elections since 1993; civil liberties are almost nonexistent; and as of 2016, thousands of Eritreans each week tried to migrate to escape persecution (Plaut 2016; UN Human Rights Council 2015). Third, the country is highly neopatrimonial (with a World Bank effectiveness score of just 13.88), a fact that undermines policy implementation. Fourth, while it has two civil society groups working on NCDs, its repressive political climate makes it unlikely that these groups have much influence in policymaking. Finally, the country has few ties to donors except Arab states, and even Saudi Arabia and Qatar have given little aid to the country (See AidData 2016). Unlike in Zambia (or to a lesser extent Ghana), donor programs do not condition state health policies.

Yet Eritrea has some attributes that push its actions on NCDs. The country's authoritarian president, Isaias Afwerki, has a long time horizon, because the state's repressive power and the country's lack of elections mean there is little chance that he will be ousted anytime soon. In the context of AIDS, Kim Dionne (2011) found that African leaders with long time horizons were more likely than executives with short time horizons to allocate budgetary resources to AIDS. Long time horizons are particularly important for actions on NCDs, since these chronic diseases often have long durations. A long time horizon empowers President Afwerki to act on a severe health issue: 37 percent of deaths in Eritrea result from NCDs. In addition, Eritrea is a developmental authoritarian state, or one in which the state has a "longstanding and genuine" commitment to socioeconomic improvement but also staunchly insists on autonomous control of its development processes. Developmental authoritarianism has led the country to improve health indicators, such as maternal mortality rates (Wrong 2006; Africa Research Institute 2011; see Matfess 2015 on developmental authoritarianism).

South Africa, Ghana, Zambia, and Eritrea illustrate the complicated and inconclusive relationship between, on the one hand, state-level characteristics like democracy, state capacity, neopatrimonialism, and disease burden and, on the other hand, the adoption and implementation of actions on NCDs. These cases show that country-level factors matter: democracy, disease burden, and state resources in South Africa; disease burden and epistemic community in Ghana; leadership and donor priorities in Zambia; and developmental authoritarianism in Eritrea. Does an aggregate-level analysis demonstrate any relation between these state-level factors and policy implementation on NCDs? To investigate this question, I use states' reported adoption of the nine indicators listed in the Global Action Plan on NCDs. I then classify states into three categories: high policy adopters (states that have adopted six or more indicators), low policy adopters (states that have adopted one to five policies), and zero policy adopters (states that have adopted no indicators). I divide states into these categories because if states adopted any policies, they tended to adopt more than more than one. (For example, a national strategy on NCDs often included an operational plan on tobacco control, physical activity, nutrition, or alcohol control.) However, adoption of more than five indicators demonstrated commitment to the issue.

As table 4.3 shows, 16 percent of reporting democracies (four of twenty-four states) and 13 percent of reporting autocracies (two of fifteen states) adopted six or more policies. Regime type did not correlate with high levels of activities on NCDs. However, among states with between one and five indicators, autocracies did better: 67 percent of reporting autocracies (or ten of fifteen states) claimed to have at least one policy compared to 38 percent of democracies. Additionally, the percentage of democratic states that were zero policy adopters was over twice the percentage of autocratic states in that category. These results show that regime type had an ambiguous effect on policy implementation. In terms of neopatrimonialism, of the twenty-six states that had a government effectiveness score below the

TABLE 4.3 Adopters of Policies on NCDs by State Characteristics for Reporting States

Policy adoption	Percentage of democracies (N=24)	Percentage of autocracies (N=15)	Percentage of low-income* states (N=21)	Percentage of lower-middle-income states (N=12)	Percentage of upper-middle-income states (N=6)	Percentage of states below region's govt. effectiveness score** (N=26)	Percentage of states with disease severity above regional mean*** (N=18)
High policy adopter (6 or more indicators)	16	13	24	8	0****	15	21
Low policy adopter (1–5 indicators)	38	67	33	67	67	46	43
Zero policy adopter (0 indicators)	46	20	43	25	33	38	36

Source: Compiled by author from WHO 2011b, 2014b; World Bank 2015a, 2015d; Marshall and Cole 2014.

Note: N = 39 states with reports to the WHO in 2013.

* Low-income countries have a GDI/capita of $1,045 or less; lower-middle–income countries have a GDI/capita of between $1,046 and $4,125; upper-middle–income countries have a GDI/capita of $4,126 to $12,745; and high-income countries have a GDI/capita above $12,745 (World Bank 2015a).

** The average government effectiveness score for Africa is 26 on a scale of 1 to 100. Lower numbers indicate less effectiveness, as measured by corruption and state capacity indicators (see World Bank 2015d).

*** The average percentage of deaths caused by NCDs for the region is 33 (WHO 2011b, 2014b).

**** South Africa fits into this category, based on its responses to the WHO 2010 survey (see WHO 2011b).

region's average, only 15 percent were high policy adopters. In contrast, 46 percent were low adopters, and 38 percent were zero policy adopters. Using this measure, neopatrimonialism relates to foot dragging in policy implementation, perhaps because ineffective states face personnel shortages, corruption, and bureaucratic red tape.

In addition, state income level does not relate to policy adoption. Sixty-seven percent of lower-middle–income countries and 67 percent of upper-middle–income countries were low policy adopters. If we just examine low-income countries, they are more equally divided into the categories, though Togo, Eritrea, Mozambique, Guinea, Madagascar, and Côte d'Ivoire adopted six or more policy indicators. The fact that low-income African countries have adopted some policies on NCDs challenges African states' insistence at the 2011 High-Level Meeting that they needed external resources in order to act. Their extraversion seems to indicate that access to donor resources is crucial to facilitate policy action not necessarily because resources are essential but because resources enable the state to reward agencies and civil society groups and to shore up its legitimacy. As chapter 2 shows, these outcomes facilitate the acceptance of global health governance on AIDS (Hunsmann 2012). Some African leaders argued that without strong global support, state officials will face "competing interests" in the implementation of global health governance on NCDs (UNGA 2011c, 15).

Finally, there was no pattern in terms of disease burden: 21 percent of states with a high disease burden from NCDs were high policy adopters, while 43 percent were low policy adopters and 36 percent were zero policy adopters. Thus, despite the South African and Ghanaian cases, high levels of policy adoption do not always correlate with disease burden. The upshot is that regime type, neopatrimonialism, country income, and disease severity drive actions for individual states, but these factors do not fully explain ambivalence to global health governance on NCDs.

The Societal Level: Weak, Disengaged, and Misunderstood

Chapter 2 illustrated how civil society mobilization on AIDS at both the national and international levels challenged African states and donors to develop AIDS institutions that were situated around coherent issue frames and that provided substantial funding (Smith and Siplon 2006). Once the AIDS response was institutionalized, civil society groups became incorporated into the response, a fact that helped to legitimate states' continued involvement on AIDS. Chapter 3 illustrated how in Liberia, civil society groups with deep legitimacy and societal trust pushed the government to challenge global health governance patterns that downplayed traditions or undermined societal autonomy. In the case of NCDs, African civil society has been relatively disengaged from the issue. The few groups that work on NCDs face resource limitations, internal divisions, societal misunderstandings about these diseases, and competition with AIDS groups.

To begin, in Africa there are relatively few organizations that work on NCDs. The figure below shows the percentage of countries with various numbers of groups (0–3 groups, 4–6 groups, 7–9 groups, and 10 or more groups). To determine the number of organizations in each country, I looked at the NCD Alliance list of country affiliates. While not all groups in a country belong to the NCD Alliance, a large majority do. This membership list provided the most comprehensive and comparative set of organizational data on mobilization around NCDs. The figure illustrates that 67 percent of African states (thirty-three states) have between zero and three such groups. Nine states have no groups. Twelve percent of states (six states) have four to six groups; 14 percent (seven states) have seven to nine groups; and only 6 percent (three states) have ten or more groups.[10] On one hand, more groups could show the saliency of NCDs to state officials and donors, provide strong representation, and potentially increase opportunities for resource generation. One global health official remarked: "If we only had some social mobilization, it would help in getting government attention" (interview, multilateral donor official, New York, October 1, 2015). Indeed, a few states with actions on NCDs, such as Ghana, South Africa, and Togo, do have several active advocacy organizations. On the other hand, multiple groups that advocate on NCDs could face competition for resources and attention as well as problems in coordinating advocacy efforts (interviews, advocate on NCDs, Kampala, June 19, 2014; tobacco control advocate, Dar es Salaam, July 9, 2015; expert on NCDs, Accra, May 4, 2017). The result could be limited influence on policy. For example, Nigeria and Kenya have numerous advocacy groups but have adopted few aspects of global health governance on NCDs.

Groups that mobilize around NCDs face particular challenges that undermine their ability to push African states to accept global health governance on NCDs. While many African groups have transnational advocacy linkages, the global movement on NCDs faces its own obstacles which, in turn, limit African advocacy. At the international level, some groups have been excluded from policymaking. In the case of the 2011 High-Level Meeting, China, Cuba, and Venezuela prevented the participation of some advocates, effectively limiting their influence on the Political Declaration (phone interview, global advocate on NCDs, October 9, 2015). But the movement faces more than just exclusion from decision-making venues. Unlike

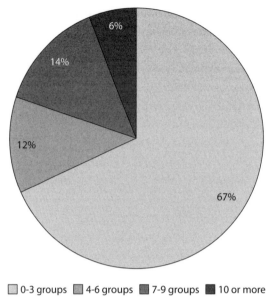

□ 0-3 groups ■ 4-6 groups ■ 7-9 groups ■ 10 or more

Figure 4.1. Percentage of African States with Select Number of NCD Groups.
Note: N = 40 states. *Source:* Compiled by author from NCD Alliance 2014c.

with AIDS mobilization in which people living with HIV have been crucial activists, there are few patient organizations to push an aggressive agenda, including a human rights frame (Bollyky 2012; on AIDS see Siplon 2002; J. Chan 2015; Gould 2009). In addition, because NCDs are a collection of diseases, the issue's complexity has led to divisions among disease groups (Editorial Board 2011; Bollyky 2012). For example, cancer groups have been more vocal and organized than diabetes groups, with cervical and breast cancer getting attention from the Forum of African First Ladies and the Pink Ribbon-Red Ribbon Initiative, an organization established in 2011 by the George W. Bush Institute (Parkhurst and Vulimiri 2013; Pink Ribbon-Red Ribbon 2016). Advocates for the four major NCDs of cancers, cardiovascular diseases, diabetes, and chronic respiratory diseases have been hesitant to include mental health in their advocacy, with the issue omitted from the 2011 High-Level Meeting (Tomlinson and Lund 2012). Some organizations that work on NCDs lack focus, wanting everything from prevention programs to treatment access. Some have worked with the food, beverage, and pharmaceutical industries, while others have not (Sturchio and Galambos 2014, 8). And unlike with AIDS, the epistemic community has been divided about aspects of the campaign against NCDs, including levels of safe alcohol use, appropriate levels of salt and sugar intake, and the level of health risk that electronic cigarettes pose (Sturchio and Galambos 2014; Schmitz 2015; Maron 2014; Barraclough 2009; Britton et al. 2016). The lack of consensus undermines advocates' efforts.

Resources and capacity are problematic for most advocates on NCDs. All of the group representatives I interviewed in Tanzania, Uganda, Zambia, Ghana, and the United States said funding was the biggest challenge they faced. Advocates mentioned the lack of money to pay for office space, phones, transportation to meetings, conference attendance, staff, workshops, photocopies, and health education messages on radio or billboards. Many advocates in Africa were not full-time employees of their organization: they were health-care workers, educators, spouses of middle- or upper-class professionals, and (in a few cases) disease survivors; most worked on NCDs in addition to having other family and job obligations. To gain resources, many groups depended heavily on international donors like WHO and transnational NGOs such as the American Cancer Society. This dependence led them to align their concerns with those of donors, "because you have to do that to get funding" (interview, advocate on NCDs, Kampala, June 26, 2014). But dependence also had the potential to delegitimize the local organization (Michael 2004), something that was particularly a problem for tobacco control groups. Because of the large sums from the Bloomberg Initiative and Gates Foundation to low-income countries to help with FCTC implementation and adjudication, tobacco control groups tend to be the most organized and best-funded groups working on NCDs in Africa (*Guardian*, March 19, 2015; Bollyky and Fidler 2015). One respondent explained how this situation created problems in advocacy:

> Anti-tobacco groups are seen as "outsiders," that they are a movement started in the United States that has just been exported to Africa. So if we are linked to this movement, then we are portrayed as just trying to stir up a problem when there really isn't one. People look around and see that tobacco users are surviving. . . . So they ask, "What is the problem? Who is lying to us? The government or you tobacco control NGOs with your foreign backing?" (Interview, tobacco control advocate, Dar es Salaam, July 4, 2015)

As the interviewee points out, when the government portrays tobacco use as a way of life and not as a health risk, people are hesitant to believe outsiders. Even scientific studies on the risks of tobacco use do not align with the population's observations. When African organizations seek linkages to global advocates, they have to be careful that those relationships do not undermine their own legitimacy (phone interview, transnational tobacco control advocate, April 27, 2017).

The lack of resources and the small number of groups mean that African organizations that work on NCDs have been somewhat disengaged from policy advocacy. According to a 2014 survey, 40 percent of the member organizations of NCD Alliance focus on service provision, not advocacy (NCD Alliance 2014a). The Zambian Cancer Society, for example, only began community awareness programs in 2014; it initially focused on treatment and palliative care (interview, advocate on NCDs, Lusaka, June 12, 2014). One respondent said, "We know we need to be working in the community to educate, but we are only at the clinic, supporting the patients. . . . There are just too many things for us to do" (interview, advocate on NCDs, Dodoma, July 2, 2015). This is not to say there is no advocacy: In Angola, tobacco control groups effectively urged the government to limit advertising, with "the tobacco industry giving in so it could look good" (interview, tobacco control advocate, Dar es Salaam, July 4, 2015). Ghanaian groups have been relatively active educating about hypertension and diabetes (PLOS Blogs 2014) and advocating for passage of the 2012 Mental Health Act (interview, mental health expert, Accra, May 18, 2017), and in South Africa, civil society has collaborated with government to write policies in the National Health Commission (phone interview, South African government official, October 13, 2015). At the global level, African civil society mobilization on NCDs was also more apparent at the 2014 High-Level Review that examined progress after the 2011 meeting. For example, Ugandan faith-based service providers participated in Africa-wide discussions that informed the 2014 meeting agenda (interview, FBO health director, Kampala, June 19, 2014). But even then such advocacy has often been done by health-care providers, not activist or patient organizations.

The efforts of these health organizations in Africa are situated in a context in which NCDs, and health more broadly, have low political saliency. An Afrobarometer survey (2012) found that only 5 percent of people in twenty-seven countries said that health should be government's top priority, compared to 20 percent who named unemployment. Even for AIDS, a health problem that has received great media attention and donor funding, few prioritized the disease. (The number was 0 percent.) The lack of resources makes it hard for advocates on NCDs to do the type of community mobilization that is needed to make these diseases politically salient. One interviewee explained: "If we had greater resources to mobilize society, then I think that the grassroots would also be pushing for this

NCD agenda—things like access to drugs and health care. There would be pressure from below" (interview, advocate on NCDs, Kampala, June 26, 2014). Resources facilitate local mobilization, education, and interest, all of which push the state to respond.

Part of the low saliency of NCDs relates to the stigma linked to some of these diseases. While some health-care providers said there was no stigma against most NCDs (interviews, physicians, Dodoma, Dar es Salaam, and Accra, July 2, 2015, July 8, 2015, and May 9, 2017), advocates and scholars were more circumspect. The view that NCDs are the result of personal choices contributes to the stigma that some people with NCDs face (informal conversation, scholar of health-related behavior, Accra, May 9, 2017). In addition, because NCDs in Africa have high mortality rates, their relation to proximate death creates a culture of hopelessness that causes people to shun diagnosis and awareness programs. One advocate explained:

> It is not uncommon for someone to say they had a brother who had AIDS [when in fact] he had cancer. I've been told that [untruth] to my face, because people live with AIDS [but] die of cancer. . . . Even the stories on the radio or in papers, it is always the worst-case. This perpetuates the [cancer is death] myth. (Interview, advocate on NCDs, Lusaka, June 12, 2014)

The speaker indicates that people in Zambia would rather be diagnosed with HIV than cancer, because in Zambia, like most African states, the majority of people with HIV can get free access to ART. In contrast, cancer treatment regimens that are rarely used in the West because they are ineffective are costly in Africa (Livingston 2012), and even hypertension medications are too expensive for many patients (Ilesanmi, Ige, and Adebiyi 2012).

Stigma also relates to the pain associated with NCDs, particularly given their lack of available treatment in Africa. For example, almost 90 percent of cancer patients in South Africa and Uganda reported pain as a prevalent symptom, and an estimated 88 percent of all cancer deaths in Africa with moderate to severe pain are not treated with pain relief medications such as opioids (Harding et al. 2013). In her ethnography of Botswana's only cancer ward, Julie Livingston (2012) details how cancer patients stoically endure profound pain and are often sent home to die with little more than acetaminophen, since morphine and codeine are highly controlled and hospital bed space is rationed. Bodies become disfigured, thin, and writhing while worried relatives jockey for medical staff members' attention and medications, both of which are in short supply. Pain is not acknowledged, despite its pervasiveness in the cancer ward. And surveys of low- and middle-income country governments indicate that policies related to palliative care and the availability of morphine are poorly designed (Camacho et al. 2015). As indicated above, inattention to the ubiquitous suffering that NCDs bring was also apparent in the speeches by African delegates at the 2011 High-Level Meeting.

In addition to the privacy of pain, cultural beliefs about the causes of some NCDs make it difficult for NCDs to become politically salient. Some Nigerian women, for example, reported that when they discovered lumps in their breasts, they turned to traditional healers (Pruitt et al. 2014). Some Zambian women who faced unusual gynecological symptoms blamed these on witchcraft (White et al. 2012). Not only did such actions delay care, but they also illustrate how NCDs are relegated to the private realm of religion, the occult, and "shyness" about the body. Gender norms also matter, as one advocate explained, "Cervical cancer, very often it is associated with promiscuity, because cervical cancer is the number one [type of women's cancer] and [it's] sexually transmitted so people think promiscuity plays a role.[11] It is not uncommon for the men to leave their wives or their partners [after diagnosis]." The advocate then said that breast and cervical cancer lead to a perceived loss of "womanhood," which in turn discourages women from seeking medical assistance:

> If you lose a breast, you no longer are a full woman . . . or worse still, you
> have a hysterectomy, or you have cancer of the vagina, or some of these shy
> cancers. [People will say], "You just need to go back to your mother's home."
> So there's a lot of stigma. . . . As an example, a few years ago the cancer hos-
> pital offered free mammograms . . . I called my friends, relatives. "Go! Go!" I
> said. Not one person went. When I asked why [they said], "You know, I'm
> busy." Or, "If I am told I have breast cancer, then what?" Or, "I don't think
> I've got any lumps or bumps." But really the excuse was fear. (Interview, ad-
> vocate on NCDs, Lusaka, June 12, 2014)

The speaker highlights the perception that if a woman is diagnosed with cancer she will not only face certain death but also lose everything that matters in life—relationships, marriage, friends, and identity. The fear associated with cancer screening, the stigma against some types of cancer, and the link between many NCDs and painful death make civil society mobilization for policy advocacy difficult. The result is a de facto disengagement from the policy process, so that the type of challenge that civil society presented to African states around AIDS in the early 2000s is not yet evident on NCDs. And unlike during Liberian's Ebola outbreak, when legitimacy and societal trust enabled traditional and religious organizations to challenge state officials, groups that advocate on NCDs lack power and legitimacy within society.

Mobilization to address NCDs must be situated temporally: It follows after the well-funded, highly institutionalized global AIDS response which led to the creation of thousands of AIDS organizations that advocate, provide services, and educate about the disease (Morfit 2011). As chapter 2 showed, donor funding for AIDS created opportunities for patronage to civil society, including food distribution for some people living with HIV and AIDS orphans, per diems to attend workshops, and NGO employment. In poor communities, these resources helped to elevate the status of local brokers, lifting them from destitution and giving them a long-term stake in AIDS programs (Burchardt 2013). This state (and societal) acceptance of global AIDS governance could cause the state to ignore or downplay other issues, including NCDs. In contrast to AIDS, there are few resources for NCDs to be distributed for patronage through inclusive policy-making institutions. Yet many communities have come to expect such benefits, leading organizations that work on NCDs to compete with AIDS groups for the community's attention. One Ugandan advocate on NCDs said that when the organization requests that community clinic workers educate their patients about NCDs, the workers ask what they will receive for this service. The respondent mimicked their questions: "Will there be a training with per diems? Will we get extra stipends?" This advocate blamed well-funded AIDS programs for making local health-care workers unwilling to engage the issue (interview, advocate on NCDs, Kampala, June 26, 2014). As another respondent said, "How do you contend with AIDS, even if you have a national disease burden [of NCDs] that greatly exceeds the programs you have in place?" (phone interview, global advocate on NCDs, October 9, 2015).

The case of Ghana supports the assertion that when AIDS is a less pressing issue, countries can focus more on NCDs. Ghana has an HIV rate of 1.3 percent (UNAIDS 2014e); it has seven groups that advocate on NCDs and a growing epistemic community. While donors still concentrate on communicable diseases (see above), some have started to focus on health system strengthening (USAID 2015). In 2008, a health official pointed out that Ghana had much bigger health challenges than AIDS: "We have diabetes, heart disease, and sickle cell that are killing so many" (interview, health advocate, Accra, August 29, 2008). In fact, six of eight states (all but Mozambique and Zambia) that reported that they had adopted a majority of the indicators from the WHO Global Action Plan had HIV rates below 3 percent

(UNAIDS 2014b). (South Africa counters this point, with its HIV rate of 18 percent. See UNAIDS 2014g.) For some countries, tensions between AIDS groups and groups that work on NCDs make it difficult for civil society to mobilize for NCDs.

In summary, many African groups that advocate on NCDs lack resources and political sway, and some represent stigmatized diseases in an environment in which populations seem to not prioritize health. Some disengage from policy, overwhelmed with providing care for and support to the increasing number of people suffering from NCDs and their dependents. As one respondent said, "We are overwhelmed with the numbers we are trying to serve" (interview, advocate on NCDs, Dodoma, July 2, 2015). In the context of low levels of international funding, competing issue frames, and weak global institutions, civil society faces an uphill battle to move most African states from ambivalence to acceptance of global health governance on NCDs.

Conclusion

This chapter has illustrated the ambivalent position of many African states toward the emerging global health governance of NCDs. In global health diplomacy, African states played a minor role in the run-up to the 2011 High-Level Meeting, and African leaders' speeches at the meeting often illustrated disinterest in or confusion about these complex health issues. At the policy implementation stage, many African states have adopted few, if any, policies to address these health concerns. Reasons for this ambivalence include the international community's lack of commitment to building institutions to govern and fund the response to NCDs, contested frames about NCDs, weak civil society mobilization at the global and state levels, and social attitudes of fear and stigma. In short, African states can remain ambivalent because they lack "a push from the top" or "pressure from the bottom."

While ambivalent, African states are not without agency. Hedging their bets for the future (for NCDs might be the next health issue to receive substantial funding), they used the 2011 High-Level Meeting to engage in extraversion and performances of compliance. Their adoption of minimal WHO recommendations illustrates how African states utilize their sovereignty to respond to policy suggestions. In such a context, unique state characteristics matter, such as South Africa's income status, democracy, and disease severity, Zambian elites' personal experiences with NCDs, Ghana's disease severity and epistemic community, and Eritrea's authoritarian developmentalist regime. Indeed, the eight states of Ghana, Côte d'Ivoire,

Eritrea, Mozambique, Togo, Zambia, Guinea, and Madagascar that reported adopting a majority of WHO Global Action Plan indicators in 2013 vary politically, economically, historically, geographically, and in terms of disease burden. As the final chapter argues, the dynamic nature of global health governance will influence African states' engagement with the emerging issue of NCDs in the future.

African Agency and Health for All

African states' engagement with global health governance provides a window into analyzing the role of weak states in international relations. Lacking military and economic might, weak states often depend on international actors and their resources to drive global action (Hey 2003; Ólafsson 1998). Being reactive, not proactive, they are incorporated into or required to accept processes and policies they did not design, envision, or even want (Callaghy and Ravenhill 1993; Andreasson 2013). Yet this volume illustrates that the picture is more complicated than this view of weak-state dependency, particularly in the realm of global health governance, which involves complex interactions among states, IGOs, NGOs, civil society organizations, and epistemic communities, all of which seek to address health issues (Youde 2012; Fidler 2010). In the post–cold war era, global health politics presents a new site for African agency, one in which traditionally weaker states bring unique perspectives and experiences (Brown and Harman 2013, 13). Approaching health issues from a variety of disciplines and sometimes with divergent end goals, the complicated webs of global health governance provide arenas in which African states can exert agency. In short, there are spaces for action in the sometimes confusing morass of norms, institutions, funding mechanisms, and nonstate actors. As this volume has demonstrated, African states have crucial roles to play in the messy processes of designing and implementing global health policies. For example, their speeches at the UN Special Session on HIV/AIDS created urgency for global health governance on AIDS, as did Ebola-affected states' manipulation of the West's fear of Ebola. They shape how health issues are discussed, they avoid or implement the policy suggestions of global health experts, and they incorporate, downplay, ignore, or feel threatened by health advocates in civil society. In the process, they advance or hinder cooperation to address major health issues like AIDS, infectious disease outbreaks, and the increasing morbidity and mortality related to different NCDs.

This volume has analyzed factors at the international, state, and societal levels to illustrate the conditions that shape African states' role in global health governance of the AIDS pandemic, the rising crisis of NCDs, and the 2014–2015 Ebola outbreak in West Africa. The choice of disease cases enabled me to see state reactions over time (AIDS), in moments of crisis (the 2014–2015 Ebola outbreak), and with an emerging health problem (NCDs). While it is tempting to explain state reactions based on the crisis nature of the health condition or the length of time the health issue has been discussed globally, this temporal factor provides an incomplete explanation. Instead, I question how this factor might create political opportunities in which international, state, and societal variables then determine state action. For AIDS, increased global interest in a post–9/11 world and the long-term maturation of AIDS groups in the West provided unique openings around which state actions occurred. Ebola created opportunities for crisis-oriented extraversion, while the newness of the crisis in NCDs means that international policy and civil society groups are underdeveloped. These conditions create a context, but they are not sufficient for explaining why African states have accepted, challenged, or remained ambivalent to global health governance on certain issues.

This book demonstrates that at the international level, African states find it more difficult to challenge or ignore global health governance when that governance includes strong institutions rooted in accepted norms and accompanied by significant monetary resources. While states accept such governance partially because they want resources, they also follow because there are reputational costs if they do not adhere to norms. The norm that the human right to health must be protected for the "innocent" and "deserving" members of society drove donor states in the early 2000s to develop programs like the Global Fund and PEPFAR that seek to provide universal access to ART (Kapstein and Busby 2013; Siplon 2013; Keck and Sikkink 1998). Similarly, wide support for The Vaccine Alliance (GAVI), a public-private partnership among states, the Gates Foundation, and pharmaceutical companies that supports immunization efforts, is rooted in the normative human right to health for children (Tarantola, Ferguson, and Gruskin 2011). When Nigeria failed to immunize children against polio in 2003, global health officials and other states questioned its commitment to this norm. The country's reputation suffered, a factor that then pushed the Nigerian national government to work closely with religious leaders to alleviate fears over vaccine safety (Renne 2011; Jegede 2007).

Yet global health governance is not always characterized by coherent norms, strong global institutions, and significant monetary resources, as the case of infectious disease control and the 2014–2015 Ebola outbreak illustrated. One of the primary goals since states first began to cooperate on health issues with the International Sanitary Conferences in the nineteenth century has been to control the spread of infectious diseases such as yellow fever, cholera, and plague, and to ensure that states not affected by outbreaks do not unnecessarily limit travelers from or trade with affected states (Kamradt-Scott 2015). The revised International Health Regulations (WHO 2005), an international agreement signed by all WHO member-states, creates a decision-making rule for when a state must report outbreaks to WHO; the WHO then can decide to declare a Public Health Emergency of International Concern which may (or may not) include a recommendation on travel or trade restrictions. States are supposed to follow these WHO recommendations. In addition, the IHR requires that states establish surveillance, control, and reporting mechanisms for outbreaks (Youde 2012; WHO 2005).

On one hand, the IHR presents strong institutions for outbreak prevention and control; states experience reputational pressure to report outbreaks or at least to justify their inaction when they do not report outbreaks (Davies, Kamradt-Scott, and Rushton 2015). On the other hand, as the Ebola crisis showed, *de jure* institutional strength is not necessarily synonymous with *de facto* institutional strength. Before the outbreak, low- and middle-income countries had done little to develop their capacity for infectious disease surveillance, control, and reporting. The WHO's own Global Outbreak Alert and Response Network was woefully understaffed and underfinanced, and the WHO structure, with its autonomous regional offices, created few incentives for early action on cases (Garrett 2015b). When the WHO recommended against travel or trade restrictions on Ebola-affected states, over half of African states ignored the recommendation. The WHO then did not criticize or shame violators, meaning there was little (if any) cost to reneging on global cooperation. Without a continued commitment of funding from the donor states and autonomy to enforce the IHR, the formal institutions of the IHR and WHO could not engage in strong action on the Ebola outbreak. The WHO's political, financial, and administrative weakness created space for African states to challenge global health governance: nonaffected states adopted travel restrictions, and the affected state of Liberia used the issue frames of neglect and crisis to mobilize global action and demanded autonomous control over the response.

Unlike infectious disease outbreaks, as a disparate collection of chronic diseases, NCDs lack strong global institutions to guide a response. Issue frames compete, epistemic communities are divided about the danger of some risk factors and the appropriateness of some policy responses, and global advocates lack resources and unity. Funding is insufficient for the magnitude of the problem, with NCDs being the biggest cause of morbidity and mortality in all regions of the world except Africa (*Lancet* 2012). Advocates have struggled to frame access to treatment or protection from risk factors like alcohol and tobacco marketing as a human right (Geneau et al. 2010; Ferguson, Tarantola, Hoffman, and Gruskin 2016; Cassell 2016). These diseases also face an image problem: they are perceived to be a health problem only in high-income countries, and they are thought to necessitate high-cost, technological solutions (phone interview, global advocate on NCDs, October 9, 2015; see Bollyky 2012; Sturchio and Galambos 2014). As a result, donors have yet to develop many programs beyond those linked to AIDS or child and maternal health (e.g., cervical and breast cancer screening and HPV immunizations). This lack of strong global institutions and adequate funding enables African states to remain ambivalent.

Beyond the ideational factor of norms, the aspirational identities of states also matter for their reaction to global health governance (Ruggie 1998), particularly for those states that seek to move beyond unflattering characterizations that negatively influence foreign investment, tourism, and, more broadly, their global position. Since colonialism, Africa has been portrayed as a primitive place, with chaotic and underdeveloped political institutions, an uneducated population, and cultural practices (from patron-client relations to traditional healers to patriarchal gender norms) that hinder the continent's socioeconomic development (Keim 1999; Iliffe 1995). The conventional wisdom asserts that highly contagious diseases that endanger the West often originate in Africa (Wald 2008; Gostin 2014; Wilkinson and Leach 2014). But African states and their populations aspire for greater respect than such tropes bestow. The region includes states that have accomplished a variety of milestones: some have rebuilt from war, almost all have experienced a decline in poverty, many have established multiparty democracy, and several have increased foreign trade and investment (Radelet 2010; Rotberg 2013; Cheeseman 2015). At times, such as during the early years of the AIDS epidemic, the Thabo Mbeki era in South Africa, or the 2014–2015 Ebola crisis, aspirational hope drove states to challenge patterns of global health governance that seemed to blame Africans for their suffering, morbidity, and mortality. At other times, African state leaders capitalized on these simplistic characterizations of the region. For example, Liberian officials stressed how the transnational spread of Ebola meant that "not even people in their nice suburban homes in the United States were safe." This framing motivated donor states and the UN Security Council to act (interview, government official, Monrovia, May 18, 2016). In this process, African state agency was facilitated by the ways that outsiders have constructed and understood Africa (Harrison 2010, 16–17).

Attributes of the African state also influence how states engage with global health governance. This volume focused on democracy and neopatrimonialism, though chapter 3 also investigated how geography and tourist revenue affected states' actions on Ebola travel bans, and chapter 4 explored how a country's income level and the severity of its epidemic of NCDs shaped state actions. The relationship between democracy and state actions in global health governance was mixed. Many democratic states with elections in 2014 or 2015 implemented Ebola-related travel restrictions in a challenge to global health governance, and citizen distrust of Liberia's nascent democratic government pushed the state to act autonomously in order to increase its own legitimacy. Democracy did not correlate with states' adoption of AIDS institutions or development of national AIDS strategies. However, autocratic states were less likely to have AIDS policies to protect key populations like men who have sex with men or people who inject drugs from discrimination. In the case of NCDs, an aggregate-level comparison showed that in 2013 more autocracies than democracies had adopted the policies and structures that the WHO recommended. Yet the case studies of South Africa and Ghana illustrate that democracies have established some policies to respond to this health crisis. Thus, the effect of democracy on state actions was inconsistent.

This book took as a starting point the assumption that African states have some neopatrimonial elements, though it did not assume that neopatrimonialism always has a negative effect on social policies or economic development (Kelsall 2011; Mkandawire 2015; Goldsmith 2000). It also recognized that patronage-based politics is not unique to Africa (Kitschelt and Wilkinson 2007). As with democracy, neopatrimonialism had mixed effects on how African states interacted with global health governance. In the case of AIDS, neopatrimonial states seeking global resources adopted global AIDS governance; in turn, the structures and policies of global health governance encouraged the development of centralized, inclusive institutions that incorporated many stakeholders in decision-making and patronage distribution. These institutions fostered state legitimacy, led to more effective policies, enabled the state to claim credit, and promoted the AIDS response (see Kelsall 2011 on centralized, inclusive neopatrimonial institutions). Initially pushed by donors but now embraced by states, national AIDS commissions and country coordinating mechanisms exemplify such institutions. Ultimately, these structures gave state officials a long-term interest in global AIDS governance and, more crucially, the people the disease infects and affects. This does not mean that HIV prevention, care, and treatment services reach all individuals who need them or that the AIDS problem has been solved. But these structures do help states get closer to the goal of zero new HIV infections, zero AIDS deaths, and zero discrimination (UNAIDS 2010). Citizens have perceived these efforts to be relatively successful in their service delivery (Fox 2014; Afrobarometer 2012).

In the case of NCDs, neopatrimonialism had an unclear effect. At the aggregate level, when I operationalized neopatrimonial states as those with low government effectiveness scores from the World Bank (2015d), then neopatrimonial states tended to adopt fewer policies on NCDs than states with higher effectiveness scores. Ghana and South Africa illustrate this pattern, though Eritrea does not. In addition, donor activities shaped neopatrimonial states' activities on NCDs, as the Zambia case illustrated. Global health governance on NCDs is characterized by weak institutions, contested norms, and few resources, providing states with few incentives to be proactive on these diseases. Technocrats in what tend to be somewhat politically powerless ministries of health make policies, often without the inclusion of civil society actors. (South Africa is an exceptional case. See de-Graft Aikins et al. 2010, 5). Resources (if they exist) are not centrally controlled, creating little political incentive for patronage-based state officials to develop policies and programs. With time, though, this situation could change. Global health governance on NCDs could strengthen, generating political and material reasons for neopatrimonial states to act. In addition, African state leaders themselves could begin to believe that the future tsunami of high health-care costs, disability, morbidity, and death associated with NCDs will undermine their own state resources. (Such a realization has started to occur in South Africa, Ghana, and Zambia.) But because they are not now "sufficiently scared," many state officials remain ambivalent about NCDs (*Quartz Africa*, July 13, 2015).

Ebola created opportunities for the affected states to benefit, though the crisis nature of the outbreak meant donors did not commit long-term funding and, thus, state officials did not have a long time horizon that pushed them to develop rent-management institutions that could incorporate stakeholders and build state legitimacy. As chapter 3 showed with the case of Liberia, decision-making was situated in existing decentralized neopatrimonial networks, whose fluidity led to a free-for-all in accessing resources. Network politics necessitated that Liberians challenge the framing of global health governance through strategies of extraversion; the country's leaders manipulated the neglect and crisis frames in order to gain donor attention and resources. Because they were the only ones rooted in the fluid networks of governance and the "shadow state," Liberians needed to control policy implementation (see Reno 2000; Utas 2008). The outcome was Ebola activities that reflected local context but also created opportunities for resource gains and, in some cases, corruption.

Throughout the three cases, international-level variables interact with state-level conditions to make adopting global health governance possible or impossible. The availability of international resources and well-developed global health institutions, as exist with AIDS, gave state officials long time horizons that helped them to build inclusive, centralized institutions. Their actions then increased state legitimacy and showed that the state could be responsive to the concerns of the population (Fox 2014). In contrast, minimal financial and political commitment among donors and IGOs has meant that African state elites see little need to construct centralized institutions to make policies or distribute resources on NCDs. Without institutions, states gain no opportunities to forge civil society ties or to use the issue to increase their domestic legitimacy. Indeed, civil society groups often remain outside policymaking on NCDs. In the case of Liberia and the Ebola crisis, international-level factors—particularly the Western perception that Ebola would spread to the West—enabled state leaders to lobby for global funding and demand that they control the response. In turn, this response—the Incident Management System—was situated in the broad neopatrimonial networks that influence Liberian politics.

Societal-level factors also have influenced African states' role in global health governance. Some civil society groups in Africa have historically provided essential social services like education and health care (van de Walle 2001; Michael 2004; Scherz 2014; on FBOs, see Haynes 2007), while other associations have engaged in advocacy and protest politics to demand the end of colonial rule, the establishment of multiparty democracy, the promotion of gender equality, and the end of neoliberal economic policies (Bratton and van de Walle 1987; Cheeseman 2015; Kevane 2004; Tripp 2000; Branch and Mamphilly 2015). Despite this mobilization, many civil society organizations lack resources, unity, internal accountability, autonomy, clear objectives, and political clout (Michael 2004; Gyimah-Boadi 2004; Fatton 1995; Patterson 1998). Because the African state has faced legitimacy challenges, citizen distrust, and low capacity (Bayart 1993; Englebert 2009; Bratton 2013), it has sought to control civil society. The state–civil society relationship has vacillated: civil society has disengaged from the state, it has challenged or opposed the state, and it has been incorporated into state decision-making processes (Azarya 1988; Rothchild and Chazan 1988).

This book has illustrated civil society's disengagement, opposition, and incorporation, all of which lead the African state to interact with global health governance in different ways. In the case of AIDS during the 1980s and 1990s, or more recently NCDs, civil society groups disengaged. This did not mean there are no organizations or health-related activities: TASO in Uganda, for example, established caregiving activities in the late 1980s. For NCDs, in 2017 there were organizations that worked on this issue in a majority of African countries. But as with the early AIDS groups, many of these groups involved with NCDs do not engage in advocacy. In addition, they face stigma and public skepticism, and they are under-resourced (Bollyky 2012; phone interview, global advocate on NCDs, October 9, 2015). With the exception of a few states like South Africa or select issues like cigarette package warning labels, groups have been unable to push most states beyond ambivalence (interviews, tobacco control advocates, Lusaka and Dar es Salaam, June 13, 2014 and July 4, 2015; Drope 2011). These organizations' disengagement contrasts with the challenge that AIDS advocates presented during the early 2000s or, more recently, the pressure that traditional and religious organizations put on the Liberian state to address Ebola in culturally appropriate ways. Because of the longevity of global health governance on AIDS, it is possible to see the dynamic nature of the state–civil society relationship, as civil society groups have moved from disengagement, to challenge, to incorporation into state decision-making processes. As was the case with the international and state levels of analysis, the international and societal levels intertwine. Global networks with resources and the support of a relatively unified epistemic community helped African AIDS groups challenge the state in the early 2000s, while divisions among the different groups that work on various NCDs and within epistemic communities that study these health conditions mean that African groups have insufficient transnational allies and resources. In the case of Ebola, transnational actors such as MSF or faith-based development groups assisted African societal actors, who had the legitimacy to shape local actions (e-mail conversation, United Methodist Church official, Tennessee, June 30, 2016).

Through its bottom-up view of international relations, an angle often discounted in scholarship (Clapham 1996), this book has argued that the African state demonstrates agency in global health governance. State officials have used institutions, frames, extraversion, and sovereignty as tools of agency in many ways. First, African state leaders have accepted donor-driven AIDS institutions like the country coordinating mechanisms and expanded them to incorporate more stakeholders. In the process, this institutionalization helps to coopt civil society, reward allies, and foster state legitimacy. Second, African actors have used particular images or rhetoric to generate resources or downplay obligations. Aware that populations in donor states were panicked over Ebola, Liberia emphasized the crisis frame, with its focus on fear, globalization, and gruesome, unstoppable death, to motivate donor states. Groups of people living with HIV in Malawi and Zambia speak of their empowerment through donor-funded ART programs in order to validate the continuance of such programs (Anderson and Patterson 2017). Third, African state leaders have practiced performances of compliance and extraversion. At the 2011 UN High-Level Meeting on NCDs, state officials conveyed their deep concern about NCDs but stressed their lack of resources to address these health problems. Fourth, states have exercised their sovereign right to recognize and approve donor programs on politically acceptable health issues, like malaria or childhood immunizations, while they dissuade donors from establishing in-country programs on issues that state elites find politically difficult, like tobacco taxation or HIV prevention programs for men who have sex with men (interviews, tobacco control advocate, Dar es Salaam, July 9, 2015; multilateral donor official, Kampala, June 30, 2014; AIDS NGO official, Kampala, June 24, 2014; and NAC official, Lusaka, June 13, 2014; on states and sovereignty, see Englebert 2009). Fifth, African state and civil society leaders have challenged the very biomedical foundations of global health governance. Mbeki's questioning of the link between HIV and AIDS, Yahya Jammeh's "AIDS cure," and societal leaders' belief that Ebola was a spiritual curse or a US government creation necessitated that global health governance react. Agency enables African actors to choose different paths in relation to global health governance.

The Impact of Agency

It is crucial to conclude with some discussion of the implications of African state agency for global health governance, the zero-sum nature of vertical health programs, and, ultimately, the health of millions of Africans. First, African agency has an effect on global health governance, because governance itself is a dynamic and dialectical process. The impact of African states in these processes echoes findings about the continent's role in negotiations on the small arms trade or African states' ability to sway resolution outcomes in the UN General Assembly (Cornelissen 2009; Shaw, Cheru, and Cornelissen 2012). The success that several African states have had with the AIDS response has helped to justify global AIDS institutions and has led some African state officials to call for similar institutions for other health issues like NCDs (see chapter 4). But the internal politics of a state—its legitimacy and neopatrimonial rent-managing institutions, as well as its state–civil society relations—affect its agency in the international realm: "For all African states, questions of internal strength . . . play a key role in enabling participation in, and influence over, external relations" (Brown and Harman 2013, 9).

The challenge that Liberia presented when it insisted on controlling the Ebola response led both to stopping Ebola infections and to making international health experts recognize the necessity of cultural awareness in outbreak control (interviews, government official and international NGO official, Monrovia, May 18, 2016, and May 19, 2016; WHO 2015d). In addition, African states have specific expertise on some health issues which then enables those states to design global health governance (Price-Smith 2009; Wald 2008). South Africa provides an example on the issue of TB control. In 2014, it had over 500,000 active TB cases, with 12 percent of the country's deaths being attributed to TB. Additionally, South Africa has witnessed the rapid rise of multidrug-resistant TB and extremely drug-resistant TB (SANTA 2016). This experience means other states widely consult with South Africa for advice on TB (interview, multilateral donor official, New York, October 1, 2015). One respondent said, "South Africa has influence on global health: look at how our community efforts have become a model in other countries, even in TB-affected communities in the United States" (phone interview, South African government official, October 13, 2015).

Analyzing the role of African states in global health governance enables us to see how African states are not merely "acted on" in international structures but also "actors in" these structures (Brown and Harman 2013). They help to shape agendas and frame issues. In the process, they affect "what might be possible" in future policy bargaining or donor assistance programs, though this realm of possibilities may be somewhat constrained (Chabal 2014; Lonsdale 2000). This influence mirrors other studies of African state assertiveness in bilateral relations which show that Africa is not a subservient region (Fisher 2013; Killick 1998). For example, through connections to US officials and careful use of extraversion, Liberian officials pushed the Ebola outbreak to the UN Security Council's agenda. While the council had discussed another health issue—AIDS—in 2001, it had not labeled AIDS to be a security threat, and it had not established a UN emergency mission to address AIDS (Rushton 2016). As Liberia pushed for action to address its Ebola crisis, it expanded the definition of what issues can be legitimately placed in front of the council in the future. In short, it contributed to a broader discussion of health security and the purview of the council. Time will tell if other states, IGOs, or health advocates will use this precedent to push for Security Council actions on future health crises.

Could African agency help global health governance move beyond a system of vertical programs that place diseases in silos and often pit health conditions against one other in a zero-sum game? While several actors now recognize the crucial role of health system strengthening, they face challenges in terms of cohesion in their advocacy and weak evidence to inform policies (Hafner and Shiffman 2013). The 2014–2015 Ebola outbreak presented an opportunity for health system strengthening, because the spread of the virus in health-care centers called attention to the weaknesses of public health systems and the dangers of focusing on disease-specific programs. If the Ebola-affected states had had well-trained and well-supplied health-care workers, community health educators, and public trust in the health-care system, the outbreak might not have caused as much morbidity and mortality as it did (Harman 2015; Benton 2015; Alexander et al. 2015). During and after the outbreak, the WHO, NGOs, donors, and advocates spoke about the need to strengthen health systems by training more personnel, improving community-based health education, providing basic supplies, and improving logistics and management (Kieney, Evans, Schmets, and Kadandale 2014; IDS 2015; *InterPress Service*, July 7, 2015). As chapter 3 indicated, this broader focus has yet to receive sufficient political traction and substantial resources. Instead, the Ebola outbreak has led donor states to focus on outbreak surveillance, control, and reporting (interview, multilateral donor official, New York, October 1, 2015; see also Nkengasong, Maiyegun, and Moeti 2017). In response, one activist said, "I fear we have lost an opportunity" (phone interview, global advocate on NCDs, October 9, 2015). As of early 2017, global health politics appeared to be a zero-sum game, with health system strengthening losing to infectious disease outbreaks.

The lessons of this book indicate that African agency often does not contribute to the move beyond vertical health programs, because these programs enable states to incorporate civil society, claim credit, and bolster their legitimacy. In short, vertical programs have political benefits (see Hafner and Shiffman 2013). Even though strengthening health systems could help all citizens, the political benefits are less certain and the rewarded constituencies less identifiable than in a vertical program. (This is also a challenge that the response to NCDs faces, since this disease category includes so many health conditions.) Additionally, competition between different groups gives the state power to control health policymaking and funding all the way to the community level (interview, health NGO official, Dodoma, July 3, 2015). Even when disease-focused programs try to integrate with other health issues, it can be difficult. For example, many groups that work on NCDs recognize that one solution to the lack of political attention that these diseases receive is to collaborate with AIDS efforts (interview, advocate on NCDs, Lusaka, June 12, 2014). But this possibility threatens AIDS groups that fear a loss of funding and influence (interview, AIDS activist, Kampala, June 25, 2014). Without an institutionalized response like AIDS has, other health issues suffer. One Tanzanian health authority said, "We are doing quite well on HIV, with most people with access to ARVs and they are adhering. But we still have things that are killing people . . . malaria, childhood diseases, maternal mortality, hypertension, diabetes" (interview, health NGO official, Dodoma, July 3, 2015).

Ultimately, what does African agency in global health governance mean for the health of Africans? The pattern of state acceptance brings health benefits, but because of the incentive structure that undergirds this acceptance, African states do not act on issues such as mental health, neglected tropical diseases, and NCDs that have few global institutions and funding sources, limited civil society mobilization, and beneficiaries who are hard to identify. Even if they do act, states often neglect some components of global health governance because of the lack of politically acceptable stakeholders to incorporate into decision-making institutions. An example is the exclusion of men who have sex with men and people who inject drugs in the case of AIDS, women and girls who suffered rape and gender-based violence during the Ebola outbreak (Harman 2016b), and people who experience mental illnesses (interview, mental health expert, Accra, May 18, 2017). As a result, the health of these marginalized groups suffers. Men who have sex with men and people who inject drugs face much higher rates of HIV infection, and they lack access to health services (UNAIDS 2014d); teenage pregnancy rates soared during the Ebola outbreak as a result of gender-based violence (Yasmin 2016b). When states remain ambivalent on global health governance, health concerns are ignored; witness the millions of diabetics who need insulin, the 50 to 90 percent of African children with sickle cell disease who have no access to pain management and die during childhood (Grosse et al. 2011), and cancer patients whose tumors are not diagnosed until too late.

State ambivalence also leads to unique health inequalities, beyond just the fact that wealthy Africans with health problems can afford treatments or medications in high-income countries. Access to AIDS medications provides an example of these nuanced inequalities. Before the global effort to provide universal access to ART, some AIDS activists forged ties to Western AIDS groups in order to get medications from abroad. As Vinh-Kim Nguyen (2010) illustrates with AIDS activists in

West Africa, testimonies about one's life with the disease helped these individuals to forge these life-saving connections. Such testimonies and connections could become increasingly important for Africans with various NCDs, if the state lacks a commitment to health for all (personal observations of and informal conversations with cancer-affected Africans, 2014–2016). But because not all disease sufferers effectively play the role of patient in a system where such performances and connections matter for survival, some people win and some lose essential health benefits.

Promoting the human right to health for all people regardless of disease necessitates getting the politics of global health right, so that agentic states can claim credit, build legitimacy, and foster ties with civil society. The costs are clear. Without such incentives, African states ignore or downplay diseases, such as various NCDs in the 2000s or AIDS during the 1980s and 1990s, leading to suffering, disability, sickness, and death. Families and communities lose breadwinners, parents, workers, leaders, and citizens. When African states recognize the unique ways their people and civil society organizations can address health, as during the Ebola crisis, citizens survive. Acceptance of global health governance can advance both state interests and citizens' health. African states choose, ignore, challenge, pretend, and forge their own path in the politics of global health. But those actions and nonactions have consequences for the Zambian woman suffering from Stage 4 breast cancer, the young Ghanaian homosexual who is at high risk for HIV infection, and the Liberian nurse who, without any infectious disease training and at great risk to her health, gives water, food, and comfort to Ebola victims. African agency in global health governance matters for these individuals and millions of others.

African States with Ebola-Related Travel Restrictions

State (N = 32)	Health spending as % of GDP	ECOWAS member	Regime type	Election (2014 or 2015)	Tourist # above average
Angola	2.1		weak autocracy		
Botswana	3.2		strong democracy	October 2014	Yes
Cameroon	0.9		weak autocracy		
Cape Verde	3.6	Yes	strong democracy		
Chad	2.0		weak autocracy		
Côte d'Ivoire	1.7	Yes	weak democracy	October 2015	
DRC	1.6		weak democracy		
Equatorial Guinea	2.9		weak autocracy		
Gabon	2.4		weak democracy		
Gambia	5.0	Yes	weak autocracy		
Ghana	2.1	Yes	strong democracy		Yes
Guinea-Bissau	1.1	Yes	weak democracy	March 2014 May 2014	
Lesotho	8.1		strong democracy	February 2015	
Kenya	3.5		strong democracy		Yes
Madagascar	0.5		weak democracy		
Malawi	6.0		strong democracy	May 2014	
Mauritania	1.9		weak autocracy		
Mauritius	2.4		strong democracy		Yes
Mozambique	3.9		weak democracy	October 2014	Yes
Namibia	5.4		strong democracy	November 2014	Yes
Nigeria	0.9	Yes	weak democracy	March 2015	Yes
Rwanda	2.9		weak autocracy		
São Tomé and Príncipe	3.6		weak democracy		
Senegal	2.4	Yes	strong democracy		Yes
Seychelles	3.1		weak autocracy	December 2015	
South Africa	4.2		strong democracy	May 2014	Yes
South Sudan	1.1		state failure		
Swaziland	7.0		strong autocracy		Yes
Tanzania	2.6		weak autocracy	October 2015	
Togo	2.0	Yes	weak autocracy	April 2015	
Zambia	2.8		strong democracy	January 2015	Yes
Zimbabwe	2.5		weak democracy		Yes
32 total states with restrictions		8	20 democracies 12 autocracies, with South Sudan	13	12

Source: Compiled by author from World Bank (2014c); Marshall and Cole (2014); National Democratic Institute (2016); UNWTO (2013); SOS International (2015); Worsnop (2016b); Poletto et al. (2014).

Note: See chapter 3 for definitions of regime types.

APPENDIX B

Countries by Number of WHO Global Action Plan Indicators Adopted, 2013
(Sub-Saharan African Countries in Bold and Listed First)

0 of 9 indicators	1 of 9 indicators	2 of 9 indicators	3 of 9 indicators	4 of 9 indicators	5 of 9 indicators
Burundi	**Benin**	**Botswana**	**Gambia**	**Congo**	**Côte d'Ivoire**
Central African Republic	**Nigeria**	**Burkina Faso**	**Cameroon**	**São Tomé & Príncipe**	**Ghana**
Comoros	**Rwanda**	Austria	**Malawi**	**Sudan**	Algeria
Djibouti	**Swaziland**	Bulgaria	**Mauritania**		Andorra
Equatorial Guinea	**Uganda**	Egypt	**Namibia**	Bolivia	Brazil
Gabon	**Zimbabwe**	El Salvador	**Seychelles**	Brunei	Croatia
Guinea-Bissau	Bahrain	Georgia	Albania	Cook Islands	Denmark
Kenya	Honduras	Jamaica	Bhutan	Costa Rica	Dominican Republic
Liberia	Laos	Kuwait	Iceland	Cyprus	Ecuador
Lesotho	Libya	Lebanon	Iraq	France	Greece
Mali	Maldives	New Zealand	Israel	Kiribati	Hungary
Niger	Morocco	Peru	Kazakhstan	Marshall Islands	India
Senegal	Nepal	Syria	Nicaragua	Netherlands	Indonesia
Somalia	Pakistan	UAE	Romania	Moldova	Luxembourg
	St. Kitts & Nevis	Uzbekistan	Serbia		Micronesia
Afghanistan	St. Lucia		Ukraine		Monaco
Antigua & Barbuda	Tunisia		Vietnam		Montenegro
Azerbaijan	Vanuatu				Oman
Belize					Paraguay
Dominica					Philippines
Grenada					San Marino
Papua New Guinea					Saudi Arabia
Yemen					Solomon Islands
					Uruguay
					Venezuela

Source: Compiled by author from WHO 2014b; all states (*N* = 194); Sub-Saharan African states (*N* = 49).

6 of 9 indicators	7 of 9 indicators	8 of 9 indicators	9 of 9 indicators	No response to WHO survey
Eritrea	**Guinea**	Barbados	China	**Angola**
Mozambique	**Madagascar**	Canada	Lithuania	**Cape Verde**
Togo		Chile	South Korea	**Chad**
Zambia	Argentina	Czech Republic	United States	**Democratic Republic**
	Armenia	Estonia		**of Congo**
Belgium	Australia	Finland		**Ethiopia**
Cambodia	Bahrain	Germany		**Mauritius**
Colombia	Bangladesh	Iran		**Sierra Leone**
Cuba	North Korea	Japan		**South Africa**
Fiji	Italy	Latvia		**South Sudan**
Guatemala	Malta	Portugal		**Tanzania**
Ireland	Niue	Qatar		
Jordan	Norway	Trinidad & Tobago		Belarus
Kyrgyzstan	Palau	United Kingdom		Bosnia & Herzegovina
Malaysia	Panama			Guyana
Mexico	Singapore			Haiti
Mongolia	Suriname			St. Vincent & Grenadines
Myanmar	Sweden			Timor-Leste
Nauru	Thailand			
Poland	Yugoslav			
Russia	Republic of			
Samoa	Macedonia			
Slovakia	Turkmenistan			
Slovenia				
Spain				
Sri Lanka				
Switzerland				
Tajikistan				
Tonga				
Turkey				
Tuvalu				

Chapter 1. African States and Global Health Governance

1. By 2014, Nigeria had reversed this trend. Between 2014 and August 2016, it did not report any new wild polio cases. However, just as the country was about to be declared polio free in August 2016, it reported two cases. Complacency in the state's immunization campaign and violence by the terrorist organization Boko Haram were blamed for the disease's re-emergence (*Science*, August 15, 2016). No cases were reported during the first five months of 2017 (Global Polio Eradication Initiative 2017).

2. This book focuses on sub-Saharan Africa, because North African states have different cultural, historic, and socioeconomic experiences. Many North African states also have different ties to the West because of oil and geostrategic considerations. The term "Africa" is used to refer to sub-Saharan Africa.

3. I use the acronym "NCDs" to indicate more than one chronic disease or health condition. I use "NCD" when I directly quote a source or when I refer to the name of an organization, such as the advocacy group NCD Alliance.

4. As of 2015, 30 percent of global deaths from diabetes occurred in low-income countries. In southern Africa, women are at least 30 percent more likely to be diabetic than men (*Lancet* 2016). By 2010, diabetes was one of the top ten killers in southern Africa (*Lancet* 2012). In 2016, the disease also was one of the top ten causes of morbidity and mortality in Ghana (interview, NGO health-care system administrator, Accra, April 18, 2017).

5. While I use the terms "small states" and "weak states" interchangeably, the "small states" literature also includes states like Luxembourg and Iceland, which clearly have more economic resources and state capacity than African states (see Ólafsson 1998; Hey 2003).

6. For a perspective that questions leadership's importance in the AIDS response, see Parkhurst 2013.

7. Mali, Nigeria, Senegal, Italy, the United States, Spain, and the United Kingdom also had Ebola cases, but I use the term "affected states" to refer to Liberia, Guinea, and Sierra Leone, which experienced most cases (CDC 2016).

8. Many NGOs that work on NCDs in Africa do not have a specific focus, such as diabetes or cancer. Rather, they seek to shape policies and programs for NCDs as a collection of diseases and health conditions. In response, governments tend to develop blanket policies, programs, and institutions for NCDs, not for individual noncommunicable health conditions.

Chapter 2. When All Factors Align: Acceptance of Global AIDS Governance

1. Studies have demonstrated that Africans have no more sexual partners over their lifetime than individuals in the United States (Stillwaggon 2006), though they are more likely to engage in concurrent sexual relationships (Epstein 2007). While initially blamed for the spread of HIV, polygyny has complicated effects. If all partners within a polygynous relationship are HIV negative, polygyny can serve as a protective practice. Georges Reniers and Susan Watkins (2010) discover lower HIV rates in countries where polygyny is common.

2. Senegal and Uganda were exceptions because of their early AIDS efforts (Green 2003; Putzel 2006).

3. UNAIDS (2015c) asserts that prisoners, sex workers, and youth (particularly young women) are key populations. The terms "key populations" and "most-at-risk" or "at-risk" populations are used interchangeably, though the former has been viewed to be more acceptable and less stigmatizing.

4. In Ghana, the National AIDS Commission is termed the Ghana AIDS Commission (GAC).

5. Of the forty-one countries that completed the Instrument, those with HIV rates above 10 percent were Botswana, Lesotho, Malawi, Mozambique, Namibia, South Africa, Swaziland, Zambia, and Zimbabwe. Countries with HIV rates below 1 percent were Burkina Faso, Burundi, Cape Verde, Djibouti, Eritrea, Madagascar, Mali, Niger, São Tomé and Príncipe, Senegal, Somalia, and Sudan. Countries with rates between 1 and 10 percent were Angola, Benin, Cameroon, Central African Republic, Chad, Comoros, Congo, Côte d'Ivoire, Democratic Republic of Congo, Equatorial Guinea, Ethiopia, Gabon, Ghana, Kenya, Liberia, Nigeria, Rwanda, Sierra Leone, Tanzania, and Uganda (UNAIDS 2014a).

6. In 2016, Mbeki seemed to stick to his views on the science of AIDS. He asserted, "I never said HIV does not cause AIDS. . . . What I said is that a virus cannot cause a syndrome" (*News24*, March 17, 2016). Because AIDS is a syndrome, or a collection of diseases, the statement still denied the link between HIV and AIDS.

7. The level of Jammeh's corruption was evident during his 2017 exit, when he stole millions from the country's treasury before leaving the country (*Associated Press*, January 22, 2017).

Chapter 3. International Confusion, Local Demands: Challenging Global Health Governance during the 2014–2015 Ebola Outbreak

1. As Morten Bøås and Mats Utas (2014, 49) assert, "The Liberian conflict was not just one war: it was a series of local conflicts tangled up in each other." Yet for the sake of simplicity, I refer to the Liberian conflicts in the singular.

2. As a counterpoint, Helen Epstein (2014) shows that Ebola emerged in cities of over 100,000 people in previous outbreaks in Uganda and Democratic Republic of Congo (or what was formerly known as Zaire).

3. For analysis of post-Ebola proposals to reform the WHO, see Youde (2016) and Clift (2016).

4. According to the US Census Bureau (2014), there are over 70,000 Liberians in the United States.

5. In 2016, Liberians complained that they remained isolated, forced to take expensive flights through Accra, Nairobi, and Brussels to reach the United States.

6. Wendy Rhymer and Rick Speare (2016) identify eighteen African states, because of their stricter definition of travel restrictions which does not include temperature and health screenings. I use the broader definition because all restrictions can limit travel and because three other sources—Worsnop 2016b; Poletto et al. 2014; and SOS International 2015—do the same.

7. The average number of tourists for the region was 780,000 in 2010, the last year in which the most comprehensive data are available (UNWTO 2013).

8. Articles from Namibia's major newspaper *New Era* can be found at www.newera.com .na/tag/ebola.

9. Other examples of media events include President Sirleaf's speech on October 9, 2014 to the World Bank in which she blamed the world for "a slow international response" (World Bank 2014b), her letter dated September 9, 2014, to President and Mrs. Obama in which she said "the virus will overwhelm us" (*New York Times*, September 12, 2014), and a letter dated August 29, 2014, and cowritten with the presidents of Guinea and Sierra Leone to UN Secretary General Ban Ki-Moon in which they asserted that the outbreak had placed an "enormous strain on our institutions" (UN 2014).

10. Some commentators echoed her sentiment that Ebola could destabilize the country, even reporting on rumors about a coup d'état (Morrison and Streifel 2015; see Epstein 2014).

11. The Lorma are also referred to as the Loma, Loghoma, and Looma. Another wing of the NPFL was led by Prince Johnson, who reached Monrovia before Taylor and murdered Doe. Johnson and Taylor quickly split, and in 1992, Johnson left for Nigeria (Ellis 1999, 99). He returned in 2004 and was elected senator for Nimba County. As of 2017, he continued to serve in the national legislature and planned to run in the October 2017 presidential elections (*Financial Times*, April 7, 2016; *FrontPageAfrica*, April 3, 2017).

12. What Stephen Ellis (1999, 39) terms "widespread prejudice" against the Mandingo remains. One Liberian claimed: "The Mandingo are not really Liberians" (informal conversation, community leader, Monrovia, May 18, 2016).

13. One Liberian professional said that a popular rumor is that when any high-level state official meets with a foreigner, the Liberian automatically "asks for something" (informal conversation, Liberian professional, Monrovia, May 22, 2016). The statement indicated the conventional wisdom about corruption's ubiquity.

14. The same type of rumor circulated in Sierra Leone (see Wigmore 2015; Wilkinson and Leach 2014).

15. See the Ebola Response Anthropology Platform, www.ebola-anthropology.net/?post _type=evidence, for discussion of how social scientists added to knowledge about Ebola in communities.

16. The government also quarantined Dolo's Town, a highly concentrated community of 17,000 people near the airport and forty miles east of Monrovia. Dolo's Town residents did not protest, perhaps because of clear and timely communication between state and community leaders (interview, Ebola Task Force member, Dolo's Town, May 17, 2016). Sierra Leone also

implemented quarantine in several districts in November 2014 (*Mail Online*, December 2, 2014).

17. In a highly symbolic action, the prayer vigil was held at the Providence Baptist Church in Monrovia, the site of the signing of the country's declaration of independence in 1847 (see Liebenow 1987, 16).

Chapter 4. What Is the Problem? Ambivalence about Global Health Governance of NCDs

1. The other WHO departments focus on general management; outbreaks and health emergencies; HIV/AIDS, TB, and malaria; family, women's, and children's health; and health systems.

2. The NCD Alliance was formed in 2010 by the International Diabetes Federation, International Union Against Tuberculosis and Lung Disease, Union for International Cancer Control, and the World Heart Foundation; it represents over 2000 local organizations in 170 countries. The Lancet NCD Action Group is an informal group of academics, practitioners, and NGO representatives which formed around 2010. The Bloomberg Initiative to Reduce Tobacco Use was established in 2007 by then New York City mayor Michael Bloomberg. Other involved organizations include the Harvard School of Public Health and the World Economic Forum (which collaborated to produce a 2011 report about the high cost of NCDs), the Council on Foreign Relations Independent Task Force on NCDs (formed in 2014 and led by US politicians and policy analysts), and the WHO Global Coordinating Mechanism on NCDs (formed in 2014 and mandated by the 2011 Political Declaration). Websites for the various organizations include NCD Alliance (www.ncdalliance.org), Lancet NCD Group (www .thelancet.com/series/noncommunicable-diseases), Bloomberg Initiative (www.tobacco controlgrants.org), the Council on Foreign Relations Task Force on NCDs (www.cfr.org /projects/world/independent-task-force-on-noncommunicable-diseases/pr1667), the World Economic Forum (www.weforum.org), the Harvard School of Public Health (www.hsph .harvard.edu), and the WHO Global Coordination Mechanism for NCDs (www.who.int/nmh /en/).

3. South Africa suffers concurrent epidemics of HIV and the NCDs of cervical cancer and Type 2 diabetes. HIV makes women more vulnerable to infection with the human papilloma-virus (HPV) that can cause cervical cancer. Because of its connection to depression and its predominance among low-income South Africans who already suffer poor nutrition, HIV has been linked to high diabetes rates (Mendenhall and Norris 2015).

4. The Harvard School of Public Health estimate ($2 billion annually) and the WHO estimate ($11 billion annually) differ greatly, because the latter includes access to more medications and because the data on NCDs needed for making such estimates are limited.

5. For example, in response to a question about taxes on tobacco products in Sierra Leone, one official wrote that the country had "completely abandoned" any excise taxes and "was not compliant" with Article 6.2(a) of the FCTC, which requires taxation of tobacco products (Sierra Leone 2014).

6. For example, at the 2001 Special Session on HIV/AIDS, the King of Swaziland tearfully and pleadingly said, "My people are dying. They are dying before their time, leaving behind their children as orphans, and a nation in a continuous state of mourning" (UNGA 2001).

7. In 2017, African states not party to the FCTC were Eritrea, Malawi, Somalia, and South Sudan. A major tobacco producer—Zimbabwe—ratified the FCTC in 2014. (On Zimbabwe's accession to the FCTC, see Lown, McDaniel, and Malone 2016).

8. One observer commented that the general health of African leaders should make them care about NCDs: "All of these guys have hypertension, diabetes . . . They don't eat well and ride around in cars all day" (interview, multilateral donor official, New York, October 1, 2015).

9. Because of their relative isolation from international actors, Eritrean officials could misreport policy adoption on NCDs. The country's lack of reliance on donors makes it less likely that it seeks to paint a positive picture to gain donor funds. In addition, because African citizens tend to not prioritize health, it is unlikely that the government has painted a positive picture in order to increase its legitimacy with its citizens. All of this does not deny that authoritarian regimes can and do manipulate socioeconomic data (see *East Africa Monitor*, November 4, 2015).

10. Countries with zero to three groups were Angola (1), Botswana (2), Burundi (2), Central African Republic (1), Chad (1), Cape Verde (0), Comoros (0), Côte d'Ivoire (3), Djibouti (0), Equatorial Guinea (1), Eritrea (2), Gabon (1), Gambia (0), Guinea (2), Guinea Bissau (1), Lesotho (1), Liberia (1), Madagascar (1), Malawi (1), Mauritania (0), Mauritius (1), Mozambique (3), Namibia (2), Niger (3), Rwanda (1), Seychelles (2), São Tomé and Príncipe (0), Sierra Leone (1), Somalia (0), South Sudan (0), Sudan (1), Swaziland (0), and Zimbabwe (2). Countries with four to six groups were Benin (5), Burkina Faso (6), Republic of Congo (5), Ethiopia (4), Mali (4), and Zambia (4). Countries with seven to nine groups were Cameroon (8), Democratic Republic of Congo (7), Ghana (7), Senegal (9), Tanzania (7), Togo (8), and Uganda (8). Those with ten or more groups were Kenya (13), Nigeria (17), and South Africa (10).

11. Cancer itself is not sexually transmitted, but HPV, which can cause cervical cancer, is.

Interviews Cited (in Chronological Order)

multilateral donor official, New York	October 15, 2002
bilateral donor, Washington, DC	October 22, 2002
international NGO official, Washington, DC	March 18, 2005
bilateral donor official, Lusaka	August 13, 2007
leader of group of people living with HIV, Lusaka	August 14, 2007
NAC official, Lusaka	August 14, 2007
AIDS NGO official, Lusaka	August 14, 2007
bilateral donor official, Lusaka	August 15, 2007
NAC official, Lusaka	August 15, 2007
CHAZ official, Lusaka	August 16, 2007
AIDS NGO official, Lusaka	August 17, 2007
leader of group of people living with HIV, Lusaka	August 19, 2007
AIDS NGO official, Lusaka	August 20, 2007
advocate for people living with HIV, Lusaka	August 20, 2007
AIDS expert, Lusaka	August 20, 2007
health advocate, Accra	August 29, 2008
international NGO official, Accra	September 23, 2008
AIDS NGO official, Accra	September 24, 2008
GAC official, Accra	October 1, 2008
multilateral donor official, Accra	October 8, 2008
GAC official, Accra	October 10, 2008
leader of group of people living with HIV, Accra	October 10, 2008
advocate for people living with HIV, Accra	October 14, 2008
AIDS NGO official, Accra	October 22, 2008
health FBO official, Accra	November 10, 2008
advocate for people living with HIV, Accra	November 18, 2008
advocate for people living with HIV, Kampala	July 8, 2010
AIDS expert, Lusaka	February 14, 2011
NAC member, Lusaka	February 17, 2011
multilateral donor official, Lusaka	February 23, 2011
person living with HIV, Lusaka	March 2, 2011
advocate for people living with HIV, Lusaka	March 7, 2011

person living with HIV, Chawama	March 23, 2011
leader of group of people living with HIV, Lusaka	May 10, 2011
AIDS NGO official, Kitwe, Zambia	May 19, 2011
advocate on NCDs, Lusaka	June 12, 2014
CCM member, Lusaka	June 12, 2014
tobacco control advocate, Lusaka	June 13, 2014
NAC official, Lusaka	June 13, 2014
advocate on NCDs, Kampala	June 19, 2014
FBO health director, Kampala	June 19, 2014
leader of group of people living with HIV, Kampala	June 19, 2014
health NGO official, Kampala	June 20, 2014
AIDS NGO official, Kampala	June 24, 2014
AIDS activist, Kampala	June 25, 2014
FBO official, Kampala	June 25, 2014
FBO official, Kampala	June 27, 2014
multilateral donor official, Kampala	June 30, 2014
advocate on NCDs, Kampala	June 26, 2014
advocate on NCDs, Dodoma	July 2, 2015
physician, Dodoma	July 2, 2015
health NGO official, Dodoma	July 3, 2015
government official, Dodoma	July 3, 2015
tobacco control advocate, Dar es Salaam	July 4, 2015
AIDS NGO official, Dar es Salaam	July 6, 2015
physician, Dar es Salaam	July 8, 2015
advocate on NCDs, Dar es Salaam	July 9, 2015
multilateral donor official, New York	October 1, 2015
UN Security Council delegate, New York	October 5, 2015
African state UN representative, New York	October 6, 2015
Namibian government official, New York	October 6, 2015
global advocate on NCDs	October 9, 2015
South African government official	October 13, 2015
African UN representative	October 15, 2015
Liberian community leader, Tennessee	March 14, 2016
hospital official, Harbel	May 16, 2016
hospital official, Kakata	May 16, 2016
hospital senior nurse, Kakata	May 16, 2016
hospital nursing assistant, Kakata	May 16, 2016
Ebola Task Force member, Dolo's Town	May 17, 2016
Ebola survivor, Monrovia	May 17, 2016
church official, Monrovia	May 17, 2016
government official, Monrovia	May 18, 2016
church relief agency official, Monrovia	May 18, 2016
humanitarian relief agency official, Monrovia	May 18, 2016

government official, Monrovia	May 19, 2016
international humanitarian NGO official, Monrovia	May 19, 2016
international NGO official, Monrovia	May 19, 2016
psychosocial team member, Gbargna	May 20, 2016
priest, Gbargna	May 20, 2016
pastor, Gbargna	May 21, 2016
psychosocial team member, Gbargna	May 21, 2016
government official, Monrovia	May 21, 2016
health-care workers, Margibi, Montserrado, and Bong Counties	May 16, 2016, May 20, 2016, and May 22, 2016
Christian Council of Ghana official, Accra	March 17, 2017
NGO health-care system administrator, Accra	April 18, 2017
tobacco control advocate, Accra	April 6, 2017
transnational tobacco control advocate	April 27, 2017
Rwandan tobacco control advocate	May 3, 2017
expert on NCDs, Accra	May 4, 2017
transnational tobacco control advocate	May 5, 2017
physician, Accra	May 9, 2017
bilateral donor, Accra	May 18, 2017
mental health expert, Accra	May 18, 2017

Other Fieldwork Cited (in Chronological Order)

e-mail conversation, UN representative from EU state	October 1, 2002
informal conversation, bilateral donor official, Lusaka	April 14, 2009
focus group discussion, group of people living with HIV, Lusaka	March 23, 2011
focus group discussion, group of people living with HIV, Mumbwa, Zambia	April 15, 2011
focus group discussion, group of people living with HIV, Kabwe, Zambia	April 18, 2011
focus group discussion, group of people living with HIV, Lusaka	May 5, 2011
focus group discussion, group of people living with HIV, Lusaka	May 10, 2011
participant observations, three Lusaka AIDS clinics	February–April 2011
focus group discussion, group of people living with HIV, Livingstone, Zambia	June 20, 2011
informal discussion, TAC activist, Guguletu, South Africa	August 7, 2014
informal conversation, Kenyan health activist, Cape Town	August 8, 2014
informal conversation, Liberian priest, Tennessee	December 5, 2015
informal conversation, Liberian professional, Monrovia	May 15, 2016
participant observations, public hospital, Kakata	May 16, 2016
informal conversation, community leader, Monrovia	May 18, 2016
informal conversation, Liberians with family in United States, Harbel	May 22, 2016

informal conversation, two health-care workers, Harbel	May 22, 2016
informal conversation, Liberian professional, Monrovia	May 22, 2016
e-mail conversation, United Methodist Church official, Tennessee	June 30, 2016
personal observations of and informal conversations with cancer-affected Africans	2014–2016
personal observations of health messages, Zambia, Tanzania, South Africa, Ghana, Liberia, and Uganda	2007–2017
personal observations of health-related behaviors, Accra	January–May 2017
informal conversation, international NGO official, Accra	February 4, 2017
focus group discussion, university students, Accra	April 26, 2017
informal conversation, scholar of health-related behavior, Accra	May 9, 2017

Aantjes, Carolien J., Tim K. C. Quinlan, and Joske F. G. Bunders. 2014. "Practicalities and Challenges in Re-Orienting the Health System in Zambia for Treating Chronic Conditions." *BMC Health Services Research* 414: 295.

Abeysinghe, Sudeepa. 2016. "Ebola at the Borders: Newspaper Representation and the Politics of Border Control." *Third World Quarterly* 37(3): 452–467.

Abrahamsen, Rita. 2004. "The Power of Partnerships in Global Governance." *Third World Quarterly* 25(3): 1453–1467.

Adler, Emanuel. 2012. "Constructivism in International Relations: Sources, Contributions, and Debates." In *Handbook of International Relations*, 2nd edition, edited by Walter Carlnaes, Thomas Risse, and Beth Simmons, 112–144. New York: Sage.

Africa Research Institute. 2011. "Princes' Progress: Reconstruction and Authority in Eritrea and Rwanda." Newsletter, March 28. www.africaresearchinstitute.org/newsite/public ations/briefing-notes/princes-progress-reconstruction-and-authority-in-eritrea-and -rwanda/.

African Development Bank. 2016. "Zambia Economic Outlook." www.afdb.org/en/countries /southern-africa/zambia/zambia-economic-outlook.

African Union. 2012. *The Roadmap: Shared Responsibility and Global Solidarity for AIDS, TB and Malaria in Africa.* www.unaids.org/sites/default/files/media_asset/20120715_TheRoadmap _AU_en_0.pdf.

———. 2015. "Fact Sheet: African Union Response to the Ebola Epidemic in West Africa, as of 1/26/15." http://pages.au.int/sites/default/files/FACT%20SHEET_as%20of%2026%20 Jan%202015.pdf.

Afrobarometer. 2012. *Afrobarometer Round 5 (2010–2012).* www.afrobarometer-online-analysis .com/aj/AJBrowserAB.jsp.

———. 2013. *Zambia Round 5 Summary of Results.* www.afrobarometer.org/publications/zambia -round-5-summary-results-2013.

Agyei-Mensah, S., and Ama de-Graft Aikins. 2010. "Epidemiological Transition and the Double Burden of Disease in Accra, Ghana." *Journal of Urban Health* 87(5): 879–897.

AidData. 2016. "Donor Datasets." http://aiddata.org/donor-datasets.

Ajulu, Rok. 2001. "Thabo Mbeki's African Renaissance in a Globalising World Economy: The Struggle for the Soul of the Continent." *Review of African Political Economy* 28(87): 27–42.

Ake, Claude. 1996. *Democracy and Development in Africa.* Washington, DC: Brookings Institution.

Alexander, Kathleen A., Claire E. Sanderson, Madav Marathe, Bryan L. Lewis, Caitlin M. Rivers, Jeffrey Shaman, John M. Drake, Eric Lofgren, Virginia M. Dato, Marisa C. Eisenberg, and Stephen Eubank. 2015. "What Factors Might Have Led to the Emergency of Ebola in West Africa?" *PLoS Neglected Tropical Diseases* 9(6): e0003652.

Alleyne, George, and Sania Nishtar. 2014. "Sectoral Cooperation for the Prevention and Control of NCDs." In *Noncommunicable Diseases in the Developing World: Addressing Gaps in Global Policy and Research*, edited by Louis Galambos and Jeffrey L. Sturchio, 133–151. Baltimore, MD: Johns Hopkins University Press.

AMFAR. *See* The Foundation for AIDS Research.

Ammann, Theresa. 2014. "Ebola in Liberia: A Threat to Human Security and Peace." *Cultural Anthropology*, October 7. https://culanth.org/fieldsights/597-ebola-in-liberia-a-threat-to-human-security-and-peace.

Amon, Joseph. 2008. "Dangerous Medicines: Unproven AIDS Cures and Counterfeit Antiretroviral Drugs." *Globalization and Health* 4(5): 1–10.

Anderson, Emma-Louise. 2015. *Gender, Risk and HIV: Navigating Structural Violence*. New York: Palgrave Macmillan.

Anderson, Emma-Louise, and Alex Beresford. 2016. "Infectious Injustice: The Political Foundations of the Ebola Crisis in Sierra Leone." *Third World Quarterly* 37(3): 468–486.

Anderson, Emma-Louise, and Amy S. Patterson. 2017. *Dependent Agency in the Global Health Regime: Local African Responses to Donor AIDS Efforts*. New York: Palgrave Macmillan.

Andreasson, Stefan. 2011. "Africa's Prospects and South Africa's Leadership Potential in the Emerging Markets Century." *Third World Quarterly* 32(6): 1165–1181.

———. 2013. "Elusive Agency: Africa's Persistently Peripheral Role in International Relations." In *African Agency in International Politics*, edited by William Brown and Sophie Harman, 143–157. New York: Routledge.

Arriola, Leonardo. 2009. "Patronage and Political Stability in Africa." *Comparative Political Studies* 42(10): 1339–1362.

Arriola, Leonardo, and Martha Johnson. 2014. "Ethnic Politics and Women's Empowerment in Africa: Ministerial Appointments to Executive Cabinets." *American Journal of Political Science* 58(2): 495–510.

Asunka, Joseph. 2013. "What People Want from Government. Basic Services Performance Ratings, 34 Countries." Report for Afrobarometer, December 11. http://afrobarometer.org/sites/default/files/publications/Briefing%20paper/ab_r5_policypaperno5.pdf.

Austin, James, Diana Barrett, and James Weber. 2001. *Merck Global Health Initiatives: Botswana*. Boston: Harvard Business School.

Azarya, Victor. 1988. "Reordering State Society Relations: Incorporation and Disengagement." In *The Precarious Balance: State and Society in Africa*, edited by Donald Rothchild and Naomi Chazan, 3–21. Boulder, CO: Westview Press.

Bach, Daniel, and Mamadou Gazibo, editors. 2012. *Neopatrimonialism in Africa and Beyond*. New York: Routledge.

Baize, Sylvain, Delphine Pannetier, Lisa Oestereich, Toni Rieger, Lamine Koivogui, N'Faly Magassouba, Barrè Soropogui, Mamadou Saliou Sow, Sakoba Keïta, Hilde De Clerck, et al. 2014. "Ebola Virus Disease in Guinea." *New England Journal of Medicine* 371(October 9): 1418–1425.

Barkan, Joel. 1994. "Divergence and Convergence in Kenya and Tanzania: Pressures for Reform." In *Beyond Capitalism vs Socialism in Kenya and Tanzania*, edited by Joel Barkan, 1–46. Boulder, CO: Lynne Rienner.

Barnes, Amy, Garrett Brown, and Sophie Harman. 2015. *Global Politics of Health Reform in Africa*. New York: Palgrave.

Barnett, Michael, and Martha Finnemore. 2004. *Rules for the World: International Organizations in Global Politics*. Ithaca, NY: Cornell University Press.

Barnett, Tony. 2006. "A Long-Wave Event. HIV/AIDS, Politics, Governance and 'Security': Sundering the Intergenerational Bond?" *International Affairs* 8(2): 297–313.

Barraclough, Simon. 2009. "Chronic Disease and Global Health Governance: The Contrasting Cases of Food and Tobacco." In *Global Health Governance: Crisis, Institutions and Political Economy*, edited by Adrian Kay and Owain Williams, 102–128. London: Palgrave Macmillan.

Bates, Robert. 1981. *Markets and States in Tropical Africa: The Political Basis of Agricultural Policies*. Berkeley, CA: University of California Press.

Bayart, Jean-Francois. 1993. *The State in Africa: The Politics of the Belly*. London: Longman.

———. 2000. "Africa and the World: A History of Extraversion." *African Affairs* 99(395): 217–267.

Beaglehole, Robert, and the Lancet Action Group. 2011a. "Priority Actions on the Non-Communicable Disease Crisis." *Lancet* 377(April 23): 1438–1447.

———. 2011b. "UN High-Level Meeting on Non-Communicable Diseases: Addressing Four Questions." *Lancet* 378(July 30): 449–455.

Behrman, Greg. 2004. *The Invisible People: How the US Has Slept through the Global AIDS Pandemic, the Greatest Humanitarian Catastrophe of Our Time*. New York: Free Press.

Benko, Jessica. 2016. "He Survived Ebola. Now He's Fighting to Keep It From Spreading." *New York Times Magazine*, May 26.

Benton, Adia. 2015. *HIV Exceptionalism: Development through Disease in Sierra Leone*. Minneapolis, MN: University of Minnesota Press.

Benton, Adia, and Kim Yi Dionne. 2015a. "5 Things You Should Read Before Saying the IMF is Blameless in the 2014 Ebola Outbreak." *Washington Post*, January 5. www.washington-post.com/blogs/monkey-cage/wp/2015/01/05/5-things-you-should-read-before-saying-the-imf-is-blameless-in-the-2014-ebola-outbreak.

———. 2015b. "International Political Economy and the 2014 West Africa Ebola Outbreak." *African Studies Review* 58(1): 223–236.

Beresford, Alexander. 2015. "Power, Patronage, and Gatekeeper Politics in South Africa." *African Affairs* 114(455): 226–248.

Beyrer, Chris, and Stefan D. Baral. 2011. "MSM, HIV and the Law: The Case of Gay, Bisexual and Other Men Who Have Sex with Men (MSM)." Working Paper for the Third Meeting of the Technical Advisory Group of the Global Commission on HIV and the Law, July 7–9.

Bird, Philippa, Maye Omar, Victor Doku, Crick Lund, James Rogers Nsereko, Jason Mwanza, and the MHaPP Research Programme Consortium. 2011. "Increasing the

Priority of Mental Health in Africa: Findings from Qualitative Research in Ghana, South Africa, Uganda and Zambia." *Health Policy and Planning* 26(5): 357–365.

Bøås, Morten. 2005. "The Liberian Civil War: New War/Old War?" *Global Society* 19(1): 73–88.

———. 2009. "'New' Nationalism and Autochthony—Tales of Origin as Political Cleavage." *African Spectrum* 44(1): 19–38.

Bøås, Morten, and Anne Hatløy. 2008. "Getting In, Getting Out: Militia Membership and Prospects for Reintegration in Post-War Liberia." *Journal of Modern African Studies* 46(1): 33–53.

Bøås, Morten, and Mats Utas. 2014. "The Political Landscape of Postwar Liberia: Reflections on National Reconciliation and Elections." *Africa Today* 60(4): 47–65.

Boesten, Jelke. 2011. "Navigating the AIDS Industry: Being Positive and Poor in Tanzania." *Development and Change* 42(3): 781–803.

Bollyky, Thomas. 2012. "Developing Symptoms: Noncommunicable Diseases Go Global." *Foreign Affairs* (May/June). www.foreignaffairs.com/articles/137536/thomas-j-bollyky /developing-symptoms.

Bollyky, Thomas, and David Fidler. 2015. "The Tobacco Treaty Turns Ten." Council on Foreign Relations Post, February 27. www.cfr.org/health-policy-and-initiatives/tobacco-treaty -turns-ten/p36192.

Bolten, Catherine. 2014. "Articulating the Invisible: Ebola Beyond Witchcraft in Sierra Leone." *Ebola in Perspective*, October 7. www.culanth.org/fieldsights/585-ebola-in -perspective.

Boone, Catherine. 1992. *Merchant Capital and the Roots of State Power in Senegal: 1930–1985*. New York: Cambridge University Press.

Bor, Jacob. 2007. "The Political Economy of AIDS Leadership in Developing Countries: An Exploratory Analysis." *Social Science and Medicine* 64(8): 1585–1599.

Boutayeb, Abdesslam, and Saber Boutayeb. 2005. "The Burden of Non Communicable Diseases in Developing Countries." *International Journal of Equity in Health* 4(2): 1–8.

Branch, Adam, and Zachariah Mampilly. 2015. *Africa Uprising: Popular Protest and Political Change*. London: ZED.

Bratton, Michael, editor. 2013. *Voting and Democratic Citizenship in Africa*. Boulder, CO: Lynne Rienner.

Bratton, Michael, and Nicolas van de Walle. 1997. *Democratic Experiments in Africa: Regime Transitions in Comparative Perspective*. New York: Cambridge University Press.

Brett, E. A. 2006. "State Failure and Success in Uganda and Zimbabwe: The Logic of Political Decay and Reconstruction in Africa." Crisis States Research Centre Working Paper 78, February. http://citeseerx.ist.psu.edu/viewdoc/download?doi=10.1.1.602.1452&rep =rep1&type=pdf.

Bridle-Fitzpatrick, Susan. 2015. "Food Deserts or Food Swamps? A Mixed-Methods Study of Local Food Environments in a Mexican City." *Social Science and Medicine* 142(October): 202–213.

Britton, John, Deborah Arnott, Ann McNeill, Nicholas Hopkinson, and the Tobacco Advisory Group of the Royal College of Physicians. 2016. "Nicotine without Smoke—Putting

Electronic Cigarettes in Context." *British Medical Journal* 353(April 27): i1745. http://dx.doi
.org/10.1136/bmj.i1745.

Brown, William. 2012. "A Question of Agency: Africa in International Politics." *Third World
Quarterly* 33(10): 1889–1898.

———. 2013. "Sovereignty Matters: Africa, Donors and the Aid Relationship." *African Affairs*
112(447): 262–282.

Brown, William, and Sophie Harman. 2013. *African Agency in International Politics*. New York:
Routledge.

Bunker, Stephen. 1987. *Peasants against the State: The Politics of Market Control in Bugisu,
Uganda, 1900–1983*. Chicago, IL: University of Chicago Press.

Burchardt, Marian. 2013. "Faith-Based Humanitarianism: Organizational Change and
Everyday Meanings in South Africa." *Sociology of Religion* 74(1): 30–55.

Burgess, Rochelle, and Catherine Campbell. 2014. "Contextualising Women's Mental Distress
and Coping Strategies in the Time of AIDS: A Rural South African Case Study." *Transcul-
tural Psychiatry* 51(6): 875–903.

Busby, Joshua, Karen Grépin, and Jeremy Youde. 2016. "Introduction. Ebola: Implications for
Global Health Governance." *Global Health Governance* 10(1): 3–10.

Bush, George W. 2003. State of the Union address, January 28. www.washingtonpost.com/wp
-srv/onpolitics/transcripts/bushtext_012803.html.

Butler, Anthony. 2005. "South Africa's AIDS Policy, 1994–2004: How Can It Be Explained?"
African Affairs 104(417): 591–614.

Calain, Philippe. 2007. "From the Field Side of the Binoculars: A Different View on Global
Public Health Surveillance." *Health Policy and Planning* 22(1): 13–20.

Caldwell, John, Pat Caldwell, and Pat Quiggin. 1989. "The Social Context of AIDS in
Sub-Saharan Africa." *Population and Development Review* 14(2): 185–234.

Callaghy, Tom. 1988. "The State and the Development of Capitalism in Africa." In *The
Precarious Balance: State and Society in Africa*, edited by Naomi Chazan and Donald
Rothchild, 67–99. Boulder, CO: Westview Press.

Callaghy, Tom, and John Ravenhill, editors. 1993. *Hemmed In: Responses to Africa's Economic
Decline*. New York: Columbia University Press.

Camacho, Rolando, Cecilia Sepúlveda, Diogo Neves, Marion Piñeros, Maria Villanueva,
Jean-Marie Dangou, Ibtihal Fadhil, Gauden Galea, Renu Garg, and Silvana Luciani. 2015.
"Cancer Control Capacity in 50 Low- and Middle-Income Countries." *Global Public Health*
10(9): 1017–1031.

Caribbean Community. 2007. "Declaration of Port-of-Spain: Uniting to Stop the Epidemic of
Chronic NCDs." www.caricom.org/jsp/communications/meetings_statements/declaration
_port_of_spain_chronic_ncds.jsp.

CARICOM. *See* Caribbean Community.

Carter Center. 2011. *National Elections in Liberia, Fall 2011*. Final Report. www.cartercenter
.org/resources/pdfs/news/peace_publications/election_reports/liberia2011-finalrpt
.pdf.

Cassidy, Rebecca, and Melissa Leach. 2009. "Science, Politics, and the Presidential AIDS
'Cure.'" *African Affairs* 108(433): 559–580.

Casswell, Sally. 2016. "Chronic Diseases—The Social Justice Issue of Our Time." *Lancet* 387(March 5): 942–943.

CDC. *See* Centers for Disease Control and Prevention.

Centers for Disease Control and Prevention. 2015a. "African Union and U.S. CDC Partner to Launch African CDC." Press release, April 13. www.cdc.gov/media/releases/2015/p0413 -african-union.html.

———. 2015b. "Global Health Security Agenda." www.cdc.gov/globalhealth/security /ghsagenda.htm.

———. 2015c. "The Road to Zero: CDC's Response to the West African Ebola Epidemic." www.cdc.gov/about/pdf/ebola/ebola-photobook-070915.pdf.

———. 2015d. "Zambia." www.cdc.gov/globalhealth/countries/zambia.

———. 2016. "2014 Ebola Outbreak in West Africa—Case Counts." www.cdc.gov/vhf/ebola /outbreaks/2014-west-africa/case-counts.html.

Chabal, Patrick. 2014. "Foreword." In *Civic Agency in Africa: Arts of Resistance in the 21st Century*, edited by Ebenezer Obadare and Wendy Willems, xii–xviii. London: James Currey.

Chabal, Patrick, and Jean-Pascal Daloz. 1999. *Africa Works: Disorder as Political Instrument.* Bloomington, IN: Indiana University Press.

Chan, Jennifer. 2015. *Politics in the Corridor of Dying: AIDS Activism and Global Health Governance.* Baltimore, MD: Johns Hopkins University Press.

Chan, Margaret. 2014. "WHO Director-General Addresses High-Level Meeting on Noncom-municable Diseases." New York, July 10. www.who.int/dg/speeches/2014 /noncommunicable-diseases/en/.

Chandra, Kanchan. 2007. "Monopoly and Monitoring: An Approach to Political Clientelism." In *Patrons, Clients, and Policies: Patterns of Democratic Policies and Political Competition*, edited by Herbert Kitschelt and Steven I. Wilkinson, 84–109. New York: Cambridge University Press.

Chapman, Audrey. 2012. "The Contributions of a Human Rights Approach to Health." In *The Ashgate Research Companion to the Globalization of Health*, edited by Ted Schrecker, 261–276. Aldershot, UK: Ashgate.

Chayes, Abram, and Antonia Handler Chayes. 1998. *The New Sovereignty: Compliance with International Regulatory Agreements.* Cambridge, MA: Harvard University Press.

Chazan, May. 2015. *The Grandmothers' Movement: Solidarity and Survival in the Time of AIDS.* Montreal: McGill-Queen's University Press.

Cheeseman, Nic. 2015. *Democracy in Africa.* New York: Cambridge University Press.

Chigwedere, P., and M. Essex. 2010. "AIDS Denialism and Public Health Practice." *AIDS Behavior* 14(2): 237–247.

Ciment, James. 2013. *Another America: The Story of Liberia and the Former Slaves Who Ruled It.* New York: Hill and Wang.

Clapham, Christopher. 1982. "Clientelism and the State." In *Private Patronage and Public Power: Political Clientelism and the Modern State*, edited by Christopher Clapham, 1–35. London: Pinter.

———. 1985. *Third World Politics: An Introduction.* London: Croom Helm.

————1996. *Africa and the International System: The Politics of State Survival.* New York: Cambridge University Press.

Clift, Charles. 2016. "Commentary: Ebola and WHO Reform." *Global Health Governance* 10(1): 36–40.

Coetzee, David, Katherine Hildebrand, Andrew Boulle, Gary Maartens, Francoise Louis, Veliswa Labatala, Hermann Reuter, Nonthutuzelo Ntwana, and Eric Goemaere. 2004. "Outcomes after Two Years of Providing Antiretroviral Treatment in Khayelitsha, South Africa." *AIDS* 18(6): 887–895.

Cohen, Myron, Ying Q. Chen, Marybeth McCauley, Theresa Gamble, Mina C. Hosseinipour, Nagalingeswaran Kumarasamy, James G. Hakim, Johnstone Kumwenda, Beatriz Grinsztejn, Jose H. S. Pilotto, Sheela V. Godbole, et al. 2011. "Prevention of HIV-1 Infection with Early Antiretroviral Therapy." *New England Journal of Medicine* 365(August): 493–505.

Collier, David. 2011. "Understanding Process Tracing." *PS: Political Science and Politics* 44(4): 823–830.

Confortini, Catia, and Briana Krong. 2015. "Breast Cancer in the Global South and the Limitations of a Biomedical Framing: A Critical Review of the Literature." *Health Policy and Planning* 30(10): 1350–1361.

Cooper, Andrew, John Kirton, Franklyn List, and Hany Besada, editors. 2013. *Africa's Health Challenges: Sovereignty, Mobility of People and Healthcare Governance.* Burlington, VT: Ashgate.

Cooper, Andrew, John Kirton, and Ted Schrecker. 2007. *Governing Global Health: Challenge, Response, Innovation.* Burlington, VT: Ashgate.

Cornelissen, Scarlet. 2009. "Awkward Embraces: Emerging and Established Powers and the Shifting Fortunes of Africa's International Relations in the Twenty-First Century." *Politikon* 36(1): 5–26.

"The Cost of Silence." 2008. *Nature* 456(545). December 4.

Crane, Johanna Tayloe. 2013. *Scrambling for Africa: AIDS, Expertise and the Rise of American Global Health Science.* Washington, DC: Georgetown University Press.

Cross, Mai'a K. Davis. 2013. "Rethinking Epistemic Communities Twenty Years Later." *Review of International Studies* 39(1): 137–160.

Csete, Joanne. 2007. "Rhetoric and Reality: HIV/AIDS as a Human Rights Issue." In *The Global Politics of AIDS*, edited by Paul Harris and Patricia Siplon, 247–261. Boulder, CO: Lynne Rienner.

Dalal, Shona, Juan Jose Beunza, Jimmy Volmink, Clement Adebamowo, Francis Bajunirwe, Marina Njelekela, Dariush Mozaffarian, Wafaie Fawzi, Walter Willett, Hans-Olov Adami, and Michelle D. Holmes. 2011. "Non-Communicable Diseases in Sub-Saharan Africa: What We Know Now." *International Journal of Epidemiology* 40(4): 885–901.

Daniels, Mitchell, Thomas Donilon, and Thomas Bollyky. 2014. *The Emerging Global Health Crisis: Noncommunicable Diseases in Low and Middle Income Countries.* Independent Task Force Report No. 72. Council on Foreign Relations. www.cfr.org/diseases-noncom municable/emerging-global-health-crisis/p33883.

Davies, Sara. 2010. *Global Politics of Health.* Malden, MA: Polity.

Davies, Sara, Adam Kamradt-Scott, and Simon Rushton. 2015. *Disease Diplomacy: International Norms and Global Health Security.* Baltimore, MD: Johns Hopkins University Press.

Davies, Sara, and Simon Rushton. 2016. "Public Health Emergencies: A New Peacekeeping Mission? Insights from UNMIL's Role in the Liberia Ebola Outbreak." *Third World Quarterly* 37(3): 419–435.

de Grassi, Aaron. 2008. "Neopatrimonialism and Agricultural Development in Africa: Contributions and Limitations on a Contested Concept." *African Studies Review* 51(3): 107–133.

de Haan, Arjan. 2009. *How the Aid Industry Works.* Boulder, CO: Kumarian.

de Waal, Alex, and Alan Whiteside. 2003. "New Variant Famine: AIDS and the Food Crisis in Southern Africa." *Lancet* 362(9391): 1234–1237.

de-Graft Aikins, Ama, A. Anum, C. Agyemang, and O. Ogedegbe. 2012. "Lay Representations of Chronic Diseases in Ghana: Implications for Primary Prevention." *Ghana Medical Journal* 46(Supplement 2): 59–68.

de-Graft Aikins, Ama, Nigel Unwin, Charles Agyemang, Pascale Allotey, Catherine Campbell, and Daniel Arhinful. 2010. "Tackling Africa's Chronic Disease Burden: From the Local to the Global." *Globalization and Health* 6(5). www.globalizationandhealth.com /content/pdf/1744-8603-6-5.pdf.

Democratic Turnhalle Alliance. 2014. "Venaani Calls for Ebola Travel Ban." October 1. www .dtaofnamibia.org/category/from-the-press/page/2/.

Des Forges, Alison Liebhafsky. 1999. *Leave None to Tell the Story: Genocide in Rwanda.* New York: Human Rights Watch.

Dionne, Kim Yi. 2011. "The Role of Executive Time Horizons in State Response to AIDS in Africa." *Comparative Political Studies* 44(1): 55–77.

———. 2012. "Local Demand for a Global Intervention: Policy Priorities in the Time of AIDS." *World Development* 40(12): 2468–2477.

———. 2017. *Doomed Interventions: The Failure of Global Responses to AIDS in Africa.* New York: Cambridge University Press.

Dionne, Kim Yi, Patrick Gerland, and Susan Watkins. 2013. "AIDS Exceptionalism: Another Constituency Heard From." *AIDS Behavior* 17(3): 825–831.

Dorman, Sara Rich. 2002. "'Rocking the Boat?' Churches, NGOs and Democratization in Zimbabwe." *African Affairs* 101(402): 75–92.

Downie, Richard. 2012. *The Road to Recovery: Rebuilding Liberia's Health System.* Report for the CSIS Global Health Policy Center, August. https://csis-prod.s3.amazonaws.com/s3fs -public/legacy_files/files/publication/120822_Downie_RoadtoRecovery_web.pdf.

Drope, Jeffrey. 2011. *Tobacco Control in Africa: People, Politics and Policies.* Anthem Studies in Development and Globalization. http://idl-bnc.idrc.ca/dspace/bitstream/10625/47373/1 /IDL-47373.pdf.

DTA. *See* Democratic Turnhalle Alliance.

Dunn, Elwood. 2009. *Liberia and the United States during the Cold War: Limits of Reciprocity.* New York: Palgrave Macmillan.

Dunn, Kevin, and Timothy Shaw. 2001. *Africa's Challenge to International Relations Theory.* New York: Palgrave.

Economic Community of West African States. 2016. "Member States." www.ecowas.int /member-states.

Economist. 2013. "A Hopeful Continent." Special Report, March 2, 1–14.

ECOWAS. *See* Economic Community of West African States.

Editorial Board. 2011. "Global Response to Non-Communicable Diseases: Analysis." *British Medical Journal* 342: 1–6.

Eggertsson, Thráinn. 2005. *Imperfect Institutions: Possibilities and Limits of Reform.* Ann Arbor, MI: University of Michigan Press.

Ekeh, Peter. 1975. "Colonialism and the Two Publics in Africa: Theoretical Statement." *Comparative Studies in Society and History* 17(1): 91–112.

Elbe, Stefan. 2006. "Should HIV/AIDS Be Securitized? The Ethical Dilemmas of Linking HIV/AIDS and Security." *International Studies Quarterly* 50(1): 119–144.

Ellis, Stephen. 1995. "Liberia 1989–1994: A Study of Ethnic and Spiritual Violence." *African Affairs* 94(365): 165–197.

———. 1999. *The Mask of Anarchy: The Destruction of Liberia and the Religious Dimension of an African Civil War.* London: Hurst.

———. 2013. *Season of Rains.* Chicago, IL: University of Chicago Press.

Ellis, Stephen, and Gerrie ter Haar. 1998. "Religion and Politics in Sub-Saharan Africa." *Journal of Modern African Studies* 36(2): 175–201.

Englebert, Pierre. 2009. *Unity, Sovereignty, Sorrow.* Boulder, CO: Lynne Rienner.

Englebert, Pierre, and Kevin Dunn. 2013. *Inside African Politics.* Boulder, CO: Lynne Rienner.

Epp, Charles. 1998. *The Rights Revolution: Lawyers, Activists, and Supreme Courts in Comparative Perspectives.* Chicago, IL: University of Chicago Press.

Epstein, Helen. 2000. "The Mystery of AIDS in South Africa." *New York Review of Books,* July 20. www.nybooks.com/articles/2000/07/20/the-mystery-of-aids-in-south-africa/.

———. 2007. *The Invisible Cure: Why We Are Losing the Fight Against AIDS in Africa.* New York: Picador.

———. 2014. "Ebola in Liberia: An Epidemic of Rumors." *New York Review of Books,* December 18. www.nybooks.com/articles/2014/12/18/ebola-liberia-epidemic-rumors/.

Evans, David, Markus Goldstein, and Anna Popova. 2015. "Health-Worker Mortality and the Legacy of the Ebola Epidemic." *Lancet* 3(8): e439–e440.

Farmer, Paul. 2005. *Pathologies of Power: Health, Human Rights and the New War on the Poor.* Berkeley, CA: University of California Press.

Fassin, Didier. 2007. *When Bodies Remember: Experiences and Politics of AIDS in South Africa.* Berkeley, CA: University of California Press.

Fatton, Robert. 1995. "Africa in the Age of Democratization: The Civic Limits of Civil Society." *African Studies Review* 38(2): 67–110.

Fearon, James, Macartan Humphreys, and Jeremy Weinstein. 2007. *Community-Driven Reconstruction in Lofa County.* Baseline Survey Preliminary Report for International Rescue Committee. www.columbia.edu/~mh2245/FHW/FHW_baseline.pdf.

Ferguson, James. 1994. *The Anti-Politics Machine: Development, Depoliticization, and Bureau-cratic Power in Lesotho*. Minneapolis, MN: University of Minnesota Press.

———. 2006. *Global Shadows: Africa in the Neoliberal World Order*. Durham, NC: Duke University Press.

———. 2009. "The Uses of Neoliberalism." *Antipode* 41(S1): 166–184.

Ferguson, Laura, Daniel Tarantola, Michael Hoffmann, and Sofia Gruskin. 2016. "Non-Communicable Diseases and Human Rights: Global Synergies, Gaps and Opportunities." *Global Public Health*. doi: 10.1080/17441692.2016.1158847.

Fidler, David. 2010. "The Challenges of Global Health Governance." Working Paper. Council on Foreign Relations International Institutions and Global Governance Program. www.cfr.org/global-governance/challenges-global-health-governance/p22202.

Finnemore, Martha. 1993. "International Organizations as Teachers of Norms: The United Nations Educational, Scientific and Cultural Organization and Science Policy." *International Organization* 47(4): 565–597.

———. 2003. *The Purpose of Intervention: Changing Beliefs about the Use of Force*. Ithaca, NY: Cornell University Press.

———. 2009. "Legitimacy, Hypocrisy, and the Social Structure of Unipolarity." *World Politics* 61(1): 58–85.

Finnemore, Martha, and Kathryn Sikkink. 1998. "International Norm Dynamics and Political Change." *International Organization* 52(4): 887–917.

Fisher, Jonathan. 2013. "'Image Management' and African Agency: Ugandan Regional Diplomacy and Donor Relations under Museveni." In *African Agency in International Politics*, edited by William Brown and Sophie Harman, 97–113. New York: Routledge.

Florini, Ann. 1996. "The Evolution of International Norms." *International Studies Quarterly* 40(3): 363–389.

Fortin, Alfred. 1987. "The Politics of AIDS in Kenya." *Third World Quarterly* 9(3): 906–919.

Foundation for AIDS Research. 2015. "Statistics Worldwide." www.amfar.org/worldwide-aids-stats/.

Fourie, Pieter. 2015. "AIDS as a Security Threat: The Emergence and the Decline of an Idea." In *Routledge Handbook of Global Health Security*, edited by Simon Rushton and Jeremy Youde, 105–117. New York: Routledge.

Fox, Ashley. 2014. "AIDS Policy Responsiveness in Africa: Evidence from Opinion Surveys." *Global Public Health* 9(1–2): 224–248.

Freedom House. 2016a. "Ghana." https://freedomhouse.org/report/freedom-world/2016/ghana.

———. 2016b. "Sub-Saharan Africa." https://freedomhouse.org/regions/sub-saharan-africa.

———. 2016c. "Zambia." https://freedomhouse.org/report/freedom-world/2016/zambia.

Frenk, Julio, and Octavio Gomez-Dantes. 2011. "The Triple Burden: Disease in Developing Nations." *Harvard International Review* 33(3): 36–41.

Frenk, Julio, and Suerie Moon. 2013. "Governance Challenges in Global Health." *New England Journal of Medicine* 368(10): 936–942.

Friedman, Steven, and Shauna Mottiar. 2004. "A Moral to the Tale: The Treatment Action Campaign and the Politics of HIV/AIDS." Paper for the Centre for Policy Studies,

University of Kwa-Zulu Natal, Durban, South Africa. www.escr-net.org/sites/default/files
/Friedman_Mottier_-__A__Moral_to_the_Tale.pdf.

Friedman, Willa. 2015. "Corruption and Averting AIDS Deaths." Working Paper 395. Center
for Global Development, February. www.cgdev.org/publication/corruption-and-averting
-aids-deaths-working-paper-395.

Friends of the Global Fight. 2017. "How the Global Fund Encourages Increased Domestic
Financing." www.theglobalfight.org/global-fund-encourages-increased-domestic
-financing.

Frontline. 2014. "Firestone and the Warlord," November 18. www.pbs.org/wgbh/frontline/film
/firestone-and-the-warlord/.

Frueh, Jamie. 2014. "Global Messages and Local Spaces: Creativity and Ownership in the
Prevention of HIV." Paper presented at the 2014 International Studies Association
Conference, Toronto, March 26–29.

Furlong, Patrick, and Karen Ball. 2005. "The More Things Change: AIDS and the State in
South Africa, 1987–2003." In *The African State and the AIDS Crisis*, edited by Amy S.
Patterson, 155–170. Aldershot, UK: Ashgate.

Gailmard, Sean. 2014. "Accountability and Principal-Agent Theory." In *The Oxford Handbook
of Accountability*, edited by Mark Bovens, Robert Goodin, and Thomas Schillemans,
90–105. New York: Oxford University Press.

Garrett, Laurie. 2015a. "Ahead in 2015: Viruses, Epidemics and United Nations Haggling—
Part Three: Racing to Meet the MDGs (and Create SDGs)." Blog post. http://lauriegarrett.
com/blog/ahead-in-2015-part-three.

———. 2015b. "Ebola's Lessons: How the WHO Mishandled the Crisis." *Foreign Affairs*,
August 18.

Gberie, Lansan. 2008. "Briefing: Truth and Justice on Trial in Liberia." *African Affairs*
107(428): 455–465.

Geffen, Nathan. 2010. *Debunking Delusions: The Inside Story of the Treatment Action Campaign*.
Cape Town, South Africa: Jacana.

Geneau, R., D. Stuckler, S. Stachenko, M. McKee, S. Ebrahim, S. Basu, A. Chockalingham,
M. Mwatsama, R. Jamal, A. Alwan, and R. Beaglehole. 2010. "Raising the
Priority of Preventing Chronic Diseases: A Political Process." *Lancet* 376(9753):
1689–1698.

Gibson, Lucy, and Anne Mills. 1995. "Health Sector Reforms in Sub-Saharan Africa: Lessons
of the Last 10 Years." *Health Policy* 32(1–3): 215–243.

Gifford, Paul. 2009. *Christianity, Politics and Public Life in Kenya*. New York: Columbia
University Press.

Giles-Vernick, Tamara, and James Webb, editors. 2013. *Global Health in Africa: Historical
Perspectives on Disease Control*. Athens, OH: Ohio University Press.

Glasgow, Sara. 2012. "The Politics of Non-Communicable Disease Policy." In *Ashgate Research
Companion to the Globalization of Health*, edited by Ted Schrecker, 61–77. Aldershot, UK:
Ashgate.

Global Fund. *See* Global Fund to Fight AIDS, Tuberculosis and Malaria.

Global Fund to Fight AIDS, Tuberculosis and Malaria. 2013. "Guidelines and Requirements for Country Coordinating Mechanisms." 16th Board Meeting. www.theglobalfund.org/en /ccm/guidelines.

———. 2015a. "CCM Composition Reports." Excel file. Available at www.theglobalfund.org /en/ccm/data/.

———. 2015b. "Results Report 2015." www.theglobalfund.org/en/fundingmodel.

———. 2016a. "Global Fund Overview." www.theglobalfund.org/en/overview/.

———. 2016b. "Financials: Where We Invest." www.theglobalfund.org/en/financials/.

———. 2016c. "Office of the Inspector General—Updates." www.theglobalfund.org/en/oig /updates/.

Global Polio Eradication Initiative. 2017. "Nigeria." http://polioeradication.org/where-we -work/nigeria/.

Global Witness. 2015. *The New Snake Oil? The Violence, Threats and False Promises Driving Rapid Palm Oil Expansion in Liberia.* Online Report, July 23. www.globalwitness.org/en /campaigns/land-deals/new-snake-oil/

Goldsmith, Arthur. 2000. "Sizing up the African State." *Journal of Modern African Studies* 38(1): 1–20.

Goodchild, Mark, Nigar Nargis, and Edouart Tursan d'Espaignet. 2017. "Global Economic Cost of Smoking-Attributable Diseases." *Tobacco Control.* Published online January 30. doi: 10.1136/tobaccocontrol-2016-053305.

Goodliffe, Jay, and Darren Hawkins. 2009. "A Funny Thing Happened on the Way to Rome: Explaining International Criminal Court Negotiations." *Journal of Politics* 71(3): 977–997.

Gordenker, Leon, Roger Coate, Christer Jönsson, and Peter Söderholm. 1995. *International Cooperation in Response to AIDS.* New York: Pinter Press.

Gostin, Lawrence. 2014. *Global Health Law.* Cambridge, MA: Harvard University Press.

———. 2016. "AIDS: How Far the World Has Come and How Far It Needs to Go to Get to Zero." *The Conversation*, February 16.

Gostin, Lawrence, and Eric Friedman. 2015. "A Retrospective and Prospective Analysis of the West African Ebola Virus Disease Epidemic: Robust National Health Systems at the Foundation and an Empowered WHO at the Apex." *Lancet* 385(May 9): 1902–1909.

Gould, Deborah. 2009. *Moving Politics: Emotion and ACT UP's Fight against AIDS.* Chicago, IL: University of Chicago Press.

Government of Liberia. 2014. Executive Order No. 65. "Prohibition on Mass Movement of People Including Rallies, Parades, and Demonstrations on the Streets of Monrovia." www. emansion.gov.lr/doc/EONo65.pdf.

———. 2015. "Kicking Ebola Out of Liberia." *Executive Horn: Magazine of the President of the Republic of Liberia* 2(3): 14–22.

Gray, Julia. 2014. "Domestic Capacity and the Implementation Gap in Regional Trade Agreements." *Comparative Political Studies* 47(1): 55–84.

Green, Edward. 2003. *Rethinking AIDS Prevention: Learning from Successes in Developing Countries.* Westport, CT: Praeger.

Green, Edward, and Allison Herling Ruark. 2011. *AIDS, Behavior and Culture: Understanding Evidence-Based Prevention.* Walnut Creek, CA: West Coast Press.

Grosse, Scott D., Isaac Odame, Hani K. Atrash, Djesika D. Amendah, Frédéric B. Piel, and Thomas N. Williams. 2011. "Sickle Cell Disease in Africa: A Neglected Cause of Early Childhood Mortality." *American Journal of Preventative Medicine* 41(4): S398–S405.

Gruskin, Sofia, editor. 2005. *Perspectives on Health and Human Rights*. New York: Routledge.

Gruskin, Sofia, Laura Ferguson, Daniel Tarantola, and Robert Beaglehole. 2014. "Noncommunicable Diseases and Human Rights: A Promising Synergy." *American Journal of Public Health* 104(5): 773–774.

Guest, Emma. 2001. *Children of AIDS: Africa's Orphan Crisis*. London: Pluto.

Gyimah-Boadi, Emmanuel, editor. 2004. *Democratic Reform in Africa: The Quality of Progress*. Boulder, CO: Lynne Rienner.

Haas, Peter. 1992. "Introduction: Epistemic Communities and International Policy Coordination." *International Organization* 46(1): 1–35.

Hafner, Tamara, and Jeremy Shiffman. 2013. "The Emergence of Global Attention to Health Systems Strengthening." *Health Policy and Planning* 28(1): 41–50.

Hamel, Liz, Jamie Firth, and Mollyann Brodie. 2014. "Kaiser Health Policy News Index: Special Focus on Ebola," October 16. http://kff.org/global-health-policy/poll-finding/kaiser-health-policy-news-index-special-focus-on-ebola.

Hamilton, Kimberly, and Jennifer Yau. 2004. *The Global Tug-of-War for Health-Care Workers*. Migration Policy Institute Paper. www.migrationpolicy.org/article/global-tug-war-health-care-workers.

Harding, Richard, Lucy Selman, Richard Powell, Eve Namisango, Julia Downing, Anne Merriman, Zipporah Ali, Nancy Gikaara, Liz Gwyther, and Irene Higginson. 2013. "Research into Palliative Care in Sub-Saharan Africa." *Lancet Oncology* 14(April): e183–e188.

Harman, Sophie. 2009. "Fighting HIV and AIDS: Reconfiguring the State." *Review of African Political Economy* 35(121): 343–367.

———. 2015. "Why Billions in Foreign Aid Failed to Prevent Ebola Outbreak." *NOVA Next*, October 21. www.pbs.org/wgbh/nova/next/body/vertical-health-funding/.

———. 2016a. "Commentary: Norms Won't Save You: Ebola and the Norm of Global Health Security." *Global Health Governance* 10(1): 11–16.

———. 2016b. "Ebola, Gender and Conspicuously Invisible Women in Global Health Governance." *Third World Quarterly* 37(3): 524–541.

Harris, Paul, and Patricia Siplon. 2006. "International Relations and Global Ethics of HIV/AIDS." In *The Global Politics of AIDS*, edited by Paul Harris and Patricia Siplon, 263–293. Boulder, CO: Lynne Rienner.

Harrison, Graham. 2010. *Neoliberal Africa: The Impact of Global Social Engineering*. London: Zed.

Harvard School of Public Health and World Economic Forum. 2011. *The Global Economic Burden of Non-Communicable Diseases*. Online Report. www3.weforum.org/docs/WEF_Harvard_HE_GlobalEconomicBurdenNonCommunicableDiseases_2011.pdf.

Haven, Ben, and Amy S. Patterson. 2007. "The Government-NGO Disconnect: AIDS Policy in Ghana." In *The Global Politics of AIDS*, edited by Paul Harris and Patricia Siplon, 65–85. Boulder, CO: Lynne Rienner.

Hawkins, Benjamin, Chris Holden, Jappe Eckhardt, and Kelley Lee. 2016. "Reassessing Policy Paradigms: A Comparison of the Global Tobacco and Alcohol Industries." *Global Public Health*. doi: 10.1080/17441692.2016.1161815.

Haynes, Jeffrey. 2007. *Religion and Development: Conflict or Cooperation?* New York: Palgrave Macmillan.

Henrard, Kristin. 2002. *Minority Protection in Post-Apartheid South Africa: Human Rights, Minority Rights, and Self-Determination.* Westport, CT: Praeger.

Herbst, Jeffrey. 2000. *States and Power in Africa: Comparative Lessons in Authority and Control.* Princeton, NJ: Princeton University Press.

Hesse, Brian. 2015. "Africa's Intoxicating Beer Markets." *African Studies Review* 58(1): 91–111.

Hey, Jeanne. 2003. *Small States in World Politics: Explaining Foreign Policy Behavior.* Boulder, CO: Lynne Rienner.

Hilhorst, Dorothea. 2003. *The Real World of NGOs: Discourses, Diversity and Development.* London: Zed.

Hoffman, Danny. 2007. "The City as Barracks: Freetown, Monrovia and the Organization of Violence in Postcolonial African Cities." *Cultural Anthropology* 22(3): 400–428.

Honwana, Alcinda. 2005. *Child Soldiers in Africa: Ethnography of Political Violence Series.* Philadelphia: University of Pennsylvania Press.

Hotez, Peter, Oluwatoyin Asojo, and Adekunle Adesina. 2012. "Nigeria: 'Ground Zero' for the High Prevalence Neglected Tropic Diseases." *PLoS Neglected Tropical Diseases* 6(7): e1600.

Huband, Mark. 1998. *The Liberian Civil War.* London: Frank Cass.

Hunsmann, Moritz. 2012. "Limits to Evidence-Based Health Policymaking: Policy Hurdles to Structural HIV Prevention in Tanzania." *Social Science & Medicine* 74(10): 1477–1485.

———. 2015. "Global Health Initiatives in the Long Run: Donor Responsibility, African Agency and the Sustainability of Antiretroviral Treatment in Tanzania." Paper presented at the International Studies Association Conference, New Orleans, LA, February 18–21.

Hunter, Susan. 2003. *Black Death: AIDS in Africa.* New York: Palgrave Macmillan.

Huntington, Samuel. 1968. *Political Order in Changing Societies.* New Haven, CT: Yale University Press.

Huster, Karin. 2016. "WHO Says Ebola Epidemic Is Over. What Have (and Haven't) We Learned?" *National Public Radio*, March 27. www.npr.org/sections/goatsandsoda/2016/03/27/471870907/ebola-we-may-have-won-the-battle-but-we-havent-won-the-war.

Hyden, Goran. 1980. *Beyond Ujamaa in Tanzania: Underdevelopment and an Uncaptured Peasantry.* Berkeley, CA: University of California Press.

Hyden, Goran, and Kim Lanegran. 1993. "AIDS Policy and Politics: East Africa in Comparative Perspective." *Review of Policy Research* 12(1–2): 47–65.

IDS. *See* Institute of Development Studies.

Ilesanmi, Olayinka Stephen, Olusimbo Kehinde Ige, and Akindele Olupelumi Adebiyi. 2012. "The Managed Hypertensive: The Costs of Blood Pressure Control in a Nigerian Town." *Pan African Medical Journal* 12(96). www.panafrican-med-journal.com/content/article/12/96/pdf/96.pdf.

Iliffe, John. 1995. *Africans: The History of a Continent.* New York: Cambridge University Press.

———. 2006. *The African AIDS Epidemic: A History.* Athens, OH: Ohio University Press.

Institute of Development Studies. 2015. "Ebola: Time to Strengthen Health Systems and Global Health Governance." Blog post, March 10. www.ids.ac.uk/opinion/ebola-time-to -strengthen-health-systems-and-global-health-governance.

Integrated Regional Information Networks. 1999. *IRIN Background Report on Lofa County*. www.africa.upenn.edu/Newsletters/irinw_83199.html.

Inter-Agency Standing Committee. 2015. *Humanitarian Crisis in West Africa (Ebola) Gender Alert: February 2015*. News release, United Nations Women. www.unwomen.org/~ /media/headquarters/attachments/sections/library/publications/2015/iasc%20gen- der%20reference%20group%20-%20gender%20alert%20west%20africa%20ebola%20 2%20-%20february%202015.pdf.

International AIDS Society and Society for AIDS in Africa. 2007. *Statement on the Gambian Government's Unproven Claim of a Cure for AIDS*. April 24. www.iasociety.org/Web /WebContent/File/Old/PDF/1330.pdf.

International Crisis Group. 2001. *HIV/AIDS as a Security Issue*. Washington, DC: ICG.

IRIN. *See* Integrated Regional Information Networks.

Jackson, Robert. 1990. *Quasi-States: Sovereignty, International Relations and the Third World*. New York: Cambridge University Press.

Jackson, Robert, and Carl Rosberg. 1982. *Personal Rule in Black Africa*. Berkeley, CA: University of California Press.

Jegede, Ayodele Samuel. 2007. "What Led to the Nigerian Boycott of the Polio Vaccination Campaign?" *PLoS Medicine* 4(3): e73.

Jerving, Sarah. 2014. "Why Liberians Thought Ebola Was a Government Scam to Attract Western Aid." *The Nation*, September 16. www.thenation.com/article/why-liberians -thought-ebola-was-a-government-scam-attract-western-aid.

Johnson, Krista. 2006. "AIDS and the Politics of Rights in South Africa: Contested Terrain." *Human Rights Review* 7(2): 115–129.

Joint United Nations Programme on HIV/AIDS. 2004. *The Media and HIV/AIDS: Making a Difference*. http://data.unaids.org/Publications/IRC-pub06/jc1000-media_en.pdf.

———. 2010. "Getting to Zero." www.unaids.org/sites/default/files/sub_landing/files/JC2034 _UNAIDS_Strategy_en.pdf.

———. 2012a. "2012 National Commitments and Policies Instrument." www.unaids.org/en /dataanalysis/knowyourresponse/ncpi/2012countries.

———. 2012b. "AIDS Dependency Crisis: Sourcing African Solutions." www.unaids.org/sites /default/files/media_asset/JC2286_Sourcing-African-Solutions_en_1.pdf.

———. 2012c. "Mali Country Progress Report." http://files.unaids.org/en/dataanalysis /knowyourresponse/countryprogressreports/2012countries/RAPPORT_UNGASS%20 2012%20_Mali.pdf.

———. 2012d. "Value for Money in Health Programming a Key Theme at African Ministerial Conference in Tunisia." News release. www.unaids.org/en/resources/presscentre /featurestories/2012/july/20120705tunisia.

———. 2013. "Access to Antiretroviral Therapy in Africa. Status Report on Progress Towards the 2015 Targets." www.unaids.org/sites/default/files/media_asset/20131219_AccessARTA fricaStatusReportProgresstowards2015Targets_en_0.pdf.

———. 2014a. "2014 National Commitments and Policies Instrument." www.unaids.org/en
/dataanalysis/knowyourresponse/ncpi/2014countries.

———. 2014b. "2014 Progress Reports Submitted by Countries." www.unaids.org/en
/dataanalysis/knowyourresponse/countryprogressreports/2014countries.

———. 2014c. "Botswana Country Progress Report." www.unaids.org/sites/default/files/en
/dataanalysis/knowyourresponse/countryprogressreports/2014countries/BWA_narrative
_report_2014.pdf.

———. 2014d. "The Gap Report." www.unaids.org/sites/default/files/en/media/unaids
/contentassets/documents/unaidspublication/2014/UNAIDS_Gap_report_en.pdf.

———. 2014e. "Ghana Country Progress Report." www.unaids.org/sites/default/files/en
/dataanalysis/knowyourresponse/countryprogressreports/2014countries/GHA_narrative
_report_2014.pdf.

———. 2014f. "Somali HIV Epidemic and Response." http://files.unaids.org/en/dataanalysis
/knowyourresponse/countryprogressreports/2014countries/SOM_narrative_report_2014
.pdf.

———. 2014g. "South Africa Country Progress Report." http://files.unaids.org/en/dataanalysis
/knowyourresponse/countryprogressreports/2012countries/ce_ZA_Narrative_Report
.pdf.

———. 2014h. "UNAIDS Report Shows that 19 Million of the 35 Million People Living with
HIV Today Do Not Know That They Have the Virus." Press release. www.unaids.org/sites
/default/files/web_story//20140716_PR_GapReport_en.pdf.

———. 2015a. "Fact Sheet: 2014 Global Statistics." www.unaids.org/sites/default/files/media
_asset/20150714_FS_MDG6_Report_en.pdf.

———. 2015b. "The Gambia Global AIDS Response Progress Report." www.unaids.org/sites
/default/files/country/documents/GMB_narrative_report_2015.pdf.

———. 2015c. "UNAIDS Terminology Guidelines." www.unaids.org/sites/default/files/media
_asset/2015_terminology_guidelines_en.pdf.

———. 2016. "The Collapse of Global AIDS Funding." www.unaids.org/en/resources
/presscentre/featurestories/2016/july/20160719_funding.

Jones, Jared. 2014. "Ebola, Emerging: The Limitations of Culturalist Discourses in Epidemiology." *Journal of Global Health Online*, August 9. www.ghjournal.org/ebola-emerging-the
-limitations-of-culturalist-discourses-in-epidemiology.

Justesen, Mogens. 2015. "Too Poor to Care? The Salience of AIDS in Africa." *Political Research
Quarterly* 68(1): 89–103.

Kaiser Family Foundation. 2015a. "Data Note: Americans' Views on the U.S. Role in Global
Health." January 23. http://kff.org/global-health-policy/poll-finding/data-note-americans
-views-on-the-u-s-role-in-global-health/

———. 2015b. "Financing the Response to AIDS in Low- and Middle-Income Countries."
http://kff.org/report-section/financing-the-response-to-aids-in-low-and-middle-income
-countries-report.

Kaiser Family Foundation and UNAIDS. 2016. "Financing the Response to HIV in Low- and
Middle-Income Countries: International Assistance from Donor Governments in 2015."

July. http://files.kff.org/attachment/Financing-the-Response-to-HIV-in-Low-and-Middle-Income-Countries-International-Assistance-from-Donor-Governments-in-2015.

Kalichman, Seth, Lisa Eaton, and Chauncey Cherry. 2010. "'There Is No Proof that HIV Causes AIDS': AIDS Denialism Beliefs among People Living with HIV/AIDS." *Journal of Behavioral Medicine* 33(6): 432–440.

Kalipeni, Ezekiel, Susan Craddock, Joseph Oppong, and Jayati Ghosh, editors. 2004. *HIV and AIDS in Africa: Beyond Epidemiology*. Malden, MA: Blackwell.

Kalofonos, Ippolytos Andreas. 2010. "'All I Eat Is ARVs': The Paradox of AIDS Treatment Interventions in Central Mozambique." *Medical Anthropology Quarterly* 24(3): 363–380.

Kamradt-Scott, Adam. 2015. *Managing Global Health Security: The World Health Organization and Disease Outbreak Control*. New York: Palgrave Macmillan.

———. 2016. "WHO's to Blame? The World Health Organization and the 2014 Ebola Outbreak in West Africa." *Third World Quarterly* 37(3): 401–418.

Kamradt-Scott, Adam, Sophie Harman, Clare Wenham, and Frank Smith. 2015. *Saving Lives: The Civil-Military Response to the 2014 Ebola Outbreak in West Africa*. Report for University of Sydney. https://sydney.edu.au/arts/ciss/downloads/SavingLivesPDF.pdf.

Kaplan, Robert. 1994. "The Coming Anarchy." *Atlantic*, February. www.theatlantic.com/magazine/archive/1994/02/the-coming-anarchy/304670/.

Kapp, Clare. 2005. "South African Health Minister Urged to Stop Vitamin-Peddling Doctor." *Lancet* 366(9500): 1837–1838.

Kapstein, Ethan, and Joshua Busby. 2013. *AIDS Drugs for All: Social Movements and Market Transformations*. New York: Cambridge University Press.

Kasolo, Francis Chisaka, Jean-Baptiste Roungou, Florimond Kweteminga Tshioko, Benido Impouma, Ali Ahmed Yahaya, Nathan Bakyaita, Peter Gaturuku, Zabulon Yoti, Isabelle Nuttal, Stella Chungong, and Florence Fuchs. 2013. "Implementation of the International Health Regulations (2005) in the African Region." *African Health Monitor* 18: 11–13. www.aho.afro.who.int/sites/default/files/ahm/reports/746/ahm-18-03-implementation-international-health-regulations-2005.pdf.

Kata, Anna. 2012. "Anti-Vaccine Activists, Web 2.0, and the Postmodern Paradigm—An Overview of Tactics and Tropes Used Online by the Anti-Vaccination Movement." *Vaccine* 30(25): 3778–3789.

Kawachi, Ichiro, and Sarah Wamala. 2007. *Globalization and Health*. New York: Oxford University Press.

Kayima, James, Rhoda Wanyenze, Achilles Katamba, Elli Leontsini, and Fred Nuwaha. 2013. "Hypertension Awareness, Treatment and Control in Africa: A Systematic Review." *Biomed Central Cardiovascular Disorders* 13(54). www.biomedcentral.com/1471-2261/13/54.

Keck, Margaret, and Kathryn Sikkink. 1998. *Activists beyond Borders*. Ithaca, NY: Cornell University Press.

Keim, Curtis. 1999. *Mistaking Africa: Curiosities and Inventions of the American Mind*. Boulder, CO: Westview.

Kelsall, Tim. 2011. "Rethinking the Relationship between Neo-Patrimonialism and Economic Development in Africa." *IDS Bulletin* 42(2): 76–87.

Kenworthy, Nora, and Richard Parker. 2014. "HIV Scale-Up and the Politics of Global Health." *Global Public Health* 9(1–2): 1–6.

Keohane, Robert. 1984. *After Hegemony: Cooperation and Discord in the World Political Economy.* Princeton, NJ: Princeton University Press.

Kevane, Michael. 2004. *Women and Development in Africa: How Gender Works.* Boulder, CO: Lynne Rienner.

Khan, Mushtaq H. 2000. "Rents, Efficiency and Growth." In *Rents, Rent-Seeking and Economic Development: Theory and Evidence in Asia,* edited by Mushtaq H. Khan and Jomo Kwame Sundaram, 21–69. New York: Cambridge University Press.

———. 2005. "Markets, States and Democracy: Patron-Client Networks and the Case for Democracy in Developing Countries." *Democratization* 12(5): 704–724.

Kieney, Marie-Paule, David Evans, Gerard Schmets, and Sowmya Kadandale. 2014. "Health System Resilience: Reflections on the Ebola Crisis in Western Africa." *Bulletin of the World Health Organization* 92: 850.

Killick, Tony. 1998. *Aid and the Political Economy of Policy Change.* New York: Routledge.

Kim, Jim Yong, Joyce Millen, Alec Irwin, and John Gershman. 2002. *Dying for Growth: Global Inequality and the Health of the Poor.* Monroe, ME: Common Courage Press.

Kingdon, John. 1995. *Agendas, Alternatives, and Public Politics,* 2nd ed. New York: HarperCollins.

Kirkland, Anna. 2012. "The Legitimacy of Vaccine Critics: What Is Left after the Autism Hypothesis?" *Journal of Health Politics, Policy and Law* 37(1): 69–97.

Kirton, John, Andrew Cooper, Franklyn Lisk, and Hany Besada. 2014. *Moving Health Sovereignty in Africa: Disease, Governance, Climate Change.* Burlington, VT: Ashgate.

Kitschelt, Herbert, and Steven Wilkinson, editors. 2007. *Patrons, Clients, and Policies: Patterns of Democratic Accountability and Political Competition.* New York: Cambridge University Press.

Klotz, Audie. 1995. *Norms in International Relations: The Struggle against Apartheid.* Ithaca, NY: Cornell University Press.

Kupferschmidt, Kai. 2015. "In Wake of Ebola Epidemic, Margaret Chan Wants Countries to Put Their Money Where Their Mouth Is." *Science,* October 14. www.sciencemag.org/news /2015/10/wake-ebola-epidemic-margaret-chan-wants-countries-put-their-money-where -their-mouth.

Lancet. 2011. *Global Mental Health.* www.thelancet.com/series/global-mental-health-2011.

———. 2012. "Global Burden of Disease Report 2010." www.thelancet.com/global-burden-of -disease.

———. 2013. "Cancer Control in Africa: Special Series." www.thelancet.com/series/cancer -control-in-africa.

———. 2015. "Global Trends and Predictions for Tobacco Use, 1990–2025: An Analysis of Smoking Indicators from the WHO Comprehensive Information Systems for Tobacco Control." www.thelancet.com/journals/lancet/article/PIIS0140-6736(15)60264-1/fulltext.

———. 2016. "Global, Regional, and National Life Expectancy, All-Cause Mortality, and Cause-Specific Mortality for 249 Causes of Death, 1980–2015: A Systematic Analysis for

the Global Burden of Disease Study 2015." http://thelancet.com/journals/lancet/article
/PIIS0140-6736(16)31012-1/fulltext.

———. 2017. "Evolution and Patterns of Global Health Financing 1995–2014: Development
Assistance for Health, and Government, Prepaid Private, and Out-of-Pocket Health
Spending for 184 Countries." http://thelancet.com/journals/lancet/article/PIIS0140
-6736(17)30874-7/fulltext.

Lee, Jong-Wha, and Warwick McKibbin. 2004. "Globalization and Disease: The Case of
SARS." *Asian Economic Papers* 3(1): 113–131.

Legro, Jeffrey. 1997. "Which Norms Matter? Revisiting the 'Failure' of Internationalism."
International Organization 51(1): 31–63.

Lemarchand, Rene. 1972. "Political Clientelism and Ethnicity in Tropical Africa: Competing
Solidarities in Nation-Building." *American Political Science Review* 66(1): 68–90.

Leonard, David, and Scott Straus. 2003. *Africa's Stalled Development: International Causes and
Cures*. Boulder, CO: Lynne Rienner.

Levy, Brian. 2010. "Development Trajectories: An Evolutionary Approach to Integrating
Governance and Growth." *Economic Premise* 15 (May 10). Washington: World Bank.
http://siteresources.worldbank.org/INTPREMNET/Resources/EP15.pdf

Lewis, David, and David Mosse. 2006. *Brokers and Translators: The Ethnography of Aid and
Agencies*. Westport, CT: Kumarian.

Liao, John B. 2006. "Viruses and Human Cancer." *Yale Journal of Biology and Medicine*
79(3–4): 115–122.

Liebenow, Gus. 1987. *Liberia: The Quest for Democracy*. Bloomington, IN: Indiana University
Press.

Lieberman, Evan. 2012. "Descriptive Representation and AIDS Policy in South Africa."
Contemporary Politics 18(2): 156–173.

Lindberg, Steffan, editor. 2009. *Democratization by Elections: A New Model of Transition*.
Baltimore, MD: Johns Hopkins University Press.

Livingston, Julie. 2012. *Improvising Medicine*. Durham, NC: Duke University Press.

Lodge, Tom. 2003. *Politics in South Africa: From Mandela to Mbeki*. Oxford: James Currey.

———. 2014. "Neopatrimonial Politics in the ANC." *African Affairs* 113(450): 1–23.

Lonsdale, John. 2000. "Agency in Tight Corners: Narrative and Initiative in African History."
Journal of African Cultural Studies 13(1): 5–16.

Lown, E. Anne, Patricia A. McDaniel, and Ruth E. Malone. 2016. "Tobacco Is 'Our Industry
and We Must Support It': Exploring the Potential Implications of Zimbabwe's Accession to
the Framework Convention on Tobacco Control." *Globalization and Health*. doi: 10.1186/
s12922-015-0139-3.

Lundy, Brandon, and Solomon Negash. 2013. *Teaching Africa: A Guide for the 21st-Century
Classroom*. Bloomington, IN: Indiana University Press.

Lyne, Mona. 2007. "Rethinking Economics and Institutions: The Voter's Dilemma and
Democratic Accountability." In *Patrons, Clients and Policies: Patterns of Democratic
Accountability and Political Competition*, edited by Herbert Kitshelt and Steven I. Wilkin-
son, 159–181. New York: Cambridge University Press.

MacGaffey, Janet, and Rémy Bazenguissa-Ganga. 2000. *Congo-Paris: Transnational Traders on the Margins of the Law*. Bloomington, IN: Indiana University Press.

MacKenzie, John, Patrick Drury, Ray Arthur, Michael Ryan, Thomas Grein, Raphael Slattery, Sameera Suri, Christine Tiffany Domingo, and Armand Bejtullahu. 2014. "The Global Outbreak Alert and Response Network." *Global Public Health* 9(9): 1023–1039.

MacKenzie, Ross, Jappe Eckhardt, and Ade Widyati Prastyani. 2017. "Japan Tobacco International: To 'Be the Most Successful and Respected Tobacco Company in the World.'" *Global Public Health* 12(3): 281–299.

Mackey, Tim. 2016. "Lessons from Liberia: Global Health Governance in the Post-Ebola Paradigm." *Global Health Governance* 10(1): 61–71.

Mamdani, Mahmood. 2001. *When Victims Become Killers: Colonialism, Nativism and the Genocide in Rwanda*. Princeton, NJ: Princeton University Press.

Mann, Jonathan, editor. 1999. *Health and Human Rights: A Reader*. New York: Routledge.

Manyema, Mercy. 2013. "Non-Communicable Diseases in Africa: Time to Take Notice." *Report for Consultancy Africa Intelligence*, February 18. www.consultancyafrica.com/index .php?option=com_content&view=article&id=1235:non-communicable-diseases-in-africa -time-to-take-notice-&catid=61:hiv-aids-discussion-papers&Itemid=268.

Maron, Dina Fine. 2014. "Smoke Screen: Are E-Cigarettes Safe?" *Scientific American*, May 1. www.scientificamerican.com/article/smoke-screen-are-e-cigarettes-safe/.

Marquez, Patricio. 2012. "How Does Africa Fare? Findings from the Global Burden of Disease Study." Blog post. http://blogs.worldbank.org/africacan/how-does-africa-fare-findings -from-the-global-burden-of-disease-study.

Marshall, Monty, and Benjamin Cole. 2014. *Global Report 2014: Conflict, Governance, and State Fragility*. www.systemicpeace.org/globalreport.html.

Matfess, Hilary. 2015. "Rwanda and Ethiopia: Developmental Authoritarianism and the New Politics of African Strong Men." *African Studies Review* 58(2): 181–204.

Mbali, Mandisa. 2013. *South African AIDS Activism and Global Health Politics*. New York: Palgrave Macmillan.

Mbeki, Thabo. 2000. "Letter to World Leaders." April 3. www.virusmyth.com/aids/news /lettermbeki.htm.

McCauley, John. 2012. "Africa's New Big Man Rule? Pentecostalism and Patronage in Ghana." *African Affairs* 112(446): 1–21.

McCurdy, Sheryl, and Haruka Maruyama. 2013. "Heroin Use, Trafficking, and Intervention Approaches in Sub-Saharan Africa." In *Global Health in Africa: Historical Perspectives on Disease Control*, edited by Tamara Giles-Vernick and James Webb, 211–234. Athens, OH: Ohio University Press.

McDaniel, Patricia, Brie Cadman, and Ruth Malone. 2016. "African Media Coverage of Tobacco Industry Corporate Social Responsibility Initiatives." *Global Pubic Health*. doi: 10.1080/17441692.2016.1149203.

McInnes, Colin. 2016. "Crisis! What Crisis? Global Health and the 2014–15 West African Ebola Outbreak." *Third World Quarterly* 37(3): 380–400.

McInnes, Colin, Adam Kamradt-Scott, Kelley Lee, David Reubi, Anne Roemer-Mahler, Simon Rushton, Owain David Williams, and Marie Woodling. 2012. "Framing Global Health: The Governance Challenge." *Global Public Health* 7(Supplement 2): S83–S94.

McInnes, Colin, and Kelley Lee. 2012. "Framing and Global Health Governance: Key Findings." *Global Public Health* 7(Supplement 2): S191–S198.

———. 2013. *Global Health and International Relations*. New York: John Wiley.

McInnes, Colin, and Simon Rushton. 2010. "HIV, AIDS and Security: Where Are We Now?" *International Affairs* 86(1): 225–245.

McKay, Tara. 2016. "From Marginal to Marginalised: The Inclusion of Men Who Have Sex with Men in Global and National AIDS Programmes and Policy." *Global Public Health*. doi: 10.1080/17441692.2016.1143523.

Media Matters. 2014. "Report: Ebola Coverage on TV Plummeted after Mid-Terms." November 19. http://mediamatters.org/research/2014/11/19/report-ebola-coverage-on-tv -news-plummeted-afte/201619.

Médicins sans Frontières. 2014. United Nations Special Briefing on Ebola. September 2. www.doctorswithoutborders.org/news-stories/speechopen-letter/united-nations-special -briefing-ebola.

Medie, Peace. 2013. "Fighting Gender-based Violence: The Women's Movement and the Enforcement of Rape Law in Liberia." *African Affairs* 112(448): 377–397.

Meessen, Bruno, David Hercot, Mathieu Noirhomme, Valéry Ridde, Abdelmajid Tibouti, Christine Kirunga Tashobya, and Lucy Gilson. 2011. "Removing User Fees in the Health Sector: A Review of Policy Processes in Six Sub-Saharan African Countries." *Health Policy and Planning* 26(Supplement 2): ii16–ii29.

Meltzer, Martin, Charisma Atkins, Scott Santibanez, Barbara Knust, Brett Petersen, Elizabeth Ervin, Stuart Nichol, Inger Damon, and Michael Washington. 2014. "Estimating the Future Number of Cases in the Ebola Epidemic—Liberia and Sierra Leone 2014–2015." *Morbidity and Mortality Weekly Report* Supplement 63(3): 1–14.

Mendenhall, Emily, and Shane Norris. 2015. "When HIV is Ordinary and Diabetes New: Remaking Suffering in a South African Township." *Global Public Health* 10(4): 449–462.

Mendis, S., Igbal Al Bashir, Lanka Dissanayake, Cherian Varghese, Ibtihal Fadhil, Asha Marhe, Boureima Sambo, Firdosi Mehta, Hinda Elsayad, Idrisa Sow, Maltie Algoe, Herbert Tennakoon, Lai Die Troung, Le Thi Tuyet Land, Dismond Huiuinato, Neelamni Hewageegana, Naiema A. W. Fahal, Goitom Mebrhatu, Gado Tshering, and Oleg Chestnov. 2012. "Gaps in Capacity in Primary Care in Low-Resource Settings for Implementation of Essential Noncommunicable Disease Interventions." *International Journal of Hypertension* 2012 (2012). Article ID 58404. http://dx.doi.org/10.1155/2012 /584041.

Mensah, George A., and Bongani M. Mayosi. 2013. "The 2011 United Nations High-Level Meeting on Non-Communicable Diseases: The Africa Agenda Calls for a 5-by-5 Approach." *South African Medical Journal* 103(2): 77–79.

Michael, Sarah. 2004. *Undermining Development: The Absence of Power among Local NGOs in Africa*. Bloomington, IN: Indiana University Press.

Migdal, Joel. 1988. *Strong Societies and Weak States: State-Society Relations and State Capabilities in the Third World*. Princeton, NJ: Princeton University Press.

Ministry of Health. 2011. *National Policy for the Prevention and Control of Chronic Non-Communicable Diseases in Ghana*. Government of Ghana. www.alwag.org/education/courses/ncd-policy.pdf.

Mkandawire, Thandika. 2015. "Neopatrimonialism and the Political Economy of Economic Performance in Africa: Critical Reflections." *World Politics* 67(3): 563–612.

Moatti, Thomas, and Jean-Paul Moatti. 2011. "The Global Fight against HIV/AIDS: Is Corruption such a Big Deal after All?" *AIDS* 25(12): 1556–1558.

Moe, Terry. 1984. "The New Economics of Organization." *American Journal of Political Science* 28(4): 739–777.

Moeller, Susan. 2000. "Coverage of AIDS in Africa: The Media Are Silent No Longer." *Nieman Reports* 54(3): 89–94.

Mogelson, Luke. 2015. "When the Fever Breaks." *New Yorker*, January 19. www.newyorker.com/magazine/2015/01/19/when-fever-breaks.

Mold, Alex, and David Reubi. 2013. *Assembling Health Rights in Global Context: Genealogies and Anthropologies*. New York: Routledge.

Moon, Suerie, Devi Sridhar, Muhammad A. Pate, Ashish K. Jha, Chelsea Clinton, Sophie Delaunay, Valnora Edwin, Mosoka Fallah, David P. Fidler, Laurie Garrett, et al. 2015. "Will Ebola Change the Game? Ten Essential Reforms before the Next Pandemic. The Report of the Harvard-LSHTM Independent Panel on the Global Report to Ebola." *Lancet* 386 (November 18): 2204–2221.

Moore, Mick. 1998. "Death without Taxes: Democracy, State Capacity and Aid Dependence in the Fourth World." In *The Democratic Developmental State*, edited by Mark Robinson and Gordon White, 84–121. New York: Oxford University Press.

Moran, Mary. 2006. *Liberia: The Violence of Democracy*. Philadelphia: University of Pennsylvania Press.

Moran, Mary, and Daniel Hoffman. 2014. "Introduction: Ebola in Perspective." October 7. www.culanth.org/fieldsights/585-ebola-in-perspective.

Moreno, Alejandro. 2003. "Corruption and Democracy: A Cultural Assessment." In *Human Values and Social Change: Findings from the Values Surveys*, edited by Ronald Ingelhart, 265–278. Leiden, Netherlands: Brill.

Morfit, Simon. 2011. "'AIDS Is Money': How Donor Preferences Reconfigure Local Realities." *World Development* 39(2): 64–76.

Morrison, J. Stephen, and Cathryn Streifel. 2015. "After the Worst in Liberia and Sierra Leone." *Health Affairs* blog, February 9. http://healthaffairs.org/blog/2015/02/09/after-the-worst-in-liberia-and-sierra-leone/.

MSF. *See* Médicins sans Frontières.

Murphy, Elaine, Margaret E. Greene, Alexandra Mihailovic, and Peter Olupot-Olupot. 2006. "Was the 'ABC' Approach (Abstinence, Being Faithful, Using Condoms) Responsible for Uganda's Decline in HIV?" *PLoS Medicine* 3(9): e379.

Murray, Christopher, and Alan Lopez, editors. 1996. *The Global Burden of Disease*. Report for the World Health Organization. http://apps.who.int/iris/bitstream/10665/41864/1/0965546608_eng.pdf.

Mwenda, Andrew. 2007. "Personalizing Power in Uganda." *Journal of Democracy* 18(3): 23–37.

Naicker, Saraladevi, John Eastwood, Jacob Plange-Rhule, and Roger C. Tutt. 2010. "Shortage of Healthcare Workers in Sub-Saharan Africa: A Nephrological Perspective." *Clinical Nephrology* 74(S1): S129–S133.

National Democratic Institute. 2016. "Global Elections Calendar." www.ndi.org/electionscalendar/.

National Elections Commission. 2011. "2011 Presidential and Legislative Elections." www.necliberia.org/results2011/results.html.

Nattrass, Nicoli. 2007. *Mortal Combat: AIDS Denialism and the Fight for Antiretrovirals in South Africa*. Pietermaritzburg: University of Kwa-Zulu Natal Press.

———. 2012. *The AIDS Conspiracy: Science Fights Back*. New York: Columbia University Press.

NCD Alliance. 2011. "Country Commitments Made at the UN High Level Meeting on the Prevention and Control of Noncommunicable Diseases." Unpublished document.

———. 2014a. "NCD Alliance Consultation Report." UN High-Level Review on NCDs. http://ncdalliance.org/sites/default/files/rfiles/UN%20Review%20NCD%20Alliance%20Online%20Consultation%20FINAL.pdf.

———. 2014b. "NCD Alliance Statement—UN NCD Review Outcome Document." July 2014. http://ncdalliance.org/sites/default/files/rfiles/NCDA%20Statement_UN%20Review%20Outcome%20Document_July%202014%20FINAL.pdf.

———. 2014c. "Our Global Network Africa." www.ncdalliance.org/network/africa.

———. 2015. "Key Issues." www.ncdalliance.org/node/3216.

NDI. *See* National Democratic Institute.

NEC. *See* National Elections Commission.

Ng, Nora, and Jennifer Prah Ruger. 2011. "Global Health Governance at a Crossroads." *Global Health Governance* 3(2): 1–37.

Nguyen, Vinh-Kim. 2010. *The Republic of Therapy: Triage and Sovereignty in West Africa's Time of AIDS*. Raleigh, NC: Duke University Press.

———. 2014. "Ebola: How We Became Unprepared, and What Might Come Next." *Cultural Anthropology*, October 7. www.culanth.org/fieldsights/585-ebola-in-perspective.

Nkengasong, John, Olawale Maiyegun, and Matshidiso Moeti. 2017. "Establishing the Africa Centres for Disease Control and Prevention: Responding to Africa's Health Threats." *Lancet Global Health* 5(3): e247–e248.

Nulu, Shanti. 2016. "Neglected Chronic Disease: The WHO Framework on Non-Communicable Diseases and Implications for the Global Poor." *Global Public Health*. doi: 10.1080/17441692.2016.1154584.

Nunes, João. 2016. "Ebola and the Production of Neglect in Global Health." *Third World Quarterly* 37(3): 542–556.

OAU. *See* Organization of African Unity.

ODI. *See* Overseas Development Institute.

OECD. 2014. *See* Organisation for Economic Co-operation and Development.

Oelke, N. D., K. L. Rush, F. M. Goma, J. Barker, P. Marck, and C. Pedersen. 2015. "Understanding Perceptions and Practices for Zambian Adults in Western Province at Risk for Hypertension: An Exploratory Descriptive Study." *Global Journal of Health Science* 8(2): 248–259.

Oestreich, Joel. 2007. *Power and Principle: Human Rights Programming in International Organizations.* Washington, DC: Georgetown University Press.

Ofori-Asenso, Richard, and Daireen Garcia. 2016. "Cardiovascular Diseases in Ghana within the Context of Globalization." *Cardiovascular Diagnosis and Therapy* 6(1): 67–77.

Okware, S., J. Kinsman, S. Onyango, A. Opio, and P. Kaggwa. 2005. "Revisiting the ABC Strategy: HIV Prevention in Uganda in the Era of Antiretroviral Therapy." *Postgraduate Medical Journal* 81(960): 625–628.

Ólafsson, Björn. 1998. *Small States in the Global System.* Aldershot, UK: Ashgate.

Olivier de Sardan, Jean-Pierre. 1999. "A Moral Economy of Corruption in Africa?" *Journal of Modern African Studies* 37(1): 25–52.

Organisation for Economic Co-Operation and Development. 2014. "Development Aid at a Glance: Statistics by Region. Africa. 2014 Edition." www.oecd.org/dac/stats/document upload/2.%20Africa%20-%20Development%20Aid%20at%20a%20Glance%202014 .pdf.

Organization of African Unity. 2001. Abuja Declaration on HIV/AIDS, Tuberculosis and Other Related Infectious Diseases. African Summit on HIV/AIDS, Tuberculosis and Other Related Infectious Diseases, Abuja, Nigeria, April 24–27. www.un.org/ga/aids/pdf/abuja _declaration.pdf.

Overseas Development Institute. 2015. "What Ebola Exposed about Health Systems in West Africa." Blog post, October. www.odi.org/opinion/9961-infographics-ebola-health-west -africa-sierra-leone-liberia-guinea-msf.

Owusu-Dabo, E., S. Lewis, A. McNeill, A. Gilmore, and J. Britton. 2009. "Smoking Uptake and Prevalence in Ghana." *Tobacco Control* 18(5): 365–370.

Paes, Wolf-Christian. 2005. "The Challenges of Disarmament, Demobilization and Reintegration in Liberia." *International Peacekeeping* 12(2): 253–261.

PAHO. *See* Pan-American Health Organization.

Pallas, Sarah Wood, Justice Nonvignon, Moses Aikins, and Jennifer Prah Ruger. 2015. "Responses to Donor Proliferation in Ghana's Health Sector: A Qualitative Case Study." *Bulletin of the World Health Organization* 93(1): 11–18.

Pan-American Health Organization. 2015. "Americas Region Is Declared the First to Eliminate Rubella." News release. www.paho.org/hq/index.php?option=com _content&view=article&id=10798%3Aamericas-free-of-rubella&Itemid=1926&lang=en.

Parkhurst, Justin. 2011. "Evidence, Politics and Uganda's HIV Success: Moving Forward with ABC and HIV Prevention." *Journal of International Development* 23: 240–252.

———. 2012. "Framing, Ideology and Evidence: Uganda's HIV Success and the Development of PEPFAR's 'ABC' Policy for HIV Prevention." *Evidence and Policy* 8(1): 19–38.

———. 2013. "The Subtle Politics of AIDS: Values, Bias and Persistent Errors in HIV Prevention." In *Global HIV/AIDS Politics, Policy and Activism: Persistent Challenges and*

Emerging Issues, volume 1, edited by Raymond Smith, 113–139. Santa Barbara, CA: Praeger.

Parkhurst, Justin, and Madhulika Vulimiri. 2013. "Cervical Cancer and the Global Health Agenda: Insights from Multiple Policy-Analysis Frameworks." *Global Public Health* 8(10): 1093–1108.

Parkin, D. Max, Freddy Sitas, Mike Chirenje, Lara Stein, Raymond Abratt, and Henry Wabinga. 2008. "Part I: Cancer in Indigenous Africans—Burden, Distribution, and Trends." *Lancet* 9(July): 683–692.

Patterson, Amy S. 1998. "A Reappraisal of Democracy in Civil Society: Evidence from Rural Senegal." *Journal of Modern African Studies* 36(3): 423–441.

———. 2006. *The Politics of AIDS in Africa*. Boulder, CO: Lynne Rienner.

———. 2007. "The UN and the Fight against HIV/AIDS." In *The Global Politics of AIDS*, edited by Paul Harris and Patricia Siplon, 203–223. Boulder, CO: Lynne Rienner.

———. 2011. *The Church and AIDS in Africa: The Politics of Ambiguity*. Boulder, CO: FirstForum.

———. 2013. "Pastors as Leaders in Africa's Religious AIDS Mobilisation: Cases from Ghana and Zambia." *Canadian Journal of African Studies* 47(2): 207–226.

———. 2015. "Engaging Therapeutic Citizenship and Clientship: Untangling the Reasons for Therapeutic Pacifism among People Living with HIV in Urban Zambia." *Global Public Health*. http://dx.doi.org/10.1080/17441692.2015.1070053.

———. 2016. "Training Professionals, Eroding Relationships: Donors, AIDS Care, and Development in Urban Zambia." *Journal of International Development* 28(6): 827–844.

Patterson, Amy S., and David Cieminis. 2005. "Weak and Ineffective? African States and Recent International AIDS Politics." In *The African State and the AIDS Crisis*, edited by Amy S. Patterson, 171–194. Aldershot, UK: Ashgate.

Patterson, Amy S., and Tracy Kuperus. 2016. "Mobilizing the Faithful: Organizational Autonomy, Visionary Pastors, and Citizenship in South Africa and Zambia." *African Affairs* 115(459): 318–341.

Peacebuilder. 2011. *Liberia, 2011*. Data Set. www.peacebuildingdata.org/interactivemaps/liberia.

PEPFAR. *See* US President's Emergency Plan for AIDS Relief.

Percival, Valerie, and Tino Kreutzer. 2016. "Opening Up: Why the International Community Failed, and then Succeeded, in the Fight against Ebola." Paper presented at the annual International Studies Association Conference, Atlanta, GA, March 15–19.

Pew Forum. 2010. *Tolerance and Tension: Islam and Christianity in Sub-Saharan Africa*. Online Report. www.pewforum.org/2010/04/15/executive-summary-islam-and-christianity-in-sub-saharan-africa/.

Pfeiffer, James, and Rachel Chapman. 2010. "Anthropological Perspectives on Structural Adjustment and Public Health." *Annual Review of Anthropology* 39(October): 149–165.

Pink Ribbon–Red Ribbon. 2016. "Our Story." http://pinkribbonredribbon.org/our-story/.

Pitcher, Anne, Mary Moran, and Michael Johnston. 2009. "Rethinking Patrimonialism and Neopatrimonialism in Africa." *African Studies Review* 52(1): 125–156.

Plank, David. 1993. "Aid, Debt and the End of Sovereignty: Mozambique and Its Donors." *Journal of Modern African Studies* 31(3): 407–430.

Plaut, Martin. 2016. *Understanding Eritrea: Inside Africa's Most Repressive State.* London: C. Hurst.

PLOS Blogs. 2014. "Addressing NCDs in Ghana." http://blogs.plos.org/globalhealth/2013/09/ncdfree_ghana/.

Poletto, C., M. F. Gomes, A. Pastore y Piontti, L. Rossi, L. Bioglio, D. L. Chao, I. M. Longini, Jr., M. E. Halloran, V. Colizza, and A. Vespignani. 2014. "Assessing the Impact of Travel Restrictions on International Spread of the 2014 West African Ebola Epidemic." *Eurosurveillance* 19(42): October 23. www.eurosurveillance.org/ViewArticle.aspx?ArticleId=20936.

Power, Samantha. 2003. "The AIDS Rebel." *New Yorker*, May 19.

Price-Smith, Andrew. 2009. *Contagion and Chaos: Disease, Ecology and National Security in the Era of Globalization.* Cambridge, MA: MIT Press.

Price-Smith, Andrew, and Jackson Porreca. 2016. "Fear, Apathy, and the Ebola Crisis (2014–15): Psychology and Problems of Global Health Governance." *Global Health Governance* 10(1): 17–35.

Pruitt, Liese, Tolulope Mumuni, Eugene Raikhel, Adeyinka Ademola, Temidayo Ogundiran, Adeniyi Adenipekum, Imran Morhason-Bello, Oladosu Ojengbede, and Olufunmilayo Olopade. 2014. "Social Barriers to Diagnosis and Treatment of Breast Cancer in Patients Presenting at a Teaching Hospital in Ibadan, Nigeria." *Global Public Health* 10(3): 331–344.

Przeworski, Adam, Michael Alvarez, Jose Antonio Cheibub, and Fernando Limongi. 2000. *Democracy and Development: Political Institutions and Well-Being in the World, 1950–1990.* New York: Cambridge University Press.

Putnam, Robert. 1994. *Making Democracy Work.* Princeton, NJ: Princeton University Press.

Putzel, James. 2004. "The Global Fight against AIDS: How Adequate Are the National Commissions?" *Journal of International Development* 16(8): 1129–1140.

———. 2006. "A History of State Action: The Politics of AIDS in Uganda and Senegal." In *The HIV/AIDS Epidemic in Sub-Saharan Africa in a Historical Perspective,* edited by Philippe Denis and Charles Becker, 171–184. Dakar: Senegalese Network on Law, Ethics, Health.

Radelet, Steve. 2010. "Success Stories from 'Emerging Africa.'" *Journal of Democracy* 21(4): 87–101.

Ramiah, Ilavenil, and Michael Reich. 2005. "Public-Private Partnerships and Antiretroviral Drugs for HIV/AIDS: Lessons from Botswana." *Health Affairs* 24(2): 545–551.

Reniers, Georges, and Susan Watkins. 2010. "Polygyny and the Spread of HIV in Sub-Saharan Africa: A Case of Benign Concurrency." *AIDS* 24(2): 299–307.

Renne, Elisha. 2010. *The Politics of Polio in Northern Nigeria.* Bloomington, IN: Indiana University Press.

Reno, Will. 2000. "Clandestine Economies, Violence and States in Africa." *Journal of International Affairs* 53(2): 433–459.

Resnick, Danielle. 2015. "The Political Economy of Africa's Emergent Middle Class: Retrospect and Prospects." *Journal of International Development* 27(5): 573–587.

Reticker, Gini, director. 2008. *Pray the Devil Back to Hell.* New York: Fork Films.

Reubi, David. 2012. "Making a Human Right to Tobacco Control: Expert and Advocacy Networks, Framing and the Right to Health." *Global Public Health* 7(Supplement 2): S176–S190.

Rhymer, Wendy, and Rick Speare. "Countries' Response to WHO's Travel Recommendations During the 2013–2016 Ebola Outbreak." *Bulletin of the World Health Organization.* Published online October 18. www.who.int/bulletin/online_first/BLT.16.171579.pdf.

Richardson, Eugene T., Mohamed Bailor Barrie, J. Daniel Kelly, Yusupha Dibba, Songor Koedoyoma, and Paul E. Farmer. 2015. "Biosocial Approaches to the 2013–2016 Ebola Pandemic." *Health and Human Rights Journal* 18(1). www.hhrjournal.org/2015/12/biosocial-approaches-to-the-2013-2016-ebola-pandemic.

Richardson, Eugene, J. Daniel Kelly, Mohamed Bailor Barrie, Annelies W. Mesman, Sahr Karku, Komba Quiwa, Regan H. Marsh, Songor Koedoyoma, Fodei Daboh, Kathryn P. Barron, Michael Grady, Elizabeth Tucker, Kerry L. Dierberg, George W. Rutherford, Michele Barry, James Holland Jones, Megan B. Murray, and Paul E. Farmer. 2016. "Minimally Symptomatic Infection in an Ebola 'Hotspot': A Cross-Sectional Serosurvey." *PLOS Neglected Tropical Diseases* 10(11): e0005087. doi: 10.1371/journal.pntd.0005087.

Richey, Lisa-Ann. 2008. "Science Denial and Politics: 'Boundary Work' in the Provision of AIDS Treatment in South Africa." *New Political Science* 30(1): 1–21.

Riker, William. 1962. *A Theory of Political Coalitions.* New Haven, CT: Yale University Press.

Robins, Steven. 2004. "'Long Live Zackie, Long Live': AIDS Activism, Science and Citizenship after Apartheid." *Journal of Southern African Studies* 30(3): 651–672.

Rotberg, Robert. 2012. *Transformative Political Leadership: Making a Difference in the Developing World.* Chicago, IL: University of Chicago Press.

———. 2013. *Africa Emerges.* Malden, MA: Polity.

Rothchild, Donald, and Naomi Chazan, editors. 1988. *The Precarious Balance: State and Society in Africa.* Boulder, CO: Westview.

Rowden, Rick. 2014. "West Africa's Financial Immune Deficiency." *Foreign Policy,* October 30.

Ruggie, John Gerard. 1998. "What Makes the World Hang Together? Neo-Utilitarianism and the Social Constructivist Challenge." *International Organization* 52(4): 855–885.

Rushton, Simon. 2011. "Global Health Security: Security for Whom? Security from What?" *Political Studies* 59(4): 779–796.

———. 2016. "The UN Security Council and Ebola: A 'New Normal' in Responding to Global Health Emergencies?" Paper presented at the International Studies Association conference, Atlanta, GA, March 15–19.

Rushton, Simon, and Jeremy Youde, editors. 2015. *Routledge Handbook of Global Health Security.* New York: Routledge.

Saad, Lydia. 2014. "Ebola Ranks Among Americans' Top Three Health Concerns." Gallup poll, November 17. www.gallup.com/poll/179429/ebola-ranks-among-americans-top-three-healthcare-concerns.aspx.

Sacks, Audrey. 2012. *Can Donors and Non-State Actors Undermine Citizens' Legitimating Beliefs?* Afrobarometer Working Paper 140. http://afrobarometer.org/publications/can-donors-and-non-state-actors-undermine-citizens%E2%80%99-legitimating-beliefs.

Safaei, Jalil. 2006. "Is Democracy Good for Health?" *International Journal of Health Services* 36(4): 767–786.

SANTA. *See* South Africa National Tuberculosis Association.

Schartzberg, Michael. 2001. *Political Legitimacy in Middle Africa.* Bloomington, IN: Indiana University Press.

Scheckels, Theodore. 2004. "The Rhetoric of Thabo Mbeki on HIV/AIDS: Strategic Scapegoating?" *Howard Journal of Communications* 15(2): 69–82.

Scherz, China. 2014. *Having People, Having Heart: Charity, Sustainable Development, and the Problems of Dependence in Central Uganda.* Chicago, IL: University of Chicago Press.

Schmitz, Hans Peter. 2015. "The Global Health Network on Alcohol Control: Successes and Limits of Evidence-Based Advocacy." *Health Policy and Planning* 31(Supplement 1): i87–i97.

Schneider, Anne, and Helen Ingram. 1993. "Social Construction of Target Populations: Implications for Politics and Policy." *American Political Science Review* 87(2): 334–347.

Scott, Guy. 2000. "Political Will, Political Economy & the AIDS Industry in Zambia." *Review of African Political Economy* 27(86): 577–582.

Scott, James. 1990. *Domination and the Arts of Resistance.* New Haven: Yale University Press.

———. 1998. *Seeing Like a State: How Certain Schemes to Improve the Human Condition Have Failed.* New Haven, CT: Yale University Press.

Seltzer, E. K., N. S. Jean, E. Kramer-Golinkoff, D. A. Asch, and R. M. Merchant. 2015. "The Content of Social Media's Shared Images about Ebola: A Retrospective Study." *Public Health* 129(9): 1273–1277.

Sen, Amartya. 2001. "Democracy as a Universal Value." In *The Global Divergence of Democracies*, edited by Larry Diamond and Marc Plattner, 3–17. Baltimore, MD: Johns Hopkins University Press.

Shah, Sonia. 2010. *The Fever: How Malaria Has Ruled Humankind for 500,000 Years.* New York: Sarah Crichton.

Shaw, Timothy M., Fantu Cheru, and Scarlett Cornelissen. 2012. "Conclusion: What Futures for African International Relations?" In *Africa and International Relations in the 21st Century*, edited by Scarlett Cornelissen, Fantu Cheru, and Timothy Shaw, 194–209. New York: Palgrave Macmillan.

Shawar, Yusra Ribhi, Jeremy Shiffman, and David Spiegel. 2015. "Generation of Political Priority for Global Surgery: A Qualitative Policy Analysis." *Lancet Global Health* 3(8): e487–e495.

Shiffman, Jeremy. 2008. "Has Donor Prioritization of HIV/AIDS Displaced Aid for Other Health Issues?" *Health Policy and Planning* 23(2): 95–100.

———. 2009. "A Social Explanation for the Rise and Fall of Global Health Issues." *Bulletin of the World Health Organization* 87: 608–613.

———. 2010. "Issue Attention in Global Health: The Case of Newborn Survival." *Lancet* 375(9730): 2045–2049.

Shiffman, Jeremy, and Stephanie Smith. 2007. "Generation of Political Priority for Global Health Initiatives: A Framework and Case Study of Maternal Mortality." *Lancet* 370(9595): 1370–1379.

Shiffman, Jeremy, David Berlan, and Tamara Hafner. 2009. "Has Aid for AIDS Raised All Health Funding Boats?" *JAIDS* 52(Supplement 1): S45–S48.

Shiffman, Jeremy, Kathryn Quissell, Hans Peter Schmitz, David Pelletier, Stephanie Smith, David Berlan, Uwe Gneiting, Dave Van Slyke, Ines Mergel, Mariela Rodriguez, and Gill Walt. 2016. "A Framework for the Emergence and Effectiveness of Global Health Networks." *Health Policy and Planning* 31(Supplement 1): i3–i16.

Sidley, Pat. 1999. "South African Public Sceptical about New AIDS 'Cure.'" *British Medical Journal* 318(7186): 757.

Sierra Leone. 2014. *Reporting Instrument of the WHO Framework Convention on Tobacco Control.* http://apps.who.int/fctc/implementation/database/sites/implementation/files/documents /reports/sierra_leone_2014_report_final.pdf.

Sikkink, Kathryn. 2011. *The Justice Cascade.* New York: W. W. Norton.

Simutanyi, Neo. 2013. "Zambia: Manufactured One-Party Dominance and Its Collapse." In *One-Party Dominance in African Democracies*, edited by Renske Doorenspleet and Lia Nijzink, 119–142. Boulder, CO: Lynne Rienner.

Sinding, S. W. 2005. "Does 'CNN' (Condoms, Needles and Negotiation) Work Better than 'ABC' (Abstinence, Being Faithful and Condom Use) in Attacking the AIDS Epidemic?" *International Family Planning Perspectives* 31(1): 38–40.

Siplon, Patricia. 2002. *AIDS and the Policy Struggle in the United States.* Washington, DC: Georgetown University Press.

———. 2013. "Can Charity and Rights-Based Movements Be Allies in the Fight against HIV/ AIDS? Bridging Mobilisations in the United States and Sub-Saharan Africa." *Canadian Journal of African Studies* 47(2): 187–205.

Sirleaf, Ellen Johnson. 2014. "The Long-Term Cure for Ebola: An Investment in Health Systems." Posted on Liberian Embassy website, October 20. www.liberianembassyus. org/uploads/PDFFiles/The%20long-term%20cure%20for%20Ebola%20-%20An%20 investment%20in%20health%20systems.pdf.

Slutkin, G., S. Okware, W. Naamara, D. Flanagan, M. Carael, E. Blas, P. Delay, and D. Tarantola. 2006. "How Uganda Reversed Its HIV Epidemic." *AIDS and Behaviour* 10(4): 351–361.

Smith, Daniel Jordan. 2003. "Patronage, Per Diems and the 'Workshop Mentality.'" *World Development* 31(4): 703–715.

———. 2008. *A Culture of Corruption: Everyday Deception and Popular Discontent in Nigeria.* Princeton, NJ: Princeton University Press.

———. 2014. *AIDS Doesn't Show Its Face: Inequality, Morality, and Social Change in Nigeria.* Chicago, IL: University of Chicago Press.

Smith, Julia, Sheryl Thompson, and Kelley Lee. 2016. "'Public Enemy No. 1': Tobacco Industry Funding for the AIDS Response." *SAHARA-J: Journal of Social Aspects of HIV/AIDS* 13(1): 41–52.

Smith, Julia H., and Alan Whiteside. 2010. "The History of AIDS Exceptionalism." *Journal of the International AIDS Society* 13(47). doi: 10.1186/1758-2652-13-47.

Smith, Lisa, and Prashant Yadav. 2014. "Improving Access to Medicines for Noncommuni- cable Diseases through Better Supply Chains." In *Noncommunicable Diseases in the*

Developing World, edited by Louis Galambos and Jeffrey Sturchio, 53–81. Baltimore, MD: Johns Hopkins University Press.

Smith, Raymond, and Patricia Siplon. 2006. *Drugs into Bodies: Global AIDS Treatment Activism.* Westport, CT: Praeger.

SOS International. 2015. "Ebola Restrictions." https://pandemic.internationalsos.com/ebola.

South Africa National Tuberculosis Association. 2016. "About Us." www.santa.org.za/.

Specter, Michael. 2015. "Sharing the Blame for the Ebola Crisis." *New Yorker*, May 13.

Staveteig, Sarah, Shanxiao Wang, Sara Head, Sarah Bradley, and Erica Nybro. 2013. "Demographic Patterns of HIV Testing Uptake in Sub-Saharan Africa." *DHS Comparative Reports* 30. https://dhsprogram.com/pubs/pdf/CR30/CR30.pdf.

Steen, Tore, Khumo Seipone, Florindo de la Hoz Gomez, Marina Anderson, Marble Kejelepula, Koona Keapoletswe, and Howard Moffat. 2007. "Two and a Half Years of Routine HIV Testing in Botswana." *JAIDS: Journal of Acquired Immune Deficiency Syndromes* 44(4): 484–488.

Stefan, Daniela, Ahmed Elzawawy, Hussein Khaled, Fabien Ntaganda, Anita Asiimwe, Beatrice Wiafe Addai, Seth Wiafe, and Isaac Adewole. 2013. "Developing Cancer Control Plans in Africa: Examples from Five Countries." *Lancet Oncology* 14(April): e189–e195.

Stillwaggon, Eileen. 2006. *AIDS and the Ecology of Poverty.* New York: Oxford University Press.

Stone, Deborah A. 1989. "Causal Stories and the Formation of Policy Agendas." *Political Science Quarterly* 104(2): 281–300.

Stones, Rob. 2005. *Structuration Theory.* New York: Palgrave Macmillan.

Strand, Per. 2012. "Public Opinion as Leadership Disincentive: Exploring a Governance Dilemma in the AIDS Response in Africa." *Contemporary Politics* 18(2): 174–185.

Sturchio, Jeffrey, and Louis Galambos. 2014. "Noncommunicable Diseases in the Developing World: Closing the Gap." In *Noncommunicable Diseases in the Developing World*, edited by Louis Galambos and Jeffrey Sturchio, 1–27. Baltimore, MD: Johns Hopkins University Press.

Tallberg, Jonas. 2002. "Paths to Compliance: Enforcement, Management, and the European Union." *International Organization* 56(3): 609–643.

Tanzanian Tobacco Control Forum. 2012. *Implementation of the Framework Convention on Tobacco Control in Tanzania, 2007–2012. A Shadow Report.* Unpublished document.

Tarantola, Daniel, Laura Ferguson, and Sofia Gruskin. 2011. "International Health, Global Health, and Human Rights." In *Routledge Handbook of Global Public Health*, edited by Richard Parker and Marni Sommer, 51–62. New York: Routledge.

Taylor, Ian. 2008. *China's New Role in Africa.* Boulder, CO: Lynne Rienner.

Therkilsden, Ole. 2005. "Understanding Public Management through Neopatrimonialism: A Paradigm for All African Seasons?" In *The African Exception*, edited by Ulf Engel and Gorm Rye Olsen, 35–52. Aldershot, UK: Ashgate.

Thomas-Greenfield, Linda. 2016. Remarks at African Methodist Episcopal University, Monrovia, Liberia, May 16. www.myafricanwoman.com/2016/05/linda-thomas -greenfields-tough-words-liberia/.

Tomlinson, Mark, and Crick Lund. 2012. "Why Does Mental Health Not Get the Attention It Deserves? An Application of the Shiffman and Smith Framework." *PLOS Medicine* 9(2): e1001178.

Transparency International. 2006. *Global Corruption Report 2006: Corruption and Health.* Online Report. www.transparency.org/whatwedo/publication/global_corruption_report _2006_corruption_and_health.

———. 2013. "Global Corruption Barometer: Liberia." www.transparency.org/gcb2013 /country/?country=liberia.

Trinitapoli, Jenny, and Alexander Weinreb. 2012. *Religion and AIDS in Africa.* New York: Oxford University Press.

Tripp, Aili Mary. 2000. *Women and Politics in Uganda.* Madison, WI: University of Wisconsin Press.

TTCF. *See* Tanzanian Tobacco Control Forum.

Tumwine, Jacqueline. 2011. "Implementation of the Framework Convention on Tobacco Control in Africa: Current Status of Legislation." *International Journal of Environmental Research and Public Health* 8(11): 4312–4331.

UICC. *See* Union for International Cancer Control.

UN. *See* United Nations.

UNAIDS. *See* Joint United Nations Programme on HIV/AIDS.

UNDP. *See* United Nations Development Programme.

UNFPA. *See* United Nations Population Fund.

UNGA. *See* United Nations General Assembly.

UNHRC. *See* United Nations Human Rights Office of the High Commissioner.

Union for International Cancer Control. 2016. "Adoption of Agenda 2030: A Major Victory for NCDs." www.uicc.org/adoption-agenda-2030-major-victory-ncds.

United Nations. 2001. Declaration of Commitment on HIV/AIDS. United Nations General Assembly Special Session on HIV/AIDS, June 25–27, 2001. www.unaids.org/sites/default /files/sub_landing/files/aidsdeclaration_en.pdf.

———. 2014. "Letter to the UN Secretary General from Presidents Koroma, Condé, and Sirleaf." www.un.org/en/ga/president/69/pdf/letters/180914_ebola_guinea-liberia-sierraleone.pdf.

———. 2016. "Protecting Humanity from Future Health Crises." Report of UN High-Level Panel on the Global Response to Health Crises, January 25. www.un.org/News/dh/infocus /HLP/2016-02-05_Final_Report_Global_Response_to_Health_Crises.pdf.

United Nations Development Programme. 2015. "Human Development Report." http://hdr .undp.org/sites/default/files/2015_human_development_report.pdf.

United Nations General Assembly. 2001. "Speakers at the Special Session on HIV and AIDS." www.un.org/ga/aids/statements/.

———. 2011a. Eighth Plenary Session—Transcript, September 20. New York. A/66/PV.8. http://daccess-dds-ny.un.org/doc/UNDOC/GEN/N11/505/46/PDF/N1150546.pdf ?OpenElement.

———. 2011b. Fifth Plenary Session—Transcript, September 19. New York. A/66/PV.5. http://daccess-dds-ny.un.org/doc/UNDOC/GEN/N11/505/46/PDF/N1150546.pdf ?OpenElement.

———. 2011c. Fourth Plenary Session—Transcript, September 19. New York. A/66/PV.4. http://daccess-dds-ny.un.org/doc/UNDOC/GEN/N11/505/40/PDF/N1150540.pdf ?OpenElement.

―――. 2011d. High-Level Meeting of the General Assembly on the Prevention and Control of Non-Communicable Diseases. List of Speakers. www.who.int/nmh/events/un_ncd _summit2011/speakers.pdf.

―――. 2011e. Political Declaration of the High-Level Meeting of the General Assembly on the Prevention and Control of Non-Communicable Diseases. A/RES/66/2. www.who.int/nmh /events/un_ncd_summit2011/political_declaration_en.pdf.

―――. 2011f. Seventh Plenary Session—Transcript, September 20. New York. A/66/PV.7. http://daccess-dds-ny.un.org/doc/UNDOC/GEN/N11/505/40/PDF/N1150540.pdf ?OpenElement.

―――. 2011g. Third Plenary Session—Transcript, September 19. New York. A/66/PV.3. http: //daccess-dds-ny.un.org/doc/UNDOC/GEN/N11/503/56/PDF/N1150356.pdf?Open Element.

―――. 2013. "Note by the Secretary-General Transmitting the Report of the Director-General of the World Health Organization on the Prevention and Control of Non-Communicable Diseases." A/68/650. http://ncdalliance.org/sites/default/files/rfiles/SG%20progress%20 report_January%202014.pdf.

―――. 2014. "Outcome Document of the High-Level Meeting of the General Assembly on the Comprehensive Review and Assessment of the Progress Achieved in the Prevention and Control of Non-Communicable Diseases." Draft Resolution. A/68/L.53. http://ncdalliance. org/sites/default/files/rfiles/UN%20Review%20Outcome%20Document%20-%20Adopted .pdf.

United Nations Human Rights Council. 2015. "Report of the Detailed Findings of the Commission of Inquiry on Human Rights in Eritrea." www.ohchr.org/Documents/HR Bodies/HRCouncil/CoIEritrea/A_HRC_29_CRP-1.pdf.

United Nations Human Rights Office of the High Commissioner. 2014. "A Human Rights Perspective into the Ebola Outbreak." www.globalhealth.org/wp-content/uploads/A -human-rights-perspective-into-the-Ebola-outbreak.pdf.

United Nations Population Fund. 1999. *AIDS Update 1999*. New York: United Nations.

United Nations Security Council. 2014. Resolution 2177 (2014). S/RES/2177 (2014), September 18. www.securitycouncilreport.org/atf/cf/%7B65BFCF9B-6D27-4E9C-8CD3 -CF6E4FF96FF9%7D/S_RES_2177.pdf.

United Nations World Tourism Organization. 2013. *UNWTO Tourism Highlights: 2013 Edition*. www.e-unwto.org/doi/pdf/10.18111/9789284415427.

University of Zambia, Ministry of Health, and University of Waterloo. 2014. *International Tobacco Control Policy Evaluation Project. ITC Zambia National Report*. www.itcproject.org /files/ITC_ZambiaNR-ENG-FINAL-web_May2014.pdf.

UNSC. *See* United Nations Security Council.

UNWTO. *See* United Nations World Tourism Organization.

US Agency for International Development. 2015. "Global Health Ghana." www.usaid.gov /ghana/global-health.

―――. 2016. "West Africa—Ebola Outbreak." Fact Sheet 8, Fiscal Year (FY) 2016, February 19. www.usaid.gov/sites/default/files/documents/1866/west_africa_outbreak_fs08_02 -19-2016.pdf.

US Census Bureau. 2014. "The Foreign-Born Population from Africa: 2008–2012." www
.census.gov/content/dam/Census/library/publications/2014/acs/acsbr12-16.pdf.

US Department of State. 2014. "Congressional Budget Justification." www.usaid.gov/sites
/default/files/documents/9276/222898.pdf.

US Embassy Rwanda. 2014. "New Ebola Screening Procedures for Passengers from the United
States and Spain." October 21. http://rwanda.usembassy.gov/mobile/sm-102114.html.

US President's Emergency Plan for AIDS Relief. 2011. "FY 2011 PEPFAR Country Operational
Plans." www.pepfar.gov/countries/cop/C57518.htm.

———. 2015a. "Eleventh Annual Report to Congress on PEPFAR (2015)." www.pepfar.gov
/press/eleventhannualreport/index.htm.

———. 2015b. "FY 2015 Operational Plan Strategic Direction Summaries." www.pepfar.gov
/countries/cop/c69471.htm.

———. 2015c. "Partnering to Achieve Epidemic Control in Kenya." www.pepfar.gov/countries
/kenya/.

———. 2015d. "Partnering to Achieve Epidemic Control in Nigeria." www.pepfar.gov
/countries/nigeria/.

———. 2016. "PEPFAR Funding." www.pepfar.gov/documents/organization/252516.pdf.

USAID. *See* US Agency for International Development.

Utas, Mats. 2008. "Liberia Beyond the Blueprints: Poverty Reduction Strategy Papers, Big
Men and Informal Networks." Lecture Series on African Security, No. 4. Uppsala,
Sweden: Nordic Africa Institute.

Uvin, Peter. 1998. *Aiding Violence: The Development Enterprise in Rwanda*. Westport, CT:
Kumarian.

van de Walle, Nicolas. 2001. *African Economies and the Politics of Permanent Crisis*. New York:
Cambridge University Press.

———. 2010. "US Policy towards Africa: The Bush Legacy and the Obama Administration."
African Affairs 109(434): 1–21.

van Dijk, Rijk, Hansjörg Dilger, Marian Burchardt, and Thera Rasing. 2014. *Religion and AIDS
Treatment in Africa: Saving Souls, Prolonging Lives*. Aldershot, UK: Ashgate.

Vian, Taryn, Candace Miller, Zione Themba, and Paul Bukuluki. 2012. "Perceptions of Per
Diems in the Health Sector: Evidence and Implications." *Health Policy and Planning* 28(3):
237–246.

Wakabi, W. 2006. "Condoms Still Contentious in Uganda's Struggle over AIDS." *Lancet*
367(9520): 1387–1388.

Wald, Patricia. 2008. *Contagious: Cultures, Carriers, and the Outbreak Narrative*. Durham, NC:
Duke University Press.

Warner, K. E., and J. MacKay. 2006. "The Global Tobacco Disease Pandemic: Nature, Causes
and Cures." *Global Public Health* 1(1): 65–86.

Watkins, Susan Cotts, and Ann Swidler. 2012. "Working Misunderstandings: Donors, Brokers
and Villagers in Africa's AIDS Industry." *Population and Development Review* 38(Supplement): 197–208.

Wawer, M. J., et al. 2005. "Declines in HIV Prevalence in Uganda: Not as Simple as ABC."
Twelfth Conference on Retroviruses and Opportunistic Infections, Boston, Abstract 27LB.

Webb, James. 2013. "The First Large-Scale Use of Synthetic Insecticide for Malaria Control in Tropical Africa: Lessons from Liberia, 1945–62." In *Global Health in Africa: Historical Perspectives on Disease Control*, edited by Tamara Giles-Vernick and James Webb, 42–69. Athens, OH: Ohio University Press.

Wendt, Andrew. 1999. *Social Theory of International Politics*. New York: Cambridge University Press.

Westendorf, Jasmine-Kim. 2016. "Violence and the Contestation of the State after Civil Wars." In *Violence and the State*, edited by Matt Killingsworth, Matthew Sussex, and Jan Pakulski, 128–152. Manchester, UK: Manchester University Press.

Wexler, Adam, and Allison Valentine. 2015. "The US Global Health Budget: Analysis of Fiscal Year 2016 Budget Request." March 11. http://kff.org/global-health-policy/issue-brief/the-u-s-global-health-budget-analysis-of-the-fiscal-year-2016-budget-request/.

White, Heather L., Chishimba Mulambia, Moses Sinkala, Mulindi Mwanahamuntu, Groesbeck Parham, Linda Moneyham, Diana Grimley, and Eric Chamot. 2012. "'Worse than HIV' or 'Not as Serious as Other Diseases?' Conceptualization of Cervical Cancer among Newly Screened Women in Zambia." *Social Science & Medicine* 74(10): 1485–1493.

Whiteside, Alan, Robert Mattes, Samantha Willan, and Ryann Manning. 2002. *Examining HIV/AIDS in South Africa through the Eyes of Ordinary Southern Africans*. Afrobarometer Paper 21. http://pdf.usaid.gov/pdf_docs/Pnacq910.pdf.

Whitfield, Lindsay, editor. 2009. *The Politics of Aid: African Strategies for Dealing with Donors*. New York: Oxford University Press.

WHO. *See* World Health Organization.

Wigmore, Rosie. 2015. "Contextualising Ebola Rumours from a Political, Historical and Social Perspective to Understand People's Perceptions of Ebola and the Responses to It." *Ebola Response Anthropology Platform*, October 19. www.ebola-anthropology.net/key_messages/contextualising-ebola-rumours-from-a-political-historical-and-social-perspective-to-understand-peoples-perceptions-of-ebola-and-the-responses-to-it/.

Wilkinson, Annie, and Melissa Leach. 2014. "Briefing: Ebola-Myths, Realities, and Structural Violence." *African Affairs* 114(454): 136–148.

Will, Kurt Dieter. 1991. "The Global Politics of AIDS: The World Health Organization and the International Regime for AIDS." PhD diss., University of South Carolina.

Williams, Paul. 2016. *War and Conflict in Africa*, 2nd ed. Malden, MA: Polity.

Wilson Center. 2005. *Challenges and Change in Uganda*. Online Report. www.wilsoncenter.org/sites/default/files/Uganda2.pdf.

World Bank. 2000. "Africa—Multi-Country HIV/AIDS Program." Project Appraisal Document. PID9365. www-wds.worldbank.org/external/default/WDSContentServer/WDSP/IB/2000/08/03/000094946_00080305414991/Rendered/PDF/multipage.pdf.

———. 2014a. "The Economic Impact of the 2014 Ebola Epidemic: Short and Medium Term Estimates for West Africa." www.worldbank.org/en/region/afr/publication/the-economic-impact-of-the-2014-ebola-epidemic-short-and-medium-term-estimates-for-west-africa.

———. 2014b. Transcript of Remarks at the Event: Impact of the Ebola Crisis: A Perspective from the Countries. www.worldbank.org/en/news/speech/2014/10/09/transcript-event-impact-ebola-crisis-perspective-countries.

———. 2014c. "World Databank. Development Indicators." http://databank.worldbank.org
/data/reports.aspx?source=2&series=SH.XPD.PUBL.ZS&country=.

———. 2015a. "Country and Lending Groups." http://data.worldbank.org/about/country-and
-lending-groups#Sub_Saharan_Africa.

———. 2015b. "Net ODA Received (% of GNI)." http://data.worldbank.org/indicator/DT.ODA
.ODAT.GN.ZS?locations=SM.

———. 2015c. "Urban Poverty—An Overview." http://web.worldbank.org/WBSITE
/EXTERNAL/TOPICS/EXTURBANDEVELOPMENT/EXTURBANPOVERTY/0,,content
MDK:20227679~menuPK:7173704~pagePK:148956~piPK:216618~theSitePK:341325,00.
html.

———. 2015d. "Worldwide Governance Indicators." http://info.worldbank.org/governance
/wgi/index.aspx#reports.

———. 2017. "After Ebola and Zika, Most Countries Still Not Prepared for a Pandemic." Press
release, May 25. www.worldbank.org/en/news/press-release/2017/05/25/after-ebola-zika
-most-countries-still-not-prepared-for-a-pandemic.

World Health Assembly. 1986. "WHA39.14 Tobacco or Health." www.who.int/tobacco/frame
work/wha_eb/wha39_14/en/.

World Health Organization. 1978. Declaration of Alma-Ata. www.who.int/publications/almaata
_declaration_en.pdf.

———. 2005. *International Health Regulations (2005)*. Geneva: WHO. http://apps.who.int/iris
/bitstream/10665/246107/1/9789241580496-eng.pdf?ua=1.

———. 2009. "Tobacco Factsheet." www.who.int/nmh/publications/fact_sheet_tobacco_en
.pdf.

———. 2011a. "The Abuja Declaration: Ten Years On." www.who.int/healthsystems
/publications/abuja_report_aug_2011.pdf?ua=1.

———. 2011b. "Noncommunicable Diseases Country Profiles 2011." www.who.int/nmh
/publications/ncd_profiles2011/en/.

———. 2011c. "Scaling Up Action Against Noncommunicable Diseases: How Much Will It
Cost?" WHO Report. www.who.int/nmh/publications/cost_of_inaction/en/.

———. 2011d. "Summary Report of the Discussions of the Roundtables." UN High-Level
Meeting on NCDs. www.who.int/nmh/events/moscow_ncds_2011/round_tables
_summary.pdf.

———. 2012a. "Fact Sheet on Health Spending." www.who.int/mediacentre/factsheets/fs319
/en/.

———. 2012b. "Global Burden of Disease: Executive Summary." www.who.int.pmnch/media
/news/2012/who_burdenofdisease/en/.

———. 2012c. *Programme Budget 2012–2013*. www.who.int.about/resources_planning
/HQRPR14.1_PBPA2012-2013.pdf.

———. 2013. *Global Action Plan for the Prevention and Control of Non-Communicable Disease
2013–2020*. http://apps.who.int/iris/bitstream/10665/94384/1/9789241506236_eng.pdf
?ua=1.

———. 2014a. "Ebola Challenges West African Countries." Media release, June 26. www.who
.int/mediacentre/news/notes/2014/ebola-response/en/.

———. 2014b. "Non-Communicable Diseases Country Profiles 2014." www.who.int/nmh/publications/ncd-profiles-2014/en/.

———. 2014c. "Parties to the WHO Framework Convention on Tobacco Control." www.who.int/fctc/signatories_parties/en/.

———. 2014d. *Programme Budget 2014–2015*. www.who.int.about/resources_planning/PB14-15?en.pdf.

———. 2014e. "Statement on the 1st Meeting of the IHR Emergency Committee on the 2014 Ebola Outbreak in West Africa." August 8. www.who.int/mediacentre/news/statements/2014/ebola-20140808/en/.

———. 2014f. "Statement on the 3rd Meeting of the IHR Emergency Committee regarding the 2014 Ebola Outbreak in West Africa." October 23. www.who.int/mediacentre/news/statements/2014/ebola-3rd-ihr-meeting/en/.

———. 2014g. "Statement on Travel and Transport in Relation to Ebola Virus Disease Outbreak." Media release, August 18. www.who.int/mediacentre/news/statements/2014/ebola-travel-trasport/en/.

———. 2014h. "Study Warns Swift Action Needed To Curb Exponential Climb in Ebola Outbreak." News release, September 22. www.who.int/mediacentre/news/releases/2014/ebola-study/en.

———. 2014i. "Summary of States Parties 2013 Report on IHR Core Capacity Implementation: Regional Profiles." WHO/HSE/GCR/2014.10. http://apps.who.int/iris/bitstream/10665/145084/1/WHO_HSE_GCR_2014.10_eng.pdf?ua=1.

———. 2014j. "WHA67 Main Documents." http://apps.who.int/gb/e/e_wha67.html.

———. 2014k. "WHO Ramps Up to Address Ebola Challenges, to Prevent New Infections in Guinea and Liberia." www.who.int/features/2014/preventing-ebola/en.

———. 2015a. "2014 Ebola Virus Disease Outbreak: Current Context and Challenges; Stopping the Epidemic; and Preparedness in Non-Affected Countries and Regions." Report by the Secretariat. 68th World Health Assembly. A68/24, May 15. http://apps.who.int/gb/ebwha/pdf_files/WHA68/A68_24-en.pdf.

———. 2015b. "Antiretroviral Therapy (ART) Coverage among All Age Groups. Global Health Observatory (GHO) Data." www.who.int/gho/hiv/epidemic_response/ART_text/en/.

———. 2015c. "Ebola Interim Assessment Panel Report." http://apps.who.int/gb/ebwha/pdf_files/WHA68/A68_25-en.pdf?ua=1.

———. 2015d. "Factors that Contributed to Undetected Spread of the Ebola Virus and Impeded Rapid Containment." January. www.who.int/csr/disease/ebola/one-year-report/factors/en/.

———. 2015e. "Global Mental Health Action Plan." www.who.int/mental_health/mhgap/consultation_global_mh_action_plan_2013_2020/en/.

———. 2015f. "Liberia Succeeds in Fighting Ebola with Local, Sector Response." April. www.who.int/features/2015/ebola-sector-approach/en.

———. 2015g. "Parties to the WHO Framework Convention on Tobacco Control." Parties Reports, Implementation Base. http://apps.who.int/fctc/implementation/database/.

———. 2015h. *Proposed Programme Budget 2015–2017*. 68th World Health Assembly, A68/55, May 12. http://apps.who.int/gb/ebwha/pdf_files/WHA68/A68_55-en.pdf.

———. 2015i. "WHO Country Pages. Health Data." http://apps.who.int/gho/data/node.main
.A1444?lang=en.

———. 2015j. "WHO Fact Sheet: Noncommunicable Diseases." www.who.int/mediacentre
/factsheets/fs355/en/.

———. 2015k. "WHO Report on the Global Tobacco Epidemic, 2015. Country Profile: Eritrea."
www.who.int/tobacco/surveillance/policy/country_profile/eri.pdf.

———. 2016a. "Ebola Cases: Map." http://apps.who.int/ebola/sites/default/files/thumbnails
/image/sitrep_casecount_40.png?ua=1.

———. 2016b. "Ebola Virus Disease Fact Sheet No. 103." January. www.who.int/mediacentre
/factsheets/fs103/en/.

———. 2016c. "Ebola Virus Disease Outbreak Information." www.who.int/csr/disease/ebola
/en/.

———. 2016d. "Second Report of the Advisory Group on Reform of WHO's Work on
Outbreaks and Prevention." January 18. www.who.int/about/who_reform/emergency
-capacities/advisory-group/second-report.pdf?ua=1.

———. 2016e. "Situation Report." http://apps.who.int/ebola/current-situation/ebola-situation
-report-30-march-2016.

———. 2017. "South Africa. Non-Communicable Disease Prevention and Control (NCDs)."
www.afro.who.int/en/south-africa/country-programmes/4248-non-communicable-disease
-prevention-and-control-ncds.html.

WHO, UNICEF, and UNAIDS. 2013. *Global Update on HIV Treatment: Results, Impact and
Opportunities.* www.unaids.org/sites/default/files/sub_landing/files/20130630_treatment
_report_en_3.pdf.

Worsnop, Catherine. 2016a. "Concealing Disease: The Timeliness of Outbreak Reporting and
Non-Compliance with WHO's International Health Regulations." Paper presented at the
International Studies Association Conference, Atlanta, GA, March 15–19.

———. 2016b. "Domestic Politics, the IHR, and Excessive Barriers during the 2014 Ebola
Outbreak." Paper presented at the International Studies Association Conference, Atlanta,
March 15–19.

Wrong, Michela. 2006. *I Didn't Do It for You: How the World Betrayed a Small African Nation.*
New York: HarperCollins.

Yasmin, Seema. 2016a. "Africa Starts Its Own Disease Control Agency." *Scientific American*,
June 1. www.scientificamerican.com/article/africa-starts-its-own-disease-control-agency.

———. 2016b. "The Ebola Rape Epidemic No One's Talking about." *Foreign Policy*, February 2.
http://foreignpolicy.com/2016/02/02/the-ebola-rape-epidemic-west-africa-teenage
-pregnancy/.

Youde, Jeremy. 2007. *AIDS, South Africa, and the Politics of Knowledge.* Aldershot, UK: Ashgate.

———. 2008. "Is Universal Access to Antiretroviral Drugs an Emerging International Norm?"
Journal of International Relations and Development 11(4): 415–440.

———. 2010. "Public Opinion and Support for Government AIDS Policies in Sub-Saharan
Africa." *Social Science and Medicine* 74(1): 52–57.

———. 2011. "Mediating Risk through the International Health Regulations and Bio-Political
Surveillance." *Political Studies* 59(4): 813–830.

———. 2012. *Global Health Governance*. Malden, MA: Polity.

———. 2016. "Ebola, Reforming the World Health Organization, and IO Theory." Paper presented at the International Studies Association Conference, Atlanta, GA, March 15–19.

Young, Crawford. 2009. "The Heritage of Colonialism." In *Africa in World Politics*, edited by John Harbeson and Donald Rothchild, 4th ed., 19–38. Boulder, CO: Westview.

Zondi, Siphamandla. 2014. "Assessing African Health Governance amid Global Biopolitics." In *Moving Health Sovereignty in Africa*, edited by John Kirton, Andrew Cooper, Franklyn Lisk, and Hany Besada, 57–83. Aldershot, UK: Ashgate.

Christians, 46, 105

chronic health conditions, 126

chronic neurological disorders, 121

chronic obstructive pulmonary disease, 121

chronic respiratory diseases, 3, 29, 121, 125, 128, 144, 156

Churches Health Association of Zambia (CHAZ), 72, 74–75, 149, 150–51

civil rights, 81, 151

civil society, 10, 13, 17–19, 26, 75, 76, 151, 164, 170–71, 176; and AIDS, 27, 33, 37, 43, 50, 59, 60, 63, 64, 65, 66, 67, 71–77, 154, 156–57, 160–62; defined, 18; and Ebola, 28, 83, 111–18, 154–55; incorporation of, 72–75, 76, 79, 171; and NACs, 49; and NCDs, 29, 122, 135, 143, 147, 154–62, 165, 169, 170, 175; repression of, 62; and state, 18–20, 72–76, 170, 173, 174; state incorporation of vs. disengagement by, 18–19; and vertical health programs, 174

Clinton Foundation, 59

colonialism, 1, 167, 170

constructivism, 5–6, 9

Convention on the Elimination of All Forms of Discrimination against Women, 39

Convention on the Rights of the Child, 39

corruption, 15, 16, 17, 20, 69–71, 141; and AIDS, 69–70; and Ebola, 81, 83, 93, 98, 105, 108–9, 110, 170; and NCDs, 146, 147, 154. See also neopatrimonialism

Côte d'Ivoire, 49, 95, 106, 137, 154, 162–63, 182n5

Council for the Independent Churches (Ghana), 72

Council on Foreign Relations Independent Task Force on NCDs, 184n2

country coordinating mechanism(s) (CCMs), 27, 38, 42, 62, 64–65, 66, 67, 68–69, 72, 76, 168–69

Cuba, 155

culture, 8, 28, 58, 104–5, 111, 113, 115, 117–18, 167, 173

Declaration of Port-of-Spain, 126–27

democracy, 10, 13–14, 17, 18, 19, 20, 170; and AIDS, 33, 35, 36, 59, 61–63, 68–69, 71, 168; and Ebola, 83, 95–96, 98, 99, 118; and Ebola

in Liberia, 83, 103, 105–7, 110, 119, 168; and NCDs, 29, 122, 143, 146, 147, 148, 149, 151, 152, 162, 168; and neopatrimonialism, 15. See also elections; regime

Democratic Republic of Congo, 49, 68, 86, 140, 182n2, 182n5

Democratic Turnhalle Alliance, 98

development, 18, 26, 29, 81, 152, 162, 167; and AIDS, 35, 60, 69; and Ebola, 90, 100, 108, 111; in Liberia, 81, 82, 108, 111; and NCDs, 134, 144, 147. See also economic development

diabetes, 21, 24, 123, 138, 149, 151, 156, 175; deaths from, 3, 121, 181n4; and Ghana, 148, 158, 161, 181n4; and HIV, 23; and human rights and development, 132; medications for, 130–31; and South Africa, 184n3; and UN High-Level Meeting (2011), 144, 145; WHO guidelines on, 29, 128

diarrheal diseases, 3

diet/nutrition, 123, 124–25, 126, 128, 132, 133, 138, 148, 149, 151, 152. See also food

discrimination, 14, 89. See also under acquired immunodeficiency syndrome (AIDS)

Djibouti, 49, 182n5

Doe, Samuel, 106, 183n11

donors, 2, 9, 11, 12, 18, 48, 49, 72, 74, 104, 165, 171, 172; and AIDS, 22, 38, 42, 45, 47, 51, 53, 54, 55, 60, 61, 63, 64, 65, 76, 77, 78, 79, 161, 168; and Ebola, 82, 83, 85–87, 93, 99, 102, 103, 109, 110, 114, 115, 117, 119, 166, 167–68, 169, 174; and NCDs, 125–26, 131–32, 133–34, 144, 145, 146, 148–49, 150–51, 154, 157, 167, 169, 170; and neopatrimonialism, 15, 16. See also funding

Duesberg, Peter, 57

Duncan, Thomas Eric, 91

Ebola, 7, 23–24, 26–27, 80–120, 125, 164, 165, 176, 182n2, 183n10, 183–84n16; and agency, 86, 87, 93–94, 95, 99, 103, 117, 168, 169, 172, 173; and AIDS, 33, 111, 112, 118, 120; and burial and cremation, 83, 102, 111, 112, 116, 117–18; challenges to global health governance on, 5, 9, 28, 29, 80, 81–83, 85, 90, 93–118, 105, 107, 108, 109, 110, 111, 117, 118–20, 154–55, 167, 168, 169; characteristics of, 83; and civil society, 28, 83, 111–18,

Ebola (*cont.*)
154–55; deaths from, 24, 81, 86, 90; and decision-making, 28, 102, 104, 108, 114, 169; denial of, 111–12, 113, 117, 172; and discrimination, 89, 95; global health governance on, 85–92; and Liberia, 5, 9, 24, 25, 26, 28, 80–83, 84, 86–87, 93, 96, 98, 99–119, 142, 160–61, 166, 167, 168, 169, 170, 181n7; as manufactured in West, 112; narrative about, 81, 99; and NCDs, 111, 143, 160–61; and quarantine, 81, 83, 94, 99, 102, 103, 113, 114, 183n16; and state, 28, 82, 83, 89–90, 93–99, 105–10, 111, 112, 113, 114, 115, 116–19, 120, 169–70; survival rates from, 82; and teenage pregnancy rates, 175; and travel restrictions, 28, 80, 81, 82, 83, 86, 90, 93–99, 118, 119, 166, 168, 183n5, 183n6; and violence against women, 175; and war in Liberia, 6; West African outbreak of, 84; and WHO, 28, 80, 84, 86, 87–89, 90, 91, 93, 94–95, 96, 98, 99, 102, 103–4, 118, 134, 166, 174

Ebola Treatment Units (ETUs), 83, 113

Economic Community of West African States (ECOWAS), 95, 96

economic development, 5, 15–16, 17, 35, 36, 45, 131–33, 144, 167, 168. *See also* development

economy, 170; and AIDS, 34, 38; and discrimination, 40; and Ebola, 91, 93, 96–98; and extraversion, 12; and Liberia, 84; and NCDs, 123, 130, 131–33; and neopatrimonialism, 14, 15–16, 17

elections, 13, 14, 17, 62; and AIDS, 36; and challenge to global health governance, 20; and Ebola, 28, 82, 96, 98, 99, 107, 110, 118, 168; and Eritrea, 151; and Liberia, 106; and NCDs in Ghana, 148; and Zambia, 149. *See also* democracy

elites, 106; and acceptance of global health governance, 19; and agency, 172; and AIDS, 65, 66–67, 68; and ambivalence about global health governance, 20; and challenge to global health governance, 20; and Ebola in Liberia, 28, 105, 110; and extraversion, 12; and NCDs, 29, 170; and neopatrimonialism, 14–16

epistemic communities, 8, 23, 111, 164; and AIDS, 40, 171; defined, 6; and Ebola, 111; and

issue frames, 6–7; and NCDs, 148, 152, 157, 161, 162, 166

Equatorial Guinea, 182n5

Eritrea, 4, 62, 151, 185n7; HIV in, 32, 182n5; NCDs in, 27, 137, 151–52, 154, 162, 163, 169, 185n9

Ethiopia, 3, 16, 45, 49, 182n5

ethnicity, 18, 20, 105–6, 107. *See also* race

European Union (EU): Political Declaration (2011), 131

extraversion, 11, 154; and agency, 171, 172; and AIDS, 45, 54, 55; defined, 12; and Ebola, 100, 101, 108, 110, 118, 119, 165, 169, 173; and NCDs, 122, 143, 145, 162; and UN High-Level Meeting (2011), 144, 145

faith-based organizations (FBOs), 39, 42, 46, 65, 66, 71–72, 85, 111, 158

family, 18, 34, 84, 92, 94, 117

Family Health International, 42

family planning, 133

Firestone Rubber Factory and Plantation, 84

food, 41, 127, 132, 156, 161. *See also* diet/ nutrition

foreign investment, 86, 167. *See also* donors; economic development; economy

Forum of African First Ladies, 156

Framework Convention on Tobacco Control (FCTC), 1, 126, 129, 135, 151, 185n7

France, 42

Freedom House, 81, 146

Friends of the Global Fight, 53

FrontPageAfrica, 26, 108–9

funding: and AIDS, 36, 38, 41, 60, 68, 69, 161, 175; and Ebola, 82, 86, 87, 99, 166, 170; and NCDs, 122, 126, 133–34, 141–42, 144–45, 149, 157, 162, 167. *See also* donors

Gabon, 97, 137, 182n5

Gambia, The, 17, 56, 58–59, 63; and AIDS, 27, 32, 33, 44, 59, 61, 70–71, 75, 76, 77; Ministry of Health, 71; National AIDS Council, 56, 59; National AIDS Secretariat, 70–71

Gates Foundation, 45, 140, 157, 165

gay communities, 22, 34. *See also* homo- sexuality; LGBT

George W. Bush Institute, 156

Germany, 42, 43

Ghana, 24, 25, 45, 50, 52, 79, 106; and AIDS,
51, 69, 73, 74, 79, 161; Community-Based
Health Planning and Services, 148;
democracy in, 13, 14; and diabetes, 181n4;
and Ebola, 96; and HIV, 182n5; Mental
Health Act (2012), 158; national health
insurance in, 13, 148; NCDs in
(*see* noncommunicable diseases (NCDs));
Public Health Act, 148

Ghana AIDS Commission (GAC), 47–48, 65,
69, 72, 182n4

Global AIDS Alliance, 39

Global Fund to Fight AIDS, Tuberculosis, and
Malaria (Global Fund), 4, 42, 43, 53, 55, 59,
60, 64, 66, 67, 126, 133, 165; and AIDS, 45;
and civil society groups, 72; and corruption,
69, 70; and The Gambia, 71

global health governance, 1, 2; patterns of
African involvement in, 5–10. *See also*
acquired immunodeficiency syndrome
(AIDS); Ebola; noncommunicable diseases
(NCDs)

global health governance, acceptance of, 2, 8,
10, 19, 22, 26, 30, 154, 176; and AIDS, 27, 32,
33, 43–59, 61, 64, 65, 71, 76–79, 154, 161; and
civil society, 19–20; defined, 9; and issue
frames, 11, 130; and NCDs, 130, 161, 162, 175;
and norms, 12

global health governance, ambivalence toward,
2, 21, 22, 23, 27, 165, 167, 175; and agency, 10;
and AIDS, 35; and civil society, 19, 20;
defined, 9; and democracy, 14, 17; and elites,
20; and issue frames, 20; and NCDs, 16,
29–30, 122, 135, 143, 145, 146–54, 162, 169,
171; and norms, 12–13, 20

global health governance, challenges to, 2, 11,
12, 13, 22, 25, 30, 165, 166; and agency, 10,
172, 173, 176; and AIDS, 27, 29, 32, 33,
34–37, 53, 56–59, 60, 61, 70, 75–76, 167;
and civil society, 19, 20, 28; defined, 9; and
democracy, 14, 17, 28; and disease
characteristics, 21, 23; and Ebola
(*see* Ebola); and NCDs, 142; and neopatrimonial search for rents, 16–17

Global Outbreak Alert and Response Network
(GOARN), 88

Global Programme on AIDS (GPA), 34, 36–37

Greater Involvement of People with AIDS
(GIPA) Initiative, 35–36, 39–40

Guardian, 26, 89, 92

Guinea, 82, 99, 106, 154, 163; Ebola in, 24, 28,
80, 81, 84, 85, 86, 87, 181n7; and NCDs, 137

Guinea Bissau, 95

Gwenigale, Walter, 102

health: and cost-benefit analysis, 131, 133;
education about, 34, 42, 126, 133, 141, 142,
149, 159, 174; as human right, 7, 28, 39, 89,
130, 132–33, 144, 165, 176; as personal
decision, 132–33, 134, 159

health care, 4, 104, 125, 161, 170, 174; access to,
78, 127, 167; and AIDS, 34, 43, 46, 78; and
Ebola, 84–85, 89, 90, 93, 96–97, 108, 119,
174; and NCDs, 123, 125, 127, 131, 133, 134,
141–42, 144, 159, 167, 169; primary, 7, 125,
127, 129, 149, 151; vertical programs for, 23,
30, 85, 120, 125, 126, 172, 174

health-care centers and facilities, 125, 151; and
Ebola, 85, 106, 111, 112, 114

health-care workers, 4; and Ebola, 83, 85, 93,
99, 100, 101, 106, 110, 111, 112, 115, 119–20,
174; and Guinea, 81; and NCDs, 146, 157, 161;
and Zambia, 149

Health Global Access Project (Health GAP), 39

heart disease, 21, 124, 128, 132, 133, 161. *See also*
cardiovascular disease

heterosexuality, 34, 51, 57. *See also* sexual
relations

high-income countries, 147, 167

HIV (human immunodeficiency virus).
See human immunodeficiency virus (HIV)

Hogan, Barbara, 59

homosexuality, 34, 51, 55, 57. *See also* gay
communities; men who have sex with men;
sexual relations

human immunodeficiency virus (HIV), 132,
146–47, 161–62, 169; and agency, 172; and
ART norms, 7; condoms for prevention of,
22; fear of, 1; and key populations, 182n3;
and mortality rates, 3; and NCDs, 133, 144,
154, 156–57, 159; rates of, 21, 32; and sexual
relationships, 32, 182n1; and South Africa,
162, 184n3; surveillance data on, 1–2; and

human immunodeficiency virus (HIV) (*cont.*)
Tanzania, 175; testing for, 35, 40, 46, 54, 70,
79; transmission of, 32; and UNAIDS, 1–2;
and Zambia, 150. *See also* acquired
immunodeficiency syndrome (AIDS);
antiretrovirals (ARVs); antiretroviral
treatment (ART); people living with HIV
humanitarianism, 89, 95, 98, 99
human papillomavirus (HPV), 131, 167, 184n3,
185n11
human rights, 6, 14, 19, 39–40; and AIDS, 26,
34, 36, 38, 39–41, 43, 45, 50, 62, 63, 71, 76,
130, 131; and Ebola, 7, 89, 95; and NCDs, 26,
130–33, 134, 167
Human Rights Watch, 39, 63
hypertension, 4, 21, 126, 130, 136, 138, 148, 149,
151, 158, 159, 175. *See also* cardiovascular
disease

Incident Management System, 102
India, 131
Interfaith Religious Council, Liberia, 117
intergovernmental organizations (IGOs), 2,
6–7, 8, 10–11, 23, 98, 130, 164, 170
International AIDS Conference (2016), 77
International Covenant on Economic, Social,
and Cultural Rights, 39
International Diabetes Federation,
184n2
International Monetary Fund (IMF), 8, 84
International Partnership against AIDS in
Africa, 44
International Sanitary Conferences, 166
International Union Against Tuberculosis and
Lung Disease, 184n2
Inter-Religious Council of Uganda (IRCU), 72
intravenous drug use, 32, 57. *See also* substance
abuse
Islam, 1, 56, 70, 81. *See also* Muslims
issue frames, 12, 13; and agency, 11, 171,
173; and AIDS, 27, 33, 34, 38–39, 41, 43, 47,
60; and Ebola, 85, 103, 167–68; and
epistemic communities, 6; function of,
6–7; and NCDs, 122, 126, 130–33, 143–44,
162, 166; and state ambivalence about
global health governance, 20. *See also*
narrative

issue frames, of crisis: and agency, 172; and
Ebola, 5, 28, 90–93, 98, 100, 103, 105, 114,
118, 120, 166, 169
issue frames, of development: and NCDs, 134
issue frames, of neglect: and Ebola, 28, 90, 91,
92, 98, 100, 103, 105, 114, 118, 166, 169
Italy, 181n7

Jackson, Robert, 10
Jammeh, Yahya, 27, 56, 58, 59, 60, 61, 63,
70–71, 75, 76, 172, 182n7
Japan Tobacco International, 123, 140
Johnson, Prince, 183n11
Joint United Nations Programme on HIV/AIDS
(UNAIDS), 1–2, 32, 39, 41, 43, 45, 52, 60, 63,
182n3; and ART norms, 7; Country Progress
Reports, 53; formation of, 38; and National
AIDS Commissions, 8; National Commit-
ments and Policies Instrument (2012), 44,
50; National Commitments and Policies
Instrument (2014), 44, 47, 49, 50, 77

Kaplan, Robert, "The Coming Anarchy," 35
Kenya, 35, 49, 64, 98, 155, 182n5; National
AIDS Control Council, 70
Kingdon, John, 101
Kissi, 84, 113
Kpelle, 106
Krahn, 106
Kru, 113

Lancet NCD Action Group, 127, 130, 184n2
Lassa, 103
Latin America, 4, 137
LGBT, 51. *See also* bisexuality; homosexuality;
transgender
Liberia, 5, 24, 25, 26–27, 183n5; aid dependence of, 82; Americo-Liberian elite in, 106;
aspirational identity of, 6, 104–5; Bong
County, 107, 113; chieftaincy in, 108, 115,
117; civil society in, 28, 83, 111–18, 154–55;
civil war in, 35; community Ebola Task
Forces in, 118; democracy in, 83, 103, 105–7,
110, 119, 168; development in, 81, 82, 108,
111; distrust of state in, 83, 84, 105, 106–7,
108, 109, 110, 111, 116, 119, 120; Dolo's
Town, 114, 183n16; and Ebola and agency,

103, 117, 169, 172, 173; and Ebola decision-making, 101–2, 104, 107, 109–10; Ebola in, 24, 25, 26, 28, 80–83, 84, 86–87, 93, 96, 98, 99–119, 142, 160–61, 166, 167, 168, 169, 170, 181n7; and extraversion, 173; Grand Gedeh County, 115; and Guinea, 99; and HIV, 182n5; Incident Management System, 102, 103, 109, 110, 117, 170; Lofa County, 84, 99, 106, 113; Margibi County, 107; Ministry of Health, 102; Monrovia, 106, 113–14; Montserrado County, 107; and neopatrimonialism, 17, 28, 103, 105, 107–8, 109–10, 119; Nimba County, 107, 113, 115; slow response to Ebola in, 99–100, 103, 114, 117; and United States, 92, 94, 99, 100, 101, 103, 108, 112, 118, 119; war in, 6, 28, 81, 84, 85, 100, 104, 105–6, 107, 119; West Point, 113–14

Liberian Council of Churches, 117

Liberians United for Reconciliation and Democracy (LURD), 106

Liu, Joanne, 91

liver cancer, 23, 123

Lorma, 106, 113, 183n11

low-and lower-middle-income states, 104, 123

low-and middle-income states: and Ebola, 166; medications in, 130–31; and NCDs, 24, 123, 130, 131, 133, 144

low economic groups, 72, 73

lower-middle-income states, 104; Ghana as, 148; and NCDs, 123, 147, 154; Zambia as, 149

low-income states, 104, 147, 151, 157

Lungu, Edgar, 150

Luxembourg, 137

Madagascar, 32, 137, 154, 163, 182n5

Malac, Deborah, 101

malaria, 3, 22, 42, 53, 125, 133, 138, 142, 148, 149, 172, 175

Malawi, 12, 172, 182n5, 185n7

Mali, 32, 50, 53, 95, 181n7, 182n5

Mandela, Nelson, 71, 75

Mandingo, 106, 183n12

Mann, Jonathan, 34

marginalized groups, 19; and AIDS, 32, 33, 34, 39, 40, 51, 52, 54, 55, 63, 66, 73, 76, 175; and Ebola, 112; and NCDs, 130

Maureen Mwanawasa Foundation, 70

Mauritania, 68

Mauritius, 8–9, 62, 140, 147

Mbeki, Thabo, 27, 29, 44, 53, 56–58, 59, 60, 61, 62, 71, 75, 167, 172, 182n6

Mboup, Souleymane, 56

Médecins Sans Frontières (MSF), 39, 40, 88, 91

media, 13, 26, 62; and AIDS, 45, 60; and Ebola, 24, 89, 90, 91, 92–93, 96, 100, 103, 104, 114, 118, 119, 183n9; and NCDs, 138, 148

medicine, homeopathic, 56

medicine/drugs, 12, 148, 151; generic, 127, 131, 133; human right to, 130–31, 144; and intellectual property rights, 131; and NCDs, 123, 128, 133, 148, 159–60; WHO guidelines on, 128. See also antiretrovirals (ARV); antiretroviral treatment (ART)

mental health, 129, 134, 144, 156, 175

mental illness, 3, 4, 21, 24, 121, 148, 175

men who have sex with men, 32, 40, 50–52, 55, 63, 78, 168, 172, 175. See also gay communities; homosexuality

Merck Pharmaceuticals, 45

Mexico, 124, 137

middle-and high-income states, 137

Middle East Respiratory Syndrome (MERS), 88

migrants, 4, 52, 78, 84

military, 5, 38, 41. See also security

Millennium Development Goals, 39

Moi, Daniel arap, 35

mothers, 3, 22, 57, 58, 133, 148, 149, 175. See also women

Movement for Democracy in Liberia (MODEL), 106

Mozambique, 45, 137, 144, 154, 161, 163, 182n5

Mugabe, Robert, 144

Museveni, Yoweri, 12, 46, 63

Muslim Council (Ghana), 72

Muslims, 1, 63, 76, 105, 115. See also Islam

Mwanawasa, Levi, 149

Namibia, 26, 53, 77, 94, 96, 97, 98, 118, 137, 144, 182n5

narratives, 9; and AIDS, 44, 45; and Ebola, 81, 90, 92, 99, 101, 118, 142; and NCDs, 122. See also issue frames